Contagionism and Contagious Diseases

spectrum Literaturwissenschaft/ spectrum Literature

Komparatistische Studien/Comparative Studies

Herausgegeben von/Edited by
Moritz Baßler, Werner Frick,
Monika Schmitz-Emans

Band 38

Contagionism and Contagious Diseases

Medicine and Literature 1880–1933

Edited by
Thomas Rütten and Martina King

DE GRUYTER

ISBN 978-3-11-030572-2
e-ISBN 978-3-11-030611-8
ISSN 1860-210X

Library of Congress Cataloging-in-Publication Data
A CIP catalog record for this book has been applied for at the Library of Congress.

Bibliographic information published by the Deutsche Nationalbibliothek
The Deutsche Nationalbibliothek lists this publication in the Deutsche Nationalbibliografie; detailed bibliographic data are available in the Internet at http://dnb.dnb.de.

Printing: Hubert & Co. GmbH & Co. KG, Göttingen
♾ Printed on acid-free paper
Printed in Germany

www.degruyter.com

Table of Contents

Martina King, Thomas Rütten

Introduction

The phenomenon of contagion was generally well known to premodern societies, especially to pastoralists and those in charge of animals (Conrad, Wujastyk 2000, X). But such observations including the segregation of animals practiced by veterinarians tell us nothing about the ways by which this phenomenon was conceptualised. What was actually passed on from carrier to carrier and by what means? Even when the phenomenon of contagion was observed in regards to humans, a medical context co-existed with non-medical contexts. Such ambiguity is reflected in the technical vocabulary that developed to describe the phenomenon of contagion: *contagio* and *contagium* frequently used in Latin from at least the 2nd century BC onwards, the much rarer Greek *epaphē* (touch) (Nutton 2000, 138–140), *synanachrōsis* (infecting contact; dyeing; lat. *inficio*) (Grmek 1980; 1984; Gourevitch 1984; Nutton 2000, 140–142)[1], *anapimplamenoi* (those who have been filled full of a thing), *metadidonai* or *metadosis* (give a share of; transmit) (Leven 1992) and analogous terms from Chinese and Indian antiquity could be added. They all are descriptive. They all "encompass notions of touch, transmission, and transitiveness." Even if they are employed in a clearly medical context, they convey "notions of danger of proximity, pollution, and defilement" (Wujastik, Conrad 2000, X). To put it differently, the metaphorical, religious and moral overtones are inseperable from the medical connotations of ancient terms denoting the phenomenon of contagion. Such terms seem to be signifiers applicable to a variety of phenomena rather than names for precisely defined concepts.

Almost as old as these signifiers is the normativity associated with contagionism: judging, blaming, finally stigmatizing and persecuting people who transmit contagion has been part of the intellectual and political history of the Western world well before the plague waves of the Middle Ages and Early Modern times (Stearns 2011). Before 1348, the term 'contagion' is often used by chroniclers and theologians to indicate the spread of heretical or revolutionary ideas. After the second plague pandemic in 1348, it becomes more widespread as a concept of disease transmission, not only within medical circles, but also among laymen.

1 On the danger of the 'false friend' (contagio/infectio = contagion/infection), see Nutton 2000, 162: "Because words like contagio and infectio are etymologically related to modern English or French words with a specific medical meaning, there is a great danger that the modern understanding of the process of contagion and infection is to be traced back to antiquity simply on the basis of linguistics, or that the ancients are to be dismissed as unobservant or foolish for not talking in such terms."

Primarily referring to the Black Death, 'contagion' means person-to-person transmission by touch, breath, occasionally by sight (Cohn 2008, 79 f.). At the time when the Italian doctor Fracastoro systematizes the idea of disease transmission by infectious particles in his work *De contagione et contagiosis morbis et eorum curatione* (1546) (Nutton 1990), doctors are describing several diseases as contagious, e.g. the Black Death, smallpox, typhoid fever, syphilis (Cohn 2008, 80) as opposed to phthisis, scabies, leprosy, and bleary eye, the most prominent candidates for contagious diseases in ancient times (Nutton 2000, 138). On the other hand, moralists of the eighteenth century are convinced that emotional states such as religious enthusiasm are passed on as dangerous contagions (Hume 1834 [1759]; Shaftesbury 1732 [1708]). In his major work *The History of England* (1759), David Hume uses contagion simultaneously as concept for the spread of physical (plague) and spiritual epidemics (Hume 1834 [1759], 226, 165).[2] Contagionism, at least in the medical sense, seems to have a long-standing affinity to authoritarian politics – to power, control, anti-democratic ways of governing and its tools such as excessive segregation and quarantine, isolation, punishment. This relation between contagionism and political anti-liberalism has been intensely debated among scholars since Ackerknecht's seminal article (Ackerknecht 1948; Cooter 1982; Chandavarkar 1992; Evans 1992; Dinges 1995; Reichert 1997; Watts 1997; Baldwin 1999; Weindling 2000; Briese 2003; Cohn 2012).

Given the long-standing history of the concepts 'social contagion' and 'physical contagion', it remains unclear where the boundaries between the literal and metaphorical lie, where contagion works as a concept or as a trope. Mental states were thought to be literally contagious, not only communicated person to person analogous to the spread of smallpox or plague, whatever the noxious matter of plague or smallpox was.[3] Shaftesbury for example uses contemporary epidemiological theories – disease transmission by exhalations of noxious ferments – to explain the spread of religious fanaticism in his enlightened polemic *A Letter Concerning Enthusiasm*, thereby naturalising the collective mental state:

2 As an example for spiritual epidemics, see the following passage from Hume's chapter entitled *Henry VIII., A.D. 1541:* "But though the church was thus carried by policy as well as inclination to kindle the fires of persecution, they found the success of this remedy very precarious, and observed, that the enthusiastic zeal of the reformers, inflamed by punishment, was apt to prove contagious on the compassionate minds of the spectators. The new doctrine, amidst all the dangers to which it was exposed, secretly spread itself everywhere [...]" (Hume 1834 [1759], 165).

3 The borderline between literal and metaphorical use was already being discussed around 1900, as is shown by Briese in this volume. On the difficult distinction between metaphorical and literal use, see also Pernick 2002.

> The combustible Matters lie prepar'd within, and ready to take fire at a spark; but chiefly in a Multitude seiz'd with the same Spirit. No wonder if the Blaze rises so of a sudden; when innumerable Eyes glow with the Passion, and heaving Breasts are labouring with Inspiration; when not the aspect only, but the very Breath and Exhalations of Men are infectious, and the inspiring Disease imparts itself by insensible Transpiration. (Shaftesbury 1732 [1708], 45)[4]

As long as the assumed infectious matter is not defined, as long as communication of whatever material by either touch or/and breath, clothes and further objects is the only empirical fundament of contagionism, the openness between metaphorical and conceptual use is quite evident: one does not really need positivistic explanations how the person-to-person transmission of immaterial states works in detail.

What all theories of contagious transmission therefore have in common until the end of the 19th century, is a very vague, imprecise concept of contagion. It is not concretised by an ontological substrate, not substantialised, instead, since there is no experimental proof, it depends on speculative thinking. How exactly is the contagious physical or mental state passed on – by a chemical, a poison? By "invisible bullets"?[5] By an invisible living being, an animalcule?[6] With smallpox, it might be clear since the fluid of the pustules obviously transmits the disease, but how about water borne Cholera or mosquito transmitted Yellow fever epidemics during the 19th century? These two modes of transmission were not understood then; both diseases would nowadays be classified rather as infectious than as contagious diseases, meaning that they are caused by living agents, yet not transmitted directly by touch or breath. In the 19th century, they brought about long-standing debates centred on causality and conditionality, between

4 Note that in Shaftesbury, 'infectious' is used as a synonym for 'contagious,' indicating person-to-person spread by exhalations. In the post-bacteriological era, a distinction is drawn between 'infectious' – generally indicating disease causation by infectious particles – and 'contagious,' a subunit of 'infectious' that means that the infectious particle is passed on from person to person by direct contact and not via water, excrements, blood, food or animals.

5 In *A briefe and true report of the new found land of Virginia* published in 1588, Thomas Harriot recorded that the English colonists explained the exclusive mass mortality among Alonquian Indians from diseases, which we would now call epidemic diseases, by the fact that invisible and bodyless entities in the air were "shooting invisible bullets into them" – "by our entreaty and for the love of us" (Greenblatt 1988, 36).

6 Rightly assumed as early as in 1658 by German Jesuit Athanasius Kircher in his book *Scrutinium physicomedicum contagiosae luis quae pestis dicitur*, the idea of a *contagium animatum* was however considered superstitious until the end of the 19th century. Thus, the outstanding publication of Jacob Henle *On Miasmata and Contagia* (Henle 1938 [1840]), in which the anatomist and anthropologist logically derived the existence of a specific *contagium animatum* from empirical observation, was largely ignored until Koch's spectacular findings around 1880 (Leven 1997, 91 f.).

contagionists and the so-called miasmatists (Leven 1997, 91–93). Is the epidemic caused by a complex set of local factors, polluted air, climate, corrupt morals? (This is roughly the framework of the leading miasma doctrine.) Or is there a direct person-to-person spread by droplets that have been exhaled by sick people and that adhere to walls?[7]

Such cloudy, ambiguous understandings of contagion are fundamentally reformulated and actualized during the 'laboratory revolution' of the late nineteenth century (Cunningham, 1992), when bacteriology in Germany and France established itself as the dominant biomedical science. With Koch's and Pasteur's experimental methods, the speculative contagion became ontologized and specified, since it was proven that specific microorganisms could cause specific diseases – the mystery of contagion finally had a name and a face (Gradmann 2005, 90–103; Berger 2009, 59 f.). Given this major historical shift from a broad, undefined, multi-referential concept to a concrete, materially specified term, it seems important that interdisciplinary cultural and literary studies offer close readings of this era, of the interdependence of contagionism and culture. Yet, thus far scholarly works have been mainly summaries on the subject of contagion across a wide historical and functional range; namely from Early Modern Times to the 20th century (Weinstein 2003; Schaub et al. 2005), from Fracastoro to Bataille and from 18th century vaccination fears to the AIDS paranoia (Bashford, Hooker 2001).[8] The meanings of the pre-modern concept of contagion between literature, medicine and religion have been investigated (Nutton 1983; Jarcho 2000; Conrad 2000); yet there is hardly any interdisciplinary work on contagion and contagionism at the very time when this field was being fundamentally revolutionised.[9] An excep-

7 This is the theoretical framework of the zymotic theory, represented by the influential British epidemiologist William Farr. Zymosis is a version of the so-called eclectic contingent contagionism which claims that epidemics can be primarily caused by a set of miasmatic conditions but can become contagious under certain circumstances. Then, the proximate cause or exciter is an organic poison arising within and exhaled by people that have already fallen ill. Thus, the contagion is – paradoxically – both a secondary cause and an epiphenomenon of an epidemic (Farr 1852, lxxx–lxxxiii). See also Eyler 1973.

8 A further problem – apart from the broad historical spectrum – is the tendency to omit borderlines and distinctions between metaphorical and literal contagion, and to use an unspecific technique of analogizing. Contagion tends to become a universal metaphor that applies to various subjects within cultural studies, to concepts of performativity as well as to media theories.

9 There are two important monographs that intersect with our project, yet both explore the cultural and literary dimensions of contagionism around 1900 under a specific perspective: Priscilla Wald's seminal account of the outbreak narrative traces its roots back to the healthy-carrier discourse of the early 20th century, embodied in the paradigmatic figure of 'Typhoid Mary' and then pursues it throughout the 20th century (Wald 2008). Laura Otis explores in her book *Membranes. Metaphors of Invasion in Nineteenth Century Literature, Science and Politics* a new

tion is the special issue of the journal *American Literary History* entitled *Culture and Contagion* (Wald, Tomes, Lynch 2002) which analyses – with a main focus on the United States and the early 20th century – how transmissible disease is constructed within political, social and literary discourses and what general role it plays for American culture. Given this research background, a careful reconstruction and contextualization of contagionism and its semantic dimensions between 1880 and 1933 seems crucial, especially for the European context. In this period, the term 'contagion' was not only historically substantialised with Koch's and Pasteur's laboratory methods. It also underwent new and profound transformations during the further development of bacteriology – from strictly monocausal to conditional implications of higher complexity in the first decades of the 20th century (Mendelsohn 2007).

Another important reason for a publication that focusses on this particular period in the history of contagionism is the concurrence of two different revolutions: firstly, the 'laboratory revolution' with its most spectacular achievement – the discovery of specific, living microbes that cause terrifying diseases such as tuberculosis, cholera and typhoid fever. The coincidence of bacteriological discoveries and mass media development within the postindustrial societies produced a 'media hype' that has been circumscribed as "epidemic entertainment" (Tomes 2002): people were fascinated by the idea of ubiquitous microscopic killers that no one can see, hear or smell.

While natural sciences gained a hegemonial role within the separation of the 'two cultures' and offered a new 'Weltanschauung,' the fields of humanities, arts and literature – and this is the second revolution – began to display unprecedented varieties of activities. Social sciences and humanities developed and expanded as distinct disciplines, and the pluralism of aesthetic styles and programmes ranged from late-Victorian science fiction to experimental novels of the German and British Avantgarde, from Darwinian dramas to the *Duino Elegies* and the language games of international Dadaism. The background to this unprecedented heterogeneity was the diversification of 'Weltanschauungen' (Thomé 2002) and belief systems which included, at the turn of the century, scientism as well as mysticism, scepticism as well as faith in knowledge, phenomenalism as well as a new metaphysics of art. "There were those," to quote Musil,

> who loved the overman and those who loved the underman; there were health cults and sun cults and the cults of consumptive maidens; [...] people were devout and sceptical, naturalistic and mannered, robust and morbid [...]. An analysis of that epoch might produce

---

concept of 'self', arising from Virchow's and Koch's works and describes fictional representations of this 'open self' in a selection of European texts from the *fin de siècle* (Otis 1999).

> some such nonsense as a square circle trying to consist of wooden iron, but in reality it all blended into shimmering sense. (Musil 1997 [1930], 53)

To sum up: two central aspects of a particularly vibrant epoch came together, spectacular medical discoveries and a hitherto unknown intellectual and aesthetic pluralism.

Within this twofold, scientific and cultural revolution, the spectacular object 'microbe' adds new thrills to an old discursive formation – contagionism – that has yet always been at the intersection of medicine and literature. Our volume thus not only complements culturalist research on the concept of contagion, but also the current historiography of bacteriology. Having produced a plethora of sophisticated contributions, this scholarly field is focussed on various aspects of the history of science, not on possible interactions between medical and aesthetic discourses. Our book, however, examines such interactions and combines perspectives of medical history, literary theory and cultural studies, shedding light on the relationship between scientific knowledge, symbolic forms and intellectual history during the *fin de siècle* epoch. Various cultural and literary aspects of contagionism around 1900 will become evident; it is an exemplary subject situated between science, art and the humanities, which at the time were closely intermeshed. Apart from complementing the history of contagionism, this book adds to recent research on 'Modernism and Science' in the field of cultural poetics. Referring to the seminal works of Hansjörg Rheinberger (Rheinberger 2006) and using functional analogies, this area of research investigates 'experimental cultures' or 'literature and experiment' (Krause, Pethes 2005; Gamper, Bies 2011). Given this emphasis on a rather formal, procedural category, it seems crucial to expand the field of 'Modernism and Science' to cover scientific content – for example to investigate the cultural dimensions of a leading 'working object' (Daston 2007, 115–190) of the laboratory.

The living microbe renews and reifies the old, so far elusive principle of contagionism and gives it new relevance, on the literal as well as on the metaphorical level. Firstly, the literal dimension: objectifying and defining secular diseases such as cholera, tuberculosis, typhoid fever and syphilis, the new agent microbe becomes the "logical point of intervention" (Gradmann 2009, 7) in public hygiene and the management of epidemics. Old interventional, authoritarian policies such as quarantine, compulsory desinfection and confinement, not to mention the moral stigmatising of people who were assumed to carry microbes, now could be justified on experimental grounds.[10] Furthermore, complex diseases such as syphilis and tuberculosis – so far phenomenologically classified as various maladies[11] – are now defined by a specific causative agent and thus become ontological, medical and cultural entities in an entirely new sense. The old consumption is transformed into the new entity tuberculosis and traditional notions of the 'consumptive character' are now positivistically actualized under bacteriological premises; an important example is the publication *Lungenschwindsucht und Nervensystem* [Consumption of the Lungs and the Nervous System], published in 1905 by Friedrich Jessen who later on became Thomas Mann's model for the fictional character 'Hofrat Behrens' in *The Magic Mountain*. Similarly, syphilis is no longer only constructed as the disfiguring disease of sexual sinners but also as a neurological condition: the causative microbe *Spirochaeta pallida* proves that the well-known condition of progressive paralysis is of syphilitic origin.

Such factual changes in the medical system have aesthetic consequences: progressive paralysis is the link that allows one to connect syphilis with the discourse of genius and madness, finally with myths of creativity and inspiration, which are highly popular in the literary field of the *fin de siècle* (Schonlau 2005, 90 – 130). One can see that with bacteriology, new possibilities arise to narrate diseases. The latter can be assimilated to fictional worlds in a new and colourful way, they can be transformed into hybrid constructions that one could call 'mythoscientistic.' The Eastern origin of cholera for example and the exportation of the bacillus from India – revealed by Robert Koch and his collaborators in 1884 – converges ideally with one of the cultural myths of the Occidental world which has been called upon from Hölderlin to Thomas Mann: the East-West migration of the Dionysian, and even of poetry itself (Otis 1999, 119 – 148; Rütten 2005, 165 – 167). Bacteriologically renewed contagious diseases on the one hand offer new motifs and images, on the other hand they can organise novellistic plots by providing narrative frameworks; in fictional texts such as Schnitzler's *Dying* [Sterben] (1894), Thomas Mann's *Tristan* (1903) or Annette

10 On the legal, ethical and medical dimensions of the silent-carrier discourse, see Berger 2009, 105 – 126; Walzer Leavitt 1992 and Mendelsohn 1995.

11 Virchow, following morphological criteria, drew a categorical distinction between tuberculosis which he defined by the tubercle, and consumption which was defined by its exsudation. The tubercle belonged to the system of tumors, therefore tubercle-producing forms of tuberculosis such as scrofulosis (tuberculosis of the lymph nodes) were something essentially different from consumption. Although the French doctor Théophile Laënnec had postulated the unity of exsudative and proliferative forms of tuberculosis half a century earlier, Virchow's theory was considered as authoritative doctrine – until in 1882, the newly discovered tubercle bacillus united all sorts of tuberculous manifestations into a new entity (Virchow 1864/65, 620 – 727).

Kolb's *Daphne Herbst* (1928), the narration follows the gradual physical decline within the stages of tuberculosis.

To return to the microbe, a few words remain to be said about the metaphorical level on which it gives the notion of contagionism new relevance. The new object microbe continues to transport the old metaphorical meanings which had always been attached to 'contagion': otherness, badness, person-to-person spread of physical and moral corruption. Yet while objectifying and substantialising the old paradigm of contagion, bacteriology adds a new form of strict causality[12] to its semantic field and to its metaphorical implications. Following bacteriology's aetiological doctrine, evil contagious particles necessarily cause disease in healthy bodies; therefore people who carry these evil particles necessarily spread the evil, and so are like bacteria. On the level of bacteriological theory and practise, this strict monocausality is questioned within the period we investigate and finally replaced by multi-conditional models of higher complexity which touch on general questions of epistemology and philosophy of science. Yet its metaphorical force remains relevant – until its culmination point during the Nazi era when Jews were consistently identified with pathogenic parasites that had to be exterminated (Weindling 2000).

We can see that bacteriology allows for a much more stringent analogy between contagion and contagion-transmitting human subjects than the pre-bacteriological contagionism; firstly because of the new principle of inevitable causality, and secondly because of the way germs become part of popular culture. Namely, invisible, monocellular microbes are in fact so abstract, so inaccessible to sensual perception, that representational techniques are needed to make them comprehensible. Thus, they are extensively made anthropomorphic around 1900 and as such implanted in the collective knowledge. In Koch's writings, in the expanding mass media, above all in a multitude of popular books on the microcosm (Daum 2002), contagious microbes appear as foreign invaders, enemies of the state, political anarchists (Gradmann 2000; Hänseler 2009; King 2012). This equation 'microbes are like bad humans' on the one hand increases public attention and the size of newspaper print runs; on the other hand it suggests the reverse analogy 'bad humans are like microbes' (Gradmann 2007, 344f.). For example, Jews had been denounced as "cholera germs" in the German Reichstag as early as 1895 (Weindling 2007, 368). Microbes and human subjects seem linked

12 Strict aetiological monocausality replaces former eclectic, multi-conditional systems of proximate causes – exhaled contagious droplets – and ultimate causes – the epidemic condition/miasma of a place – which were common during the pre-bacteriological era of the 19th century, triggered by the cholera pandemics and represented by leading British sanitationists such as William Farr or Thomas Southwood-Smith (Pelling 1978).

in a normative, political way that forms the 'horizon of understanding' for contemporaries and provides a perfect metaphorical setting for literary adaptions. For example, one has only to think of Herbert George Wells' short story *The Stolen Bacillus* (1894) in which deadly cholera bugs and a mad anarchist are connected by narrative, suggesting their similarity. Another example is Ibsen's drama *An Enemy of the People* (1882), in the course of which the ethical position of the main character becomes more and more iridescent. Fighting against contagious typhoid microbes and contagious political corruption, this protagonist himself is infected with unethical ideas and gradually turns into a microbe-like political radical who spreads anarchy. When he argues against parasite-like politicians, he uses the same rhetoric of exterminism as for the fight against bacilli, claiming that "all men who live upon a lie ought to be exterminated like vermin." Later, he makes clear that "it's the party leaders that must be exterminated" (Ibsen 1917 [1882], 168, 216). It is, however, remarkable that Ibsen uses the language of exterminism to create an analogy between the hunting of parasites and humans even earlier than medical bacteriology; the later focusses on eradication and extermination only around 1890 (Hänseler 2009, 126–129). In this context, Ibsen's unmistakably critical undertone can be regarded as a visionary example for literary autonomy, insofar as further voices of critical intellectuals against the reactionary potential of bacteriology are not heard until around the turn of the century.[13]

No account of the 'culture of contagionism' is complete without a reference to its contemporary counterpart – the virus. During the later 20th century, the powerful load of normative metonymical meanings, of persecution and political paranoia originally attached to bacteria, is inherited by this new agent. Yet its efficiency for creative storytelling is still the same, shown for example by the success of Steven Soderbergh's recent thriller *Contagion* (2011). Instead of exploiting the primitive horror of decomposing bodies, this film rather plays with the old suggestive analogy of contagious bugs and contagious people who spread political paranoia like an epidemic.

To conclude: bacteriologically revolutionised contagionism around 1900 has literal and metaphorical implications with far-reaching consequences. On the one hand, classical diseases such as tuberculosis and syphilis which had always been attractive for literary representations, obtain new, ontological profiles and

13 See for example Karl Kraus who mocks the hygienic practise of identifying cholera carriers by compulsory analysis of their excrements (Kraus 1913), or Arthur Schnitzler who introduces in his novel *Der Weg ins Freie* [The Road into the Open] (1908) a problematic bacteriologist as a minor character; the latter represents cutting-edge laboratory research as well as eugenic ideas of exterminating the chronically ill.

can fulfil new cultural roles. On the other hand, contagious microbes are transformed into powerful, polysemic metaphors with a strong normative potential, insofar as they connect long-standing political meanings with new notions of unconditional causality. Thus, it is evident that the discourse on contagious microbes and microbe hunters extends well beyond the boundaries of the laboratory and into every-day-culture, and more importantly, into the intellectual, literary and political life of Modernism. Its epistemological and metaphorical dimensions offer links to sociology (Wald 2002), philosophy of knowledge, mysticism and of course creative writing.

Pertinent remarks of Karl Kraus and Max Nordau, for example, illustrate how fruitful the new metonymical proximity of contagious physical and contagious social corruption can be and how relevant it is that microbes are perceived as anthropomorphic. While Kraus, the Modernist, denounces traditional journalists and poets as "carriers of bacilli" [Bazillenträger] (Kraus 1911, 4), Nordau, the Anti-Modernist, denounces conversely the modernist writer as "influenza bacillus." The appearance of these "insane who [...] have previously poisoned the Zeitgeist, weakened by fatigue, and rendered it incapable of resistance" within the social body is like the appearance of influenza germs; they stimulate ordinary symbiotic bacilli "to swarm and produce mortal suppurations" (Nordau 1895 [1892], 537). The normative equation of microbes and humans being culturally established, one can easily make verdicts in opposite directions: for example argue against modern art as well as against reactionary journalism. Exponents *and* critics of aesthetic modernism can both bathe in the same pool of contagionist metaphors in order to express contradictory positions.

The manifold subject of contagion resp. microbial infection becomes especially popular in fictional prose, from biological racism – e.g. in Lasswitz' *Auf zwei Planeten* [On two Planets] (1897) or Wells' *The War of the Worlds* (1898) – to the idea of spiritual epidemics, from Zolaism with its praise of scientific progress to decadence, new mysticism and experimental storytelling – the latter e.g. in Ernst Weiss' novel *Georg Letham: Physician and Murderer* from 1931. Narrating contagionism and contagious diseases at the end of the 19th and during the first decades of the 20th century involves various genres such as science fiction, travel writing, popular science essays, realistic and Avantgarde novels; at the same time, it supports the very differentiation of these genres. Thereby, disease-causing microbes represent anything but only the evil and foreign. Thanks to being perceived as enigmatic, spectacular, incomprehensible and doubtful, they become ambiguous metaphors conveying a broad spectrum of meanings; 'evil transmission' and 'foreign invasion' are among them but do not account for all the possibilities. Instead, during the further development of bacteriology and the emergence of immunology, ecology, epidemiology in the early 20th century, new and gradually positive meanings are attached to the metaphorical complex of microbial infection. This encodes co-existence, openness, transparence, flow of information as well as questions about identity and liminality (Mayer, Weingart 2004). This increase in complexity again converges with developments within the literary system – from the principle of causality in literary Zolaism to the radical questioning of sense, meaning and narrative coherence within the European Avantgarde movements.

Given this parallel development of bacteriology and modernist literature – an example for the co-evolution of the social histories of medicine and literature assumed by Walter Erhart in a seminal article (Erhart 2004, 121) – contagionist tropes around 1900 function as a medium of reflexion regarding the sociocultural state and the intellectual formation of the period. They fit perfectly with the general pathophilia of an epoch whose experience of disruption, abstraction and fragmentation is no longer covered by the binding aesthetic values of the 19th century – the Good, the True and the Beautiful. Aesthetic Modernism replaces this old catalogue of norms with an obsession with the deviant, the ugly and the sick; within this modern set of 'countervalues,' notions of evil, decomposing transmission or at least of abnormal, 'infected' physical or mental states seem perfectly suitable. Against this background, our volume will explore facets of contagionism at the end of the 19th and during the first decades of the 20th century and illustrate that this discourse is a constitutive part of the intellectual history of Modernism.

The essays included in this volume first took shape as papers read at an international conference hosted by the Northern Centre for the History of Medicine at Newcastle University in August 2011. We thank the Wellcome Trust for generous funding of the conference and for a Strategic Award that enabled members of the Northern Centre to develop the theme of medicine and literature as a designated research strand. We also thank Laura Cresser, the Centre's administrator, for her excellent conference organization. As editors of this volume, we particularly thank those conference participants who, within a year, successfully transformed their papers into publishable articles. But special thanks are also due to those participants whose contributions could not be included in this volume. Through their papers or as chairs and respondents, they have made substantial contributions to the conference and to our thinking about contagionism and contagious diseases in medicine and literature. Last but not least we would like to thank the editors of the book series Spectrum Literaturwissenschaft for including our collective volume into their series, an anonymous referee and Peter Singer for helpful comments and Manuela Gerlof, Lena Ebert, Susanne Rade and Kevin Göthling from de Gruyter for their untiring support in bringing this project to fruition. The result is organised as follows. Olaf Briese's paper provides a longue-durée approach to 'social contagion,' thereby fathoming the historical depth of the ideas under discussion and conceptualised during the years covered by this volume. The same appraoch is taken by George Rousseau in order to illustrate the longevity of a fictitious concept thought to be scientifically proven by doctors until the end of the 20th century: the alleged contagiousness of homosexuality. Christoph Gradmann's paper on Robert Koch sets the scene for the period under investigation in this volume by focusing on a central figure for the emergence and popularisation of bacteriology far beyond the medical sphere. Thomas Anz' paper shifts the emphasis to the realm of fiction by identifying essential characteristics in the description of contagious diseases in Literary Modernism. Martina King is likewise concerned with Modernism, this time in relation to both literature and fine art, and concentrates on the germ and how it was staged by doctors, writers and artists alike as an objective, aesthetic, mythological or artistic entity. With Nicholas Saul's article there begins a series of analyses devoted to individual authors and works of fiction, in which contagion, contagious diseases and bacteria as conceived during the *fin de siècle* play a prominent role: the science fiction novels *On Two Planets* (Kurd Laßwitz, 1897) and *War of the Worlds* (Herbert George Wells, 1898); Thomas Mann's *Doktor Faustus*, the plan of which dates back to 1904 (by Thomas Rütten), the phantastic novels of Gustav Meyrink from the first two decades of the 20th century (by Luis Montiel), Ernst Weiss' *Georg Letham: Physician and Murderer* (1931) (by Rudolf Käser), and Max Frisch's novels *I'm Not Stiller* (1954), *Homo Faber* (1957) and *Gantenbein* (1964) (by Yahya Elsaghe). Although Frisch's novels were published outside the temporal scope of this volume, the events narrated in them and the literary intertexts regarding infectious diseases evoked by them date from the period, which is at the centre of attention in this volume. Finally, Priscilla Wald kindly provided an afterword, in which she attempts to weave together the scientific, cultural and social threads spun by the preceding contributors to this volume.

Berne, Wolfenbüttel, August 2013

References

Ackerknecht, Erwin. "Anticontagionism Between 1821 and 1867." *Bulletin of the History of Medicine* 22 (1948): 562–593.

Baldwin, Peter. *Contagion and the State in Europe, 1830–1930.* Cambridge: Cambridge University Press, 1999.

Bashford, Alison, and Claire Hooker (Eds). *Contagion: Historical and Cultural Studies.* London, New York, NY: Routledge, 2001.

Berger, Silvia. *Bakterien in Krieg und Frieden. Eine Geschichte der medizinischen Bakteriologie in Deutschland 1890–1933.* Göttingen: Wallstein, 2009.

Briese, Olaf. *Angst in den Zeiten der Cholera.* 4 vols. vol. 1: *Über kulturelle Ursprünge des Bakteriums.* Berlin: Akademie Verlag, 2003.
Chandavarkar, Rajnarayan. "Plague Panic and Epidemic Politics in India, 1896–1914." *Epidemics and Ideas: Essays on the Historical Perception of Pestilence.* Eds Terence Ranger and Paul Slack. Cambridge: Cambridge University Press, 1992. 203–240.
Cohn Jr., Samuel K. "Epidemiology of the Black Death and Successive Waves of Plague." *Pestilential Complexities: Understanding Medieval Plague.* Ed. Vivian Nutton. London: Wellcome Trust Centre for the History of Medicine at UCL, 2008 (Medical History, Supplement C, 27). 74–100.
Cohn Jr., Samuel K. "Pandemics: Waves of Disease, Waves of Hate from the Plague of Athens to AIDS." *Historical Research* 85.230 (2012): 1–20.
Conrad, Lawrence I., and Dominik Wujastyk (Eds). *Contagion: Perspectives from Pre-Modern Societies.* Aldershot, U.K.: Ashgate, 2000.
Cooter, Roger. "Anticontagionism and History's Medical Record." *The Problem of Medical Knowledge: Examining the Social Construction of Medicine.* Eds Peter Wright and Andrew Treacher. Edinburgh: Edinburgh University Press, 1982. 87–108.
Cunningham, Andrew. "Transforming Plague: The Laboratory and the Identity of Infectious Diseases." *The Laboratory Revolution in Medicine.* Eds Andrew Cunningham and Perry Williams. Cambridge: Cambridge University Press, 1992. 209–245.
Daston, Lorraine, and Peter Galison. *Objectivity.* New York: Zone Books, 2007.
Daum, Andreas. *Wissenschaftspopularisierung im 19. Jahrhundert: Bürgerliche Kultur, naturwissenschaftliche Bildung und die deutsche Öffentlichkeit 1848–1914.* 2nd ed. Munich: Oldenbourg, 2002.
Dinges, Martin. "Pest und Staat: Von der Institutionengeschichte zur sozialen Konstruktion?" *Neue Wege in der Seuchengeschichte.* Eds Martin Dinges and Thomas Schlich. Stuttgart: Steiner, 1995. 71–104.
Erhart, Walter. "Medizin – Sozialgeschichte – Literatur." *Internationales Archiv für Sozialgeschichte der deutschen Literatur* 29.1 (2004): 118–128.
Evans, Richard. "Epidemics and Revolutions: Cholera in 19th-century Europe." *Epidemics and Ideas: Essays on the Historical Perception of Pestilence.* Eds Terence Ranger and Paul Slack. Cambridge: Cambridge University Press, 1992. 149–173.
Eyler, John M. "William Farr on the Cholera: The Sanitarian's Disease Theory and the Statistician's Method." *Journal of the History of Medicine and Allied Sciences* 28.2 (1973): 79–100.
Farr, William. *Report on the Mortality of Cholera in England, 1848–1849.* London: W. Clowes and Sons for Her Majesty's Stationery Office, 1852.
Gamper, Michael, and Michael Bies (Eds). *"Es ist ein Laboratorium, ein Laboratorium für Worte." Experiment und Literatur III: 1890–2010.* Göttingen: Wallstein, 2011.
Gourevitch, Danielle. "Peut-on employer le mot d'infection dans les traductions françaises de textes latins?" *Mémoires du Centre Jean Palerne. Mémoires* 5. *Textes médicaux latins antiques.* Ed. Guy Sabbah. St. Etienne: Centre Jean Palerne, 1984. 49–52.
Gradmann, Christoph. "Invisible Enemies: Bacteriology and the Language of Politics in Imperial Germany." *Science in Context* 13 (2000): 9–30.
Gradmann, Christoph. "Unsichtbare Feinde. Bakteriologie und politische Sprache im deutschen Kaiserreich." *Bakteriologie und Moderne. Studien zur Propädeutik des Unsichtbaren 1870–1920.* Eds. Philipp Sarasin, Silvia Berger, Marianne Hänseler, and Myriam Spörri. Frankfurt a. M.: Suhrkamp, 2007. 327–353.

Gradmann, Christoph. *Laboratory Disease: Robert Koch's Medical Bacteriology.* Transl. by Elborg Forster. Baltimore, MA: Johns Hopkins University Press, 2009.

Greenblatt, Stephen, "Invisible Bullets." *Shakespearean Negotiations. The Circulation of Social Energy in Renaissance England.* Ed. Stephen Greenblatt. Berkeley, Los Angeles: University of California Press, 1988. 21–65.

Grmek, Mirko D. "Le concept d'infection dans l'Antiquité et au Moyen Age." *Travaux de l'Académie jougoslave* 384 (1980): 9–55.

Grmek, Mirko D. "Les vicissitudes des notions d'infection, de contagion et de germe dans la médecine antique." *Mémoires du Centre Jean Palerne. Mémoires* 5. *Textes médicaux latins antiques.* Ed. Guy Sabbah. St. Etienne: Centre Jean Palerne, 1984. 53–70.

Hänseler, Marianne. *Metaphern unter dem Mikroskop. Die epistemische Rolle von Metaphorik in den Wissenschaften und in Robert Kochs Bakteriologie.* Zurich: Chronos, 2009.

Henle, Jacob. *On Miasmata and Contagia.* Transl. by G. Rosen. Baltimore, MA: Johns Hopkins University Press, 1938 [1840].

Hume, David. *The History of England.* 4th vol. reprinted as Vol. 3 of *The History of England by Hume and Smollett.* London: Valpy 1834 [1759].

Ibsen, Henryk. *Collected Works.* Vol. 8: *An Enemy of the People.* Transl. by William Archer. New York, N.Y.: Charles Scribner's sons, 1917 [1882].

Jarcho, Saul. *The Concept of Contagion in Medicine, Literature and Religion.* Malabar, FL: Krieger, 2000.

King, Martina. "Staatsfeind und Schönheitsgöttin. Bakteriologisches Wissen in Wilhelm Bölsches populärdarwinistischen Schriften." *"Was wir im Verstande aussähen, kommt im Traume wieder." Wilhelm Bölsche 1861–1939.* Eds Gerd-Hermann Susen and Edith Wack. Würzburg: Königshausen & Neumann, 2012. 287–319.

Kraus, Karl. "Heine und die Folgen." *Die Fackel* 13, Nr. 329–330 (August 1911): 1–33.

Kraus, Karl. "Begleiterscheinungen der Cholera." *Die Fackel* 15, Nr. 381–383 (September 1913): 5–7.

Krause, Marcus, and Nicolas Pethes (Eds). *Literarische Experimentalkulturen. Poetologien des Experiments im 19. Jahrhundert.* Würzburg: Königshausen & Neumann, 2005.

Leven, Karl-Heinz. "Miasma und Metadosis. Antike Vorstellungen von Ansteckung." *Medizin in Geschichte und Gegenwart* 11 (1992): 43–72.

Leven, Karl-Heinz. *Die Geschichte der Infektionskrankheiten. Von der Antike bis ins 20. Jahrhundert.* Landsberg am Lech: Ecomed, 1997.

Mayer, Ruth, and Brigitte Weingart. "Viren zirkulieren. Eine Einführung." *VIRUS! Mutationen einer Metapher.* Ed. Ruth Mayer. Bielefeld: Transcript, 2004. 7–41.

Mendelsohn, Andrew. "*Typhoid Mary* Strikes Again: The Social and the Scientific in the Making of Modern Public Health." *Isis* 86.2 (1995): 268–277.

Mendelsohn, Andrew. "Von der Ausrottung zum Gleichgewicht. Wie Epidemien nach dem Ersten Weltkrieg komplex wurden." *Bakteriologie und Moderne. Studien zur Biopolitik des Unsichtbaren 1870–1920.* Eds Philipp Sarasin, Silvia Berger, Marianne Hänseler, and Myriam Spörri. Frankfurt a. M.: Suhrkamp, 2007. 176–220.

Musil, Robert. *The Man without Qualities.* Trans. by Sophie Wilkins and Burton Pike. London: Picador, 1997 [1930].

Nordau, Max. *Degeneration. Translated from the Second Edition of the German Work.* New York, N.Y.: Appleton, 1895 [1892].

Nutton, Vivian. "The Reception of Fracastoro's Theory of Contagion: The Seed that Fell Among the Thorns." *Osiris*, 2nd series, 6 (1990): 196–234.

Nutton, Vivian. "Did the Greeks Have a Word for It?" *Contagion: Perspectives from Pre-Modern Societies.* Eds Lawrence I. Conrad and Dominik Wujastyk. Aldershot etc.: Ashgate, 2000. 137–162.

Otis, Laura. *Membranes. Metaphors of Invasion in Nineteenth-Century Literature, Science and Politics.* Baltimore, MA: Johns Hopkins University Press, 1999.

Pelling, Margaret. *Cholera, Fever and English Medicine, 1825–1865.* Oxford, New York, N.Y.: Oxford University Press, 1978.

Pernick, Martin S. "Contagion and Culture." *American Literary History* (Special issue *Culture and Contagion*) 14.4 (2002): 858–865.

Reichert, Ramón. *Der Diskurs der Seuche. Sozialpathologien 1700–1900.* Munich: Fink, 1997.

Rheinberger, Hans-Jörg. *Experimentalsysteme und epistemische Dinge. Eine Geschichte der Proteinsynthese im Reagenzglas.* Frankfurt a. M.: Suhrkamp, 2006.

Rütten, Thomas. "Die Cholera und Thomas Manns *Der Tod in Venedig.*" *Liebe und Tod – in Venedig und anderswo. Die Davoser Literaturtage 2004.* Ed. Thomas Sprecher. Frankfurt a. M: Klostermann, 2005. 125–170.

Schaub, Mirjam, Nicola Suthor, and Erika Fischer-Lichte (Eds). *Ansteckung. Zur Körperlichkeit eines ästhetischen Prinzips.* Munich: Fink, 2005.

Schonlau, Anja. *Syphilis in der Literatur. Über Ästhetik, Moral, Genie und Medizin (1880–2000).* Würzburg: Königshausen & Neumann, 2005.

Shaftesbury, Antony A.C. Earl of. *Characteristikcs of Men, Manners, Opinions, Times.* 5th ed. 3 vols. vol. 1: *Characteristics. Treatise I. A Letter concerning Enthusiasm to my Lord.* London: John Darby 1732. 3–55 [1708].

Stearns, Justin K. *Infectious Ideas. Contagion in Premodern Islamic and Christian Thought in the Western Mediterranean.* Baltimore, MA: Johns Hopkins University Press, 2011.

Thomé, Horst. "Weltanschauungsliteratur. Vorüberlegungen zu Funktion und Texttyp." *Wissen in Literatur im 19. Jahrhundert.* Eds Lutz Danneberg and Friedrich Vollhardt. Tübingen: Niemeyer 2002. 338–381.

Tomes, Nancy. "Epidemic Entertainments. Disease and Popular Culture in Early-Twentieth Century America." *American Literary History* (Special issue *Culture and Contagion*) 14.4 (2002): 625–652.

Virchow, Rudolf. *Die krankhaften Geschwülste. Dreissig Vorlesungen, gehalten während des Wintersemesters 1862–1863 zu Berlin.* Vol. 2, 2nd part. Berlin: August Hirschwald 1864–65.

Wald, Priscilla. "Communicable Americanism: Contagion, Geographic Fictions, and the Sociological Legacy of Robert E. Park." *American Literary History* (Special issue *Culture and Contagion*) 14.4 (2002): 653–685.

Wald, Priscilla, Nancy Tomes, and Lisa Lynch (Eds). *American Literary History* (Special issue *Culture and Contagion*) 14.4 (2002).

Wald, Priscilla. *Contagious: Cultures, Carriers, and the Outbreak Narrative.* Durham, NC: Duke University Press, 2008.

Walzer Leavitt, Judith. "*Typhoid Mary* strikes back. Bacteriological Theory and Practice in Early Twentieth-Century Public Health." *Isis* 83 (1992): 608–629.

Watts, Sheldon. *Epidemics and History: Disease, Power and Imperialism.* Yale: Yale University Press, 1997.

Weindling, Paul. *Epidemics and Genocide in Eastern Europe 1890–1945.* Oxford: Oxford University Press, 2000.

Weindling, Paul. "Ansteckungsherde. Die deutsche Bakteriologie als wissenschaftlicher Rassismus 1890–1920." *Bakteriologie und Moderne. Studien zur Biopolitik des Unsichtbaren 1870–1920.* Eds Philipp Sarasin, Silvia Berger, Marianne Hänseler, and Myriam Spörri. Frankfurt a. M.: Suhrkamp, 2007. 354–374.

Weinstein, Arnold (Ed.). *Literature and Medicine* (Special issue *Contagion and Infection*) 22.1 (2003).

Olaf Briese

'Social Contagionism': Psychology, Criminology and Sociology in the Slipstream of Infection[1]

Social processes have long been described as contagious, infectious, or epidemic. One might point to the seventeenth-century French Enlightenment thinkers Pierre Charron and Antoine Furetière, who (in 1601 and 1684/1690, respectively) labeled the spread of public prejudices and misapprehensions as well as of heretical opinions as contagious (Cheyronnaud 1998, 51–53). From the Anglophone realm, the Jesuit theologian William Darrell comes to mind; around 1700 he thought atheistic ideas were epidemic (Lund 2003). But the metaphor of contagion was not restricted to the field of religious and theological controversies. By the mid-seventeenth century, moralists in France considered the reading of imaginative literature contagious (Fournier 2005, 195–202), as well as writing – including the writing of letters – in a humorous or burlesque manner (Bertrand 2005). A more strictly epistemological discourse took up this and other models, discussing the genesis and spread of imaginative creativity (Malebranche), of enthusiasm (Shaftesbury), and of the feelings and passions (Hume) in terms of infection (Cheyronnaud 1998, 51 f., 59; Roussin 1998, 137 f.). Philippe Hecquet cultivated the discourse of epidemic for the analysis of religion in his treatise *Le Naturalisme des convulsions dans les maladies de l'épidémie convulsionnaire* (1733). There the renowned and successful physician of the University of Paris characterized the Jansenist miracles and group ecstasies that had been centered in a Paris cemetery since 1727 as a contagious epidemic brought on by hysteria (Goldstein 1984, 185–190). These examples and others provided the basis for the generalizing account of Christianity that Paul-Henri Thiry d'Holbach anonymously laid before the public in 1768 under the title *La contagion sacrée, ou Histoire naturelle de la superstition*. Religion, the work claimed, was a superstition whose degree of contagion depended on the temperament of the individual (d'Holbach 1998, 123).

Leaping now to the present, 'contagion' seems to have become a securely established and even positively connoted commonplace of sociology and psychology, of emotional, behavioural, and market research, and of aesthetic and artistic theory (Schaub et al. 2005; Busch 2007; Strowick 2009; Düllo 2010). With this in

1 I wish to thank Dr Patrick Baker for his expert translation of this essay from German into English.

mind, in my essay I would like to develop four theses, concentrating on the period around 1900. The *first thesis* is that it only became possible to speak of 'social contagion' on the basis of medical concepts of contagion. Such concepts began to emerge in the Renaissance and Early Modern Period and subsequently gained force in the nineteenth century and the era of bacteriology. The *second thesis* is that while models of 'social contagion' are certainly capable of producing knowledge and understanding, their value in this sense is nevertheless limited. For this seductive conceptual model presupposes a medical or scientific matrix for social processes; it conceives of social relationships more or less directly as natural phenomena and pretends to a level of causal clarification and explanation that the humanities and social sciences as such can never achieve. The natural and the social are conceived as a seemingly organic unit. The *third thesis* is that concepts of social contagion tend to be rather simplistic, and that some have also depended – and continue to depend – on antiquated notions long since superseded in the natural and social sciences. Indeed, most concepts of 'social contagion' still feed on the idea of an unambiguous causality – an idea that was forcefully postulated by medical concepts of contagion current around 1870, but that after 1900 had to be abandoned. Thus they have fed – and continue to feed – not uncommonly on notions entrenched in, or running through, popular culture, all the while claiming to provide plausible scientific explanations.

The object of this essay, however, is in no way to distinguish between 'correct' and 'false' concepts of contagion. Instead I would like to show that there are and have been many different concepts of contagion in the various branches of medicine and epidemiology, and also that models of contagion in the social sciences and humanities vary greatly from one to another – depending on their function, on their theoretical and cultural context, and on the state of the discipline in which they are used. The concept or the metaphor of contagion (or infection or epidemic) can have starkly different meanings in the various branches of learning, in the various arts, and even within common culture. They vary not only from field to field, but also from school to school or from individual to individual. There is no single notion of contagion – not in the concepts of medicine and epidemiology, not in the social sciences, not even in the arts. I realize that it might seem trivial to emphasize something that is so obvious, but the inflammatory potential connected to the concept or metaphor of contagion, especially as conveyed by the postmodern discourse of 'circulation', has increased conceptual imprecision. In this context it is useful to step back and survey the history of this metaphor from a position of analytical distance. Such inflammatory discourses, however – and this is the *fourth* thesis of my talk – have passed their zenith. 'Social contagion' has long since turned into a largely bloodless commonplace for characterizing social normalities. The term has lost nearly all its emotional impact, and it increasingly stands for everyday activities of social communication and even for interaction of any sort. Furthermore, a semantic shift has infused the term 'contagion' with new inflammatory and positive qualities. In theories of market analysis, advertising and social networking the goal is to *go viral*. In what follows, models of social contagion as proposed by Carl Gustav Carus, Willy Hellpach, and Sigmund Freud will be discussed with regard to the possibilities and the limits of their meaningfulness. These four theses provide the framework for the following analyses, although it will not be possible within constraints of this essay to explore all points in detail.

1 On the History of 'Contagion'

In order to test the heuristic value of the phrase 'social contagion,' one must consider the major cultural transformations that the concept of contagion has traversed in Europe from antiquity to the rather recent past. Contagion in the modern medical sense – as the transmission of infectious particles from person to person – perhaps spread through indirect means – is a relatively new concept that first arose during the Renaissance. Before that, medical theories of epidemic were dominated by the meta-paradigm of 'miasma,' whose roots can ultimately be traced back to Eastern high culture. According to the *katastasis* tradition of Hippocratic-Galenic medicine, air or atmosphere was the medium for transporting epidemics, namely in the form of pestilential vapours (Leven 1992, 48–55; Jouanna 2001, 10–19). This paradigm is substantiated above all in the Hippocratic treatise *On Airs, Waters, and Places*, but also in another work attributed to him entitled *On Breaths*. In the author's – or the authors' – view, *epidemic constitution* is determined by local climatic and geographical factors. The fact that air or atmosphere is ascribed a major influence on geo-climatic environment, on the one hand, and on the psychological and physical state of individuals, on the other, highlights the causal, deterministic approach that generally characterized Ionic natural philosophy in the 5th century BC. When searching for the origins of such causal thinking, however, it must not be ignored that models that ultimately achieved the status of purely scientific concepts were still rooted in magical premises. The epidemic constitution of a place was the secular expression for the demonic *genius loci: miasmata* and *effluvia* were secularized variants of demonic winds, vapors, and breaths. Even the word 'miasma' – pollution, staining, or defilement through sin – carried this notion within it. Similarly, the word *inficere* still partially contained magic and religious connotations: miasmas 'infect' human beings in the sense that they poison, corrupt, or stain them.

In comparison, the concept of contagion was – at least in Europe (Conrad 2000; Farber 2004) – relatively fresh and novel. In the Renaissance it began to establish itself as a competitor to the ancient miasma model, and it was based on a fundamentally different causality. First formulated by the Veronese physician and poet Girolamo Fracastoro, who drew on a few fitful, hypothetical, and exceedingly fragmentary ancient texts (Nutton 1983, 1990, 1998, 2000), this model traced epidemics to a transmission of infectious particles, so-called 'contagions,' through human beings or human artifacts. In his multi-volume treatise *De contagione*, Fracastoro, whose main interest lay in syphilis, provided the model of contagion with its first comprehensive conceptualization. In his view, contagions were certain particles and substances, *seminaria*, that transmitted diseases in three ways: (1) through direct contact (*per contactum*), (2) through indirect contact by means of what he only vaguely outlined as intermediaries (*per fomitem*), and (3) at long range through magic (*ad distans*). For Fracastoro these contagious particles achieved the status of tiny supernatural, mythical animals whose spread was facilitated, for example, by certain astrological constellations, and prophylaxis and healing could thus also be effected by spiritual antipathy – no matter whether the manner of transmission was direct, indirect, or long-range (Briese 2003, 80 – 83).

This was the model that made its name in early modern medicine and enjoyed pre-eminence from then on. It provided a new, sociomorphic means of prevention for epidemics that called externally for closing political borders and internally for a strict regime of quarantines, and confining the sick to their homes or rooms – measures that appealed all too well to an absolutist *raison d'état*. Contagionism corresponded to the logic of absolute rule, which – in the interest of building up its power – now and then was almost in need of epidemics (Dinges 1995; Reichert 1997). Indeed, such measures had been in use since the beginning of the fifteenth century – and thus about 150 years before Fracastoro – without the support of any kind of theoretical model. The upshot was that physicians had been more or less demoted to administrators of epidemic defence. Of course, they also participated in the debates over the causes and possible preventions and cures for epidemics, but their overwhelmingly miasmatic program – beginning with the famous canonical report of the University of Paris in 1348 (Sticker 1908, 60 – 62) – was in short order utterly ignored in the precautionary measures instituted by magistrates, local rulers and Renaissance potentates. Physicians had *their* discourse. State institutions maintained *another*, according to which epidemics spread mostly through direct infection. The contagionist model of infection was the doctrine favored by authoritative makers of policy – although it only received a corresponding theoretical justification by Fracastoro in 1546 – whose theory, by the way, at first remained on the margins of the medical establishment. Health magistrates and sanitation committees initiated the practices of confinement, quarantine and other regulatory measures *without* medical legitimation. By the end of the fourteenth century at the latest, the city-states had ceased to pay more than lip service to the physicians' miasmatic models. They established their own *modus operandi*, including confinement, quarantine, and isolation, and gave only marginal attention, or none at all, to medical notions.

This model of contagion – according to which the seeds of disease or particles are spread from person to person – was also the cognitive framework that ultimately opened the way to the era of bacteriology (Koch) and microbiology (Pasteur). Naturally, the path was not direct, and the fundamental differences between late-nineteenth-century laboratory science and the magico-philosophical speculations of the Renaissance cannot be ignored. Yet there was an overarching commonality: one could now proceed tactically against epidemic diseases, which had not been the case with the ominous miasmas. Indeed, Koch's initial bacterial model – his so-called "Verursachungsbakteriologie" [causal bacteriology] – made the potential for such seem quite positive. Indeed, his initially minimalistic notions of causality made the prevention of epidemics seem almost child's play: wherever a given pathogen is found, he theorized, the corresponding illness must necessarily also be found. One must then detect and "wipe out" [ausmerzen] the given pathogens. A tactical combination of bacteriology and restrictive state regulations on public hygiene would seem to make this a simple task.

The minimalism of this causal conception, which soon proved to be grossly insufficient, made models of infection in the late nineteenth and early twentieth century extremely attractive. They were attractive for makers of public policy for the restrictive way epidemic prevention was handled. But they were also attractive for various branches of learning. Social psychology, criminology, sociology, and cultural anthropology drew on them enthusiastically. These disciplines, too, hoped to find simple and plausible explanations for the behaviour of the objects of their research – namely human beings in groups or masses. The notion that social phenomena were 'contagious' was attractive because it was attended by the promise that they could be convincingly explained or even controlled or governed.

2 Suggestive Analogizing: Carus's *On Spiritual Epidemics*

Around the middle of the nineteenth century, models of mental or social contagion enjoyed a veritable boom in the field of psychology as it was then developing institutionally. Closely following the preliminary work of physicians, French and German psychologists like Lucas (1833), Calmeil (1845), and Ideler (1848) labeled mental disturbances, especially mania and hysteria, as contagious. In the heyday of research on hysteria, psychologists such as Despine (1870), Rambosson (1883), Legrand du Saulle (1883), Knittel (1884), and Régnard (1887) did likewise, although each began from highly disparate premises and thus arrived at equally disparate conclusions. A short analysis of Carl Gustav Carus's 1852 pamphlet *Ueber Geistes-Epidemien der Menschheit* [On Spiritual Epidemics of Humanity] will serve as an example to illustrate the problems that arise and must be solved when the concept of contagion is applied to psychological and social processes. Moreover it will show how tenuous the methodological basis could at times be for positing an analogy between "physical" and "spiritual" contagion – to adopt the categorical pair used by Carus.

Carus (1789–1869), an important physician, psychologist, natural philosopher, writer, and painter of the Late Romantic period was competent in various fields of learning and the arts. He was a polymath and more importantly a believer in the Romantic ideal of universal knowledge. The world and its forms of being constituted for him a divine, organic unity; even the various forms of knowledge were simply different facets of a potential universal knowledge. Inorganic, organic, man, and the realms of human culture including politics, religion, science, and art were external manifestations of a theistic-pantheistic universal principle, and thus they were harmoniously connected with one another. According to Carus, this organic, unitary being contained within itself developmental processes. Development meant first the evolution of divinely-planted seeds and principles, and second that this evolution occurred by means of "metamorphoses" – a concept that yet again strongly underlined the structural unity of being. The object of this ontological development was the refinement of the conscious out of the unconscious, the perfection of being through the return to God.

This teleological concept displayed several commonalities with the ideas of Early Romantic natural philosophy. Yet there was a clear difference: Carus – a highly successful doctor and scientific administrator in the Kingdom of Saxony, as well as the king's personal physician and a court counselor and medical advisor – while according the unconscious a great deal of significance, paid little attention to the dark sides of the soul that typically occupied Early Romanticism. Aberrant mental states, abnormalities, and deviances are treated only marginally in his work, for they had no place in his optimistic concept of natural and historical development as metamorphosis. Even the unconscious was not the qualitative 'other' of the conscious but rather its ungerminated seed. In this sense, Carus belongs more to the Enlightenment than to Romanticism. In his tract *On Spiritual Epidemics of Humanity*, however, he felt compelled to probe certain historico-psychological dark sides of man – although the whole line of argument aims at toning down their historical significance. Carus's object is to place them within a teleologico-optimistic, theistic-pantheistic plan of salvation, as well as to provide a vista onto human history as a progressive process of cultural refinement at whose conclusion such spiritual epidemics will be superfluous.

Carus was spurred by a concrete event to treat the otherwise infelicitous topic of "spiritual epidemics," namely the Revolution of 1848/1849, which also resulted in heavy fighting in the Kingdom of Saxony, for example, the May Uprising of 1849 in Dresden. Carus, whose worldview was that of a free-spirited bourgeois, who stood for a synthesis of intellect and power on the basis of a reform-minded constitutional monarchy, attempted to explain these events after the fact:

> It was mainly a critical glance at a few remarkable recent events that caused me to choose the great, remarkable subject of *spiritual epidemics* as the focus of this tract. [Es mochte wohl hauptsächlich ein prüfender Blick auf manche merkwürdige Ereignisse der jüngstvergangenen Zeit sein, der mich bestimmte, diesmal gerade den grossen merkwürdigen Gegenstand *geistiger Epidemien* zum Vorwurf eines solchen Vortrags zu wählen.] (Carus 1852, 4)

For history had not followed the harmonious, evolutionary path conceived by Carus. The deviant period of revolution required an explanation. And this explanation – the author expressly promised his readers a comforting view of events – unfolded in just such a way that it was supported by Carus's beloved unitary concept of nature and history. For Carus set physical and spiritual epidemics in relation to one another. He interpreted both kinds of epidemics as cleansing states of fever, as "developmental diseases of humanity without which the index of history [has] never progressed one bit" [Entwickelungskrankheiten der Menschheit, ohne welche nun einmal der Zeiger der Geschichte niemals und nirgends bedeutend vorgerückt ist] (Carus 1852, 55). Undermining the demonization of revolution even further, he set the events retrospectively into a line of continual historical development with aberrant states of affairs from the medieval period. Portrayed as the last remnants of the unenlightened and fanatically religious Dark Ages, political revolutions appear as the final descendents of historical phenomena like St. Vitus' dance, tarantism, the Inquisition, witchcraft, Jansenist group convulsions, belief in vampires, and the cult of Joan of Arc. Carus uses the seemingly modern ideas of group and mass – both in the singular and in the plural – in his arguments, but their meaning is descriptive rather than terminological.

So, how do spiritual epidemics spread in groups and masses? How does spiritual contagion work? The simplicity of Carus's ideas shows that 'contagion' is not used in the least as a precise heuristic tool but only as a metaphor, as a non-specific catchword. The suggestive power of the analogy took precedence over its epistemic value; metaphors bridged and concealed undeveloped theoretical terrain. For how does Carus explain the corresponding causalities? What is his argument? On the one hand he bases himself on the previously postulated equation of nature and history. On the other hand he creates an analogy between the spiritual illnesses of individuals and those of groups. This, too, is meant to emphasize that there is nothing arbitrary about social epidemics, for neither – neither the mental illnesses of individuals nor those of masses – is volitional, i.e. subject to free will.

The basis for this double analogy – first that spiritual epidemics are like physical ones, and second that they are like the mental illnesses of individuals – was thus the thesis that all three abnormal states were not random occurrences. Physical epidemics have their necessary place in history; and neither the spiritual aberrations of individuals nor masses infected with epidemics are phenomena arbitrarily determined (such as intentional delusions). According to Carus, these aberrations are always due to "life having been somehow organically changed" [irgendwie organisch veränderten Leben] (Carus 1852, 11 f.), and thus ultimately have a natural cause. Here, finally (if not earlier), the concept of contagion receives methodological significance. If individual delusions and collective epidemics have life circumstances as their preconditions that changed organically, one must then wonder: in the subject's environment or in the subject itself? And do these physico-organic changes spread contagiously, thereupon causing psychological changes? Is infection actually caused by these physico-organic changes, or must it be complemented by a psychological sensitivity or predisposition? How do spiritual epidemics *come about?* And how do they *spread?* The basic distinction between these last two aspects is skipped over by Carus with the suggestive commonplace of epidemic. And more generally: what is a "spiritual epidemic?" Is it an infection *of the* spirit – which is transmitted from individual spirit to individual spirit? Or is it an infection *through* the spirit, roaming from individual to individual on the level of the spirit and thus on that of consciousness – thus through sense perception, conception, communication, and information?

All these aspects and many others remain fuzzy in Carus's work. The metaphors of epidemic and contagion lead not to specific explanations but rather remain on the level of generality. Time and again, when it would seem proper to theoretically determine the status of these spiritual epidemics, Carus digresses into historically compelling excurses, into the enumeration of case studies. The equivalence or parallelism between physical and spiritual epidemics is the premise, and a continuous chain of examples is meant to document it. Nevertheless it explains nothing, remaining mere description. At most, overwhelming rhetoric serves to fuel the notion of epidemic and infection associatively and metaphorically. Ultimately, Carus seems to be wholly uninterested in how the "spiritual epidemics" he postulates actually *come into being*, but only in how they subside and pass away. Indeed, this is what seems important in the context of his optimistic worldview:

> Observing how in events of this kind the higher spiritual conscience and the spirit's true, beautiful freedom seem for a time wholly removed from the world [...], thus we must be seized, ever longer ever more, by a deep awe for that sure guidance of an underlying, highest divine world order. [Sehen wir denn, wie in solchen Vorgängen zeitweise das höhere geistige Bewusstsein und die wahre schöne Geistesfreiheit allerdings der Welt fast gänzlich entzogen scheint [...], so muss uns auch, je länger je mehr, eine tiefe Ehrfurcht gegen jene sichere Führung eines eigentlichen und höchsten göttlichen Weltregiments ergreifen.] (Carus 1852, 57)

Do his explanations regarding the ceasing, the extinction of such epidemics permit of conclusions regarding the cause of their coming into being or spread? On the one hand, according to Carus these epidemics (like bodily ones as well) heal themselves: *natura sanat*. Spiritual and physical epidemics have their necessary place in the plan of nature and history; they have a cleansing function. The quasi-invisible hand of history then lets them expire. In this view, epidemics of both kinds appear as purely objective events. On the other hand, factors appear on the subjective level that facilitate the subsidence of spiritual epidemics. Experience has shown that healing and palliation are possible through psychological treatment – through kindness, consolation, and earlier through religious sacraments. But much more important – again on the subjective level – are mechanisms of psychological weakening. The mass diffusion of, and mass acquaintance with, abnormal group states reduces their capacity to fascinate. The loss of novelty and thus of fascination leads to a decreasing number of new infections. But the most important factors leading to a curtailing, if not to the wholesale prevention, of spiritual epidemics are knowledge and science, learning, culture, and tolerance. Half objective and occurring on their own, half subjective and to be purposefully promoted, these are the most important guarantors of a harmonious future outlook. But this still says nothing about the mechanisms by which spiritual epidemics come into being and spread. Ultimately, the commonplace of spiritual epidemics was for Carus nothing other than an imponderable, a universal projection surface. That is what made it attractive. It dealt with nature but also with culture, with individuals but also with groups, with binding, general necessity but also with variable, individual disposition. In some way it dealt with everything. It seemed capable of providing an acceptably imprecise explanation for something that ultimately seemed unexplainable, namely: that "the kindliest citizens often transform into savage standard bearers of revolution" [die wohlwollendsten Bürger oft ganz in wilde Bannerträger der Revolution sich umwandelten] (Carus 1852, 56). Contagion was a mere metaphor, a placeholder for something that could not be explained.

3 Sceptical-Analytical Distance: Hellpach's *Spiritual Epidemics*

Around 1900, when fear of bacteria was at a fever pitch that subordinated all socio-cultural domains to the behavioural norms of social, racial, and individual hygiene, the conceptual model of 'social contagion' had reached its tentative high point. Its main exponent, next to psychology, was the new discipline of sociology. In certain sociological schools, entire social value-systems, stances, and orientations were considered *in toto* 'contagious.' This development was associated with far-reaching perspectival shifts in scientific structures, with a growing orientation toward the new leading disciplines of medicine and natural science. Even the realm of the socio-psychological and the social should, according to a nearly irresistible scientific turn, be able to be explained and controlled, or even governed in compliance with laws. This was the invisible motor of sociology. The conceptualization of social or mental contagion is exemplified by the work, among others, of Aubry (1887), Lombroso and Laschi (1890), Tarde (1890a, 1890b), Sighele (1893), Le Bon (1895), Bekhterev (1905), and Durkheim (1897, 1912). The differences among the respective concepts are major. Thus the second International Congress for Criminal Anthropology, held in Paris in 1889, erupted in conflicts between the Italian criminologists, on the one hand, who argued in a strongly naturalistic manner (and even made arguments on the basis of heredity), and French criminologists like Lacassagne and Tarde, on the other hand, who emphasized that the social realm followed its own laws even in the area of criminality (before devoting himself wholly to sociology, Tarde worked as a judge and criminologist). In turn, Tarde and Durkheim were sharp antagonists over the question of whether sociology should proceed psychologically from groups and collectives or from the social whole and its laws. The 'mass' theorist Le Bon, finally, was characterized by his severe, politically ultraconservative criticism of modernity and its culture (Moscovici 1981; Nye 1984; van Ginneken 1992; Middendorf 2009).

At this point I would like to introduce a forgotten model of the psychologist and social psychologist Willy Hellpach (1877–1955), who, in contrast to Carus, was well aware of the problems associated with the concept of social contagion. His 1906 book *Die geistigen Epidemien* [Spiritual Epidemics] constituted a mature attempt to apply the concept of contagion in a methodologically sound way. This is noteworthy, as the book – actually a pamphlet – appeared as the eleventh installment in the social psychology series *Die Gesellschaft* [Society], published by Martin Buber for a broader audience of non-specialists. Highly complex distinctions would not normally have been expected in this kind of publication. Even without them, however, Hellpach manages, colourfully and with ironic flourishes, to raise substantial awareness of the problems inherent in the contemporary contagion fad. A psychologist oriented toward the social sciences, Hellpach wrote his doctoral thesis under Wilhelm Wundt – later earning another doctorate in medicine – and inherited from him an antipathy for the bio-anthropological foundation of social psychology. Appointed professor of psychology at the Technical University of Karlsruhe in 1911 – a position he later held in Heidelberg – , Hellpach worked, in the context of a broad spectrum of interests, chiefly on now-outmoded schemes for a geo-climatically-determined social psychology (Hellpach 1991). It is worth mentioning in this context that he had contacts to the Social Democrats and collaborated on the *Sozialistische Monatshefte* [Socialist Monthly], between 1898 and 1903, incidentally under a pseudonym (Hellpach 1948, 212–214; Kaune 1991, 45). These contacts, as well as a likely sporadic reading of Marxist works, will have influenced his early intention to provide a social foundation for the social sciences. Moreover, as a member of the German Democratic Party during the Weimar Republic, Hellpach was Minister of Culture and Education in Baden, in 1924 and 1925 also President of Baden, and from 1928 to 1930 a member of the Reichstag; after 1930, however, he withdrew from politics. He concentrated on his university career and was left largely in peace by the National Socialists, with whom he more or less came to terms.

Hellpach's book on *Spiritual Epidemics* inveighs with ironic mockery against highly naturalizing and universalizing scientific models in sociology and in journalistic popularization:

> They love nothing more than to speak of an ulcer gnawing on the organism of the whole, or of an abscess ready to be opened, of a socio-pathological phenomenon and of a spiritual epidemic. [...] And it is not good when even the most harmless activities of public life are given the violent stench of iodoform and phenol. [Sie reden am meisten und liebsten von einem Geschwür, das am Organismus der Gesamtheit zehre, oder von einer Eiterbeule, die zum Aufstich reif sei, von einem sozialpathologischen Phänomen und von einer geistigen Epidemie. [...] Und es ist nicht gut, wenn auch die harmlosesten Vorgänge des öffentlichen Lebens gewaltsam jodoform und karbolrüchig gemacht werden.] (Hellpach 1906, 8)

As an antidote to this fad, the author proposes the measured restraint from hasty generalizations. He is never an enemy of theory, never pleads for a positivist theoretical vacuum. But he clearly expresses his rejection of overinflated generalizations. For him there is no skeleton key that will unlock the secrets of social phenomena – only general models that must prove their worth precisely in their ability to make distinctions:

> by the way, the desire to reduce all possible means of socio-psychological transmission to *one* explanatory factor inflicts most regrettable harm on the attempt to deal with such things. [Nebenbei bemerkt, fügt das Bestreben, alle Möglichkeiten der sozialpsychischen

> Übermittlung auf *einen* erklärenden Generalnenner zu bringen, dem Interesse an der Bearbeitung dieser Dinge den bedauerlichsten Schaden zu.] (Hellpach 1906, 44)

He consistently tests the meaningfulness of the commonplace of contagion then dominating the social sciences. For Hellpach would also like to explain how ideas, beliefs, and even delusions spread collectively. But instead of quick answers, he is always armed with questions:

> But how does this diffusion occur? Through 'contagion.' That's the rub. Was does contagion mean here? It's just a figurative expression! It *is* just a figurative expression. [Aber wie geschieht diese Ausbreitung? Durch ‚Ansteckung'. Da sitzen wir fest. Was heißt hier Ansteckung? Es ist doch nur ein bildlicher Ausdruck! Es *ist* nur ein bildlicher.] (Hellpach 1906, 29)

What, then, might contagion mean when broken down for the social sciences? Would it be an infection of a material kind? Something like the materialistic, naturalistic transmission of nervous vibrations?

In order to isolate his subject – spiritual epidemics – he delimits them as a special case in the field of socio-pathological phenomena and mass mental illnesses. He then introduces the figure of three concentric circles: the largest is composed of socio-pathological phenomena, the ordinary fashions and disturbances of life (that in a stricter sense cannot be considered morbid); the second, smaller circle is composed of mass mental illnesses that, in an expressly socially-contingent way, effectively crop up of their own accord in many groups and subjects; the third and innermost circle is composed of spiritual epidemics that spread by means of contagion. Finally, Hellpach proposes three different structural possibilities for what he labels as contagion: *Einredung* [persuasion], *Einfühlung* [empathy], and *Eingebung* [predisposition/influence]. *Einredung* is an interaction between an active transmitter and a generally passive receiver. The transmitter or sender wants to impart information, news, or messages; he has a vested interest in the receiver acting in a specific way. Press, parliaments, political organizations, demagogues – they devote themselves to these activities. *Einredung* could also be called manipulation. In *Einfühlung*, however, nearly all the activity is on the side of the receiver. He willingly or unwillingly perceives something, notices something, feels something, and develops solicitude and empathy for it. The direction of activity is changed, and the intention of the initial subject can also be changed: it *can* purposefully attract attention, but it *need* not intend to do so. *Einfühlung* creates sympathy that, according to Hellpach, is of an uncertain and unpredictable nature. For its part, *Einredung* is a relatively intellectual phenomenon; it homes in on convictions. In contrast, sympathy is an affectively borne emotional state, not to be governed from without and in part not even by the sympathizer himself. The third type of transmission and contagion, *Eingebung*, is the most difficult one to govern both from without and from within. Moods, affects, fantasies, illusions, hallucinations, obsessions, actions – all derive only qualifiedly from external causes or stimuli. They are an internal, subjective disposition. These internal dispositions can be latent, breaking out or resurfacing at a moment's notice. In any case, here external contagion is only the secondary stimulus, never the primary cause.

After the discussion of the three possible kinds of psychological states, Hellpach raises the question of how they work in practice:

> But how does the practical composition of a spiritual epidemic look? What actual structural forms emerge from the larger realm of structural possibilities? What powers of transmission are most often effective and most sustainable among the three that we have discussed? [Wie gestaltet sich aber der praktische Aufbau einer seelischen Epidemie? Welche wirklichen Strukturformen treten unter den Strukturmöglichkeiten hervor? Welche Mächte der Übertragung sind unter den dreien, die wir besprochen haben, am häufigsten und nachhaltigsten wirksam?] (Hellpach 1906, 61)

Einfühlung [empathy] seems to be the procedure that most intensively puts into effect what Hellpach "figuratively" labels as contagion. For *Einredung* [persuasion] in the main only reaches the intellect; it is still up to the receiver to decide how to respond to this persuasion and manipulation. In internal *Eingebung* [predisposition], in contrast, external stimuli are ultimately secondary, providing a mere occasion for illness. Whatever they contain that might actually be contagious (beliefs, ideas, obsessions) disappears under the power of the unfolding of internal and in this sense autarkic affects, moods, and fantasies. When looking for actual infection, in the main only *Einfühlung* [empathy] can be considered:

> and it is also primarily *Einfühlung* [...] that grips the sufferer with external moods, external stimuli, and external impulses, causing them to become elements of spiritual epidemics. [und Einfühlung ist es auch in erster Linie, [...] die den Erschöpften von fremder Stimmung, fremder Erregung, fremdem Bewegungsdrang miterfaßt und jene zu häufigen Gliedern geistiger Epidemien werden läßt.] (Hellpach 1906, 67)

Of course, as Hellpach repeatedly qualifies, the boundaries between these three processes can never be clearly drawn. He always thinks relationally; he dealt in what Ernst Cassirer some time later programmatically called functional concepts [Funktionsbegriffe] as opposed to substantial concepts [Substanzbegriffe] (Cassirer 1910). A situation presents itself differently when viewed from different perspectives; *Einfühlung* can also be classified as *Eingebung* and so forth. Combinations of the three are also possible. *Einredung*, *Einfühlung*, and *Eingebung* can accompany each other in various ways, so as for mutual reinforcement, weakening, or reciprocal transformation to take place. And if the paths of transmission are relational – for example, what in one regard could be *Einredung* would be *Einfühlung* in another – so are the categories of 'herd' and 'victim.' A herd can itself already be a victim in one and the same process, a victim in one and the same process a herd. One will search in vain in Hellpach's work for simplifying and reductive definitions of what contagion might be. He refines his concept of 'spiritual epidemics' and contagion so as to open up various relational and functional possibilities, so as to encompass social communication and social persuasion.

Two things are clear. First, whatever might be called – only figuratively, of course – contagion is always a social process. Physical waves or vibrations play no part in such processes of infection and transmission. Second, whatever it is in spiritual epidemics that appears to be contagious is morbid or provokes something morbid. To this extent, Hellpach remains true to his intention to treat epidemics. The concept or metaphor of contagion thus characterizes not solely communication, impartation, persuasion, or transmission as such, not solely normal social conditions. For Hellpach, 'epidemic' always stands for something relatively deviant, relatively abnormal, something undesirable. It thus seems perfectly natural for the book to end with a focus on hysterias. They are to be seen, it is argued, as a special case of *Eingebung* [predisposition], as a radical culmination and intensification of all the emotional potential that already finds expression in moods, affects, fantasies, illusions, hallucinations, obsessions, actions. But since Hellpach gives a dominant status to *Einfühlung* [empathy] within his concept of spiritual epidemics, he downplays the significance of hysterias. In his time they were widely known to be a pet topic, even a fetish, of medicine and psychology. Hellpach – who had shortly before published his own book on the subject – distances himself from this fashion. Hysteria, he claims, is only the most extreme form in which spiritual epidemics spread, but not the most potent or momentous. For laymen they might be the most striking phenomenon; science, however, has not been blinded by the spectacular.

Here, too, it seems that Hellpach wants to depart from the scientific mainstream. At least in this early work he shows himself to be an original theoretical thinker: critical towards then-reigning scientific fashions; sceptical and analytical where others operate unreflectively with metaphors and catchwords; a curious and productive unconventional thinker in a time when others are beholden to common social and cultural prejudices. This productive stance also comes to the fore at the end of the book. Hellpach does not adhere to the scientific and ideological commonplace that spiritual epidemics – as aberrant conditions – are generally harmful and must be fought with all available theoretical and practical means. He denies the prevalent ideological premises of his age's discourses of 'mass' and 'contagion.' If at the beginning Hellpach accepted the presupposition that epidemics are morbid aberrant conditions – after all, 'epidemic' carries the attribute of illness with it – , his perspective ultimately broadens. Are epidemics necessarily phenomena that must be controlled, governed, or avoided if possible? Are there not also socially and historically productive dimensions to spiritual epidemics? Hellpach emphasizes: "What has emerged from them can be good, beautiful, true – can be holy." [Was aus ihnen hervorgegangen ist, kann Gutes, Schönes, Wahres, kann Heiliges sein] (Hellpach 1906, 99). Was this a polemic against the ideologically-charged, downright phobic fear of contemporary science that the juggernaut of the mass, morbidly infected with delusional ideas, might plunge well-ordered society into anarchy and chaos?

4 A Conceptual Alternative: Freud's *Mass Psychology and Ego Analysis*

As mentioned earlier, models of mental or social contagion were a veritable fashion in science around 1900. To describe their influence, one might apply a now established category of modern scholarship; one might speak of a contagion *turn*. It is noteworthy that Freud only dealt with contagion models very late in his career. His work on hysteria had been composed of clinical case studies of individuals, and early psychoanalysis focused exclusively on individuals. There was no place for models of contagion. Only over the course of years and decades, with the deliberative recourse to social and cultural phenomena, did they enter Freud's field of vision. How this shift in socio-cultural perspective took place remains disputed. Scholars point to the events of the First World War, which unsettled Freud, but also to the fact that new vistas can already be noted in *Totem and Taboo* (1913). The continuing attempts within the growing Freudian school to broaden the range of issues in psychoanalysis should also be considered. But ultimately it must be assumed that a theoretical dynamic led the by-now relatively successful instrument of psychoanalysis to be applied to further fields of inquiry.

The upshot of this perspectival expansion is that mass phenomena also became a focus of Freud's research. The key work in this regard is the 1921 piece *Massenpsychologie und Ich-Analyse* [Mass Psychology and Ego Analysis]. Right at the beginning Freud announces his shift in perspective, although he emphasises the continuity of his overall work. He explains that whereas he had earlier considered the individual within his familial relationships, now he was taking larger social connections into account; and whereas he had earlier studied only drives in individuals, now he would also study a group or social drive. A focus on the individual, however, remained decisive. For Freud was interested in understanding and explaining not 'masses' themselves but rather their influence on individuals. To describe this influence, Freud drew freely on Le Bon. Freud's ultimately negative anthropology, which always emphasised the dark and destructive sides of human drives, could be reconciled quite easily with Le Bon's pejorative mass theory, which highlighted above all the negative aspects of masses and mass behaviour. Le Bon also proved fitting because he had used the concept of the unconscious – albeit in a rather colloquial way – and thus displayed a certain openness to theory. This relatively thorough use of Le Bon – and this is the object of Freud's treatment – leads up to a displacement of earlier theories of social cohesion and transmission in favour of Freud's own new mass and social theories. At their center lay the tried and true concept of libido. Earlier models of socio-psychological interaction such as contagion (Le Bon), imitation (Tarde), suggestion (McDougall) and herd instinct (Trotter) are rejected and replaced by a now established key Freudian concept.

Freud formally defines the new object of his research, distinguishing masses into homogeneous and heterogeneous, natural and artificial, primitive and highly organized. Like Hellpach, Freud also prefers functional distinctions to substantial ones. For every individual is a component of many masses, is bound variously through identification, belongs to manifold mass souls: race, class, religious denomination, political organization, and so forth. Freud's treatment, however, is devoted exclusively to artificial masses, namely churches and armies. These – and masses in general – share one basic trait: libido.

> [...] shall I attempt to apply the concept of libido, which has served us so well in the study of psychoneuroses, to the explanation of mass psychology [...werde ich den Versuch machen, zur Aufklärung der Massenpsychologie den Begriff der *Libido* zu verwenden, der uns im Studium der Psychoneurosen so gute Dienste geleistet hat]. (Freud 1921, 98)

In the process this key Freudian concept receives innovative expansion. If libido hitherto counted primarily as a sexual drive, now, with explicit reference to Plato's concept of *eros*, it becomes a striving *per se* – also in the service of social ideals. Libido becomes a social and cultural category meaning: "general love of mankind," [allgemeine Menschenliebe] and "devotion to concrete objects and to abstract ideas" [Hingebung an konkrete Gegenstände und an abstrakte Ideen] (Freud 1921, 98).

This libido has two characteristic traits, namely that

> each individual is libidinously tied on the one hand to the leader of the mass (*Führer*) [...], on the other hand to the other individuals in the mass. [jeder Einzelne einerseits an den Führer [...], anderseits [sic] an die anderen Massenindividuen libidinös gebunden ist.] (Freud 1921, 104)

The originally sexual drive has thus been socially reorientated, has sought two substitute objects: ominous leaders and other mass individuals. Libido exhausts itself in this double-attachment. Yet the most it can attain is a substitute satisfaction. For Freud steadfastly maintains that this attachment causes the original orientation to be "pushed aside from [its] sexual goal" [von diesem sexuellen Ziel abgedrängt] and "diverted from its primordial goals" [von ihren ursprünglichen Zielen abgelenkt] (Freud 1921, 98, 113). That is to say, the "ego ideal" [Ich-Ideal] postulated here can only be actualized through detours and errors – games of hide-and-seek for repressing the sexual drive. The attachment to common leaders or to other subjects and presumably common ideals is thus also a kind of delusion and self-delusion. For Freud the ego is and remains decisive. He cannot and does not want to explain 'the social;' he remains decidedly oriented towards the individual. Masses – and here the consistency of his theoretical model can be seen – are from the outset a disturbance, an aberration. They merely strengthen the potential for individual deception and repression: "the individual is fettered in the mass" [Unfreiheit des Einzelnen in der Masse] (Freud 1921, 104). In this sense the title of the tract is apropos and programmatic. It deals ostensibly with masses, but essentially with the ego and the individual. Freud has no concept of the social in his psychoanalysis (only at the end of the 1920s does he finally broaden his horizon). Thus he needs no concept of contagion either, and he rejects it. Sexuality is always at hand, is always prefigured and present in every individual as an *inner* quality. The social level turns out to be at best the extension of family life; social conflicts are extended familial conflicts. Reductive concepts like contagion, imitation, and suggestion are thus replaced by another, equally reductive principle: libido.

This was an instance of reductionism, a first instance. A further instance of reductionism was Freud's systematic minimization of learned disciplines:

> Even sociology, which concerns itself with the behaviour of human beings in society, can be nothing other than applied psychology. Strictly speaking, there are only two sciences: psychology, pure and applied, and natural history. [Denn auch die Soziologie, die vom Verhalten der Menschen in der Gesellschaft handelt, kann nichts anderes sein als angewandte Psychologie. Streng genommen gibt es ja nur zwei Wissenschaften, Psychologie, reine und angewandte, und Naturkunde.] (Freud 1933, 194)

For Freud there are only two disciplines or disciplinary branches for explaining the world: the life sciences and psychology (psychology as psychoanalysis). And in the new science of psychoanalysis, the concept of contagion had no place. Modish turns had no appeal for him. Instead he always adhered to his own turn.

5 The Meaningfulness of a Metaphorical Model

Carus's 'consolatory' model of spiritual contagion, Hellpach's scepticism, and Freud's rejection – how do they relate to today's discourses of contagion? In her critical analysis of the commonplace of 'moral contagion,' the historian Jan E. Goldstein identified the conditions that favoured the success of the social-contagion model in the eighteenth and nineteenth centuries. In her view, there were several contributing factors: (1) an anti-democratic impetus, (2) an obsession with social control, and (3) the fusion of medicine and psychology with the institutions and restrictive practices of state power (Goldstein 1984, 182–184). The role of *medical policeman* played by the discourse of contagion in the Early Modern and Enlightenment periods gave way, so this line of argument could be continued, at the end of the nineteenth century to the role of *social policeman.* Indeed, in the persons of Lombroso, Sighele, and Le Bon, the discourse of social contagion was adopted and elaborated by *criminologists* and *sociologists* who stood explicitly for the ideal of a closed society unidimensionally governed and controlled by the state. Contagion was a key concept in decidedly anti-democratic notions of society; it was the basis for authoritarian social control. Nevertheless, one must also acknowledge that a more neutral use of the metaphor or concept of contagion began to emerge around 1900, as the example of Hellpach shows.

Meanwhile the implications of the contagion commonplace have expanded. Present-day concepts of social contagion need in no way be laden with the antiliberal characteristics just mentioned. Nonetheless these more recent concepts systematically naturalize the realms of the social and the cultural and have inherited the authority of scientific and medical discourse. The social sciences travel in the slipstream of the natural sciences, participate in their hegemony and make a calculated attempt thereby to maximize their status. They willingly subject themselves to the diktat of the natural sciences. The French cultural and cognitive anthropologist Dan Sperber has created a rigorous, authoritative scientific model for how speaking of social epidemics could actually make sense. Starting from the question "Pourquoi n'existe-t-il pas à ce jour de science naturelle du social" [why does no natural science of the social exist today] (Sperber 1996, 12) he is working on just such a science. He postulates processes of contagion, of epidemic contagion, which he understands, in all their possible complexity, as a basic model of social structure and development. From the viewpoint of the anthropologist schooled in the natural sciences, social processes are primarily understandable as epidemic processes of contagion, diffusion, reception, and transformation. Guided by models of self-organization, sociobiology, and genetics, he elaborates a natural cosmos of the social that embraces reductionism. As far as Sperber is concerned, it is not *his* social and cultural model that requires justification, but rather models that, while producing no tangible results, incessantly spread ostensible non-reductionism.

The debate over the 'nature' or 'culture' of the cultural remains unresolved, even in the light of Sperber's provocative considerations. But with regard to 'contagion,' one might ask: how is the concept useful at all in medical debates? Has this concept or metaphor not long been exposed as a grandiose, loaded fake, whose epistemic value is based solely on its suggestive connotations? And is this not *a fortiori* the case when it comes to contagion commonplaces in the context of social discourses? For the contagion concept is still built on an essential fallacy, one strongly adhered to by proponents of causal bacteriology after 1870 in both Germany and France. As a commonplace and as a concept, 'contagion' was understood as monocausal. By 1900 such concepts were already being rejected, as the elegant logic of causal bacteriology – where the pathogen, there the disease – showed itself to be much too simplistic. Contagion was never conceivable without impeding, abetting, retarding, or transforming factors. The whole concept had to be overhauled in terms of endemic and epidemic, latency and virulency, predisposition and immunity, variation and mutation, the relationship between individual and environment, and so forth (Sarasin et al. 2007; Berger 2009).

The concepts changed, but the culturally influential metaphors and suggestive terms remained largely the same. What were they based on? In the medical and socio-epidemiological prevention of infection, on the level of both explanation and praxis, they were based on discovering, blocking, and controlling the path that led from the presence of pathogens to the discovery of their effect on human bodies. This was and is the normality of medical and socio-epidemiological aetiology, prevention, and therapy. But this normality vanishes in the face of an ocean of extreme abnormality: why in the same place and at the same time do some people contract epidemic diseases but others not? Or with regard to the bacteriological accomplishments of the nineteenth century: why do some individuals not get sick even though bacteria or viruses are demonstrable in their bodies on a massive scale? Why do some people pass on these pathogens, others not? Indeed, medicine and socio-epidemiology do not explain these *normal cases of non-illness* but rather automatically sort them out as irrelevant special cases. In the same breath they group *special cases of illness* with those recognised as normal, formulate rules, and seek to proceed on the basis of these rules. Medicine and epidemiology therefore always work with and on special cases, and these provide examples for a rule. Baldly stated, rules are thus derived from situations that are *eo ipso* nothing but exceptions and anomalies; scientific norm and normality are made up of nothing but aberrations. They do not make – and this is an epidemiological conundrum – exceptions to the rule; they make rules out of the exception. Is this inversive concept of 'contagion,' which does not formulate specific rules but rather only exceptions to the rule, supposed to be of use to the social sciences? Should the noble dream of formulating rules of the social be conceptually based on a term that *a priori* and *per se* deals only with vanishing irregularities?

Or – and this in conclusion – has the concept of contagion changed so fundamentally in the course of its adoption by the social sciences and humanities that it now stands primarily for the impartation and transmission of social normalities? Has the concept of contagion come to live a double life: on the one hand as a normative, emotionally charged concept denoting certain aberrant conditions; on the other hand as a descriptive, neutral concept dealing, in Sperber's sense for example, with the functioning of social normality? Much seems to speak for this double life, even for a broad normalization of the contagion commonplace of late. The fashion of speaking of social contagion may once have made concerted use of mechanisms for accumulating social attention and participated in apparently basic fears of epidemic – which fears, however, it itself discursively fed – , but now the situation is clearly different. As a result of its increasing application to many disciplines, 'contagion' is no longer tied to a demeanor of excitation and the stupefying expedition of hysteria. Rather, it would seem to have become a ubiquitous social term. It no longer explains the unsafe but the safe; it no longer explains the undesirable but – in the case of aesthetic contagion in the arts or market research – the desirable; it is devoted no longer to the extraordinary but to the ordinary.

References

Aubry, Paul. *La contagion du meurtre. Étude d'anthropologie criminelle.* Paris: Félix Alcan, 1887.

Bekhterev, Vladimir von. *Die Bedeutung der Suggestion im sozialen Leben.* Wiesbaden: J. F. Bergmann, 1905.

Berger, Silvia. *Bakterien in Krieg und Frieden. Eine Geschichte der medizinischen Bakteriologie in Deutschland 1890–1933.* Göttingen: Wallstein, 2009.

Bertrand, Dominique. "Contagious Laughter and the Burlesque: From the Literal to the Metaphorical." *Imagining Contagion in Early Modern Europe.* Ed. Claire L. Carlin. Houndmills, Basingstoke, Hampshire: Palgrave Macmillan, 2005. 177–194.

Briese, Olaf. *Angst in den Zeiten der Cholera.* 4 vols. Vol. 1: *Über kulturelle Ursprünge des Bakteriums.* Berlin: Akademie Verlag, 2003.

Busch, Kathrin. "Ansteckung und Widerfahrnis. Für eine Ästhetik des Pathischen." *'pathos'. Konturen eines kulturwissenschaftlichen Grundbegriffs.* Eds Kathrin Busch and Iris Därmann. Bielefeld: Transcript, 2007. 51–74.

Calmeil, Louis Florentin. *De la folie considérée sous le point de vue pathologique* [...]. Paris: J.-B. Baillière, London: H. Baillière, 1845.

Carus, Carl Gustav. *Ueber Geistes-Epidemien der Menschheit.* Leipzig, Meissen: F. W. Goed'sche Buchhandlung, 1852.

Cassirer, Ernst. *Substanzbegriff und Funktionsbegriff. Untersuchungen über die Grundfragen der Erkenntniskritik.* Berlin: Cassirer, 1910.

Cheyronnaud, Jacques. "'Homines pestilentes'." *La contagion.* Eds Jacques Cheyronnaud, Philippe Roussin, and Georges Vigarello. Paris: Édition du Seuil, 1998. 41–64 [*Communications* 66].

Conrad, Lawrence I. "A Ninth-Century-Muslim Scholar's Discussion of Contagion." *Contagion. Perspectives from Pre-Modern Societies.* Eds. Lawrence I. Conrad and Dominik Wujastyk. Aldershot, Burlington, Singapore: Ashgate, 2000. 163–178.

Despine, Prosper Constant. *De la Contagion morale* [...]. Marseille: Etienne Camoin, 1870.

d'Holbach, Paul-Henri Thiry. "La contagion sacrée, ou Histoire naturelle de la superstition" [1768]. *Œuvres philosophiques.* Ed. Jean Pierre Jackson. Vol. 1. Paris: Éditions Alive, 1998. 121–300.

Dinges, Martin. "Pest und Staat: Von der Institutionengeschichte zur sozialen Konstruktion?" *Neue Wege in der Seuchengeschichte.* Eds Martin Dinges and Thomas Schlich. Stuttgart: Steiner, 1995. 71–104 [*Medizin, Gesellschaft und Geschichte,* Beiheft 6].

Düllo, Thomas. "Ansteckendes Erzählen." *Ästhetik & Kommunikation* 41 (2010) No. 149/150: 30–37.

Durkheim, Émile. *Le suicide. Étude de sociologie.* Paris: Félix Alcan, 1897.

Durkheim, Émile. *Les formes élémentaires de la vie religieuse* [...]. Paris: Félix Alcan, 1912.

Farber, Walter. "How to Marry a Disease: Epidemics, Contagion, and a Magic Ritual against the 'Hand of the Ghost'." *Magic and Rationality in Ancient Near Eastern and Graeco-Roman Medicine.* Ed. Herman F. J. Horstmanshoff and Martin Stol. Leiden, Boston: Brill, 2004. 117–132.

Fournier, Michel. "The Pathology of Reading: The Novel as an Agent of Infection." *Imagining Contagion in Early Modern Europe.* Ed. Claire L. Carlin. Houndmills, Basingstoke, Hampshire: Palgrave Macmillan, 2005. 195–209.

Freud, Sigmund. "Massenpsychologie und Ich-Analyse [1921]." *Gesammelte Werke. Chronologisch geordnet.* Eds Anna Freud et al. Vol. 13. Frankfurt a. M.: Fischer Taschenbuch Verlag, 1999. 74–161.

Freud, Sigmund. "Neue Folge der Vorlesungen zur Einführung in die Psychoanalyse [1933]." *Gesammelte Werke. Chronologisch geordnet.* Eds Anna Freud et al. Vol. 15. Frankfurt a. M.: Fischer Taschenbuch Verlag, 1999.

Ginneken, Jaap van. *Crowds, Psychology, and Politics, 1871–1899.* Cambridge, New York, Victoria: Cambridge University Press, 1992.

Goldstein, Jan. "'Moral Contagion': A Professional Ideology of Medicine and Psychiatry in Eighteenth- and Nineteenth-Century France." *Professions and the French State, 1700–1900.* Ed. Gerald L. Geison. Philadelphia: University of Pennsylvania Press, 1984. 181–222.

Hellpach, Willy. *Die geistigen Epidemien.* Frankfurt a. M.: Rütten & Loening, 1906 [*Die Gesellschaft* 11].

Hellpach, Willy. *Wirken in Wirren. Lebenserinnerungen. Eine Rechenschaft über Wert und Glück, Schuld und Sturz meiner Generation. Erster Band 1877–1914.* Hamburg: Christian Wegner, 1948.

Ideler, Karl Wilhelm. *Versuch einer Theorie des religiösen Wahnsinns.* Vol. 1. Halle: C. A. Schwetscke & Sohn, 1848.

Jouanna, Jacques. “Air, miasme et contagion à l’époque d’Hippocrate.” *Air, miasmes et contagion. Les épidémies dans l’Antiquité et au Moyen Age.* Eds. Sylvie Bazin-Tacchella, Danielle Queruel, and Évelyne Samama. Langres: Dominique Guéniot, 2001. 9–28.

Kaune, Claudia-Anja. *Willy Hellpach (1877–1955). Biographie eines liberalen Politikers der Weimarer Republik.* Frankfurt a. M.: Lang, 1991.

Knittel, Michel. *Ueber sporadische psychische Ansteckung.* Med. Diss. Strassburg: Johann Heinrich Eduard Heitz, 1884.

Le Bon, Gustave: *Psychologie des foules.* Paris: Félix Alcan, 1895.

Legrand du Saulle, Henri. *Les hystériques, état physique et état mental* [...]. Paris: J.-B. Baillière, 1883.

Leven, Karl-Heinz. “Miasma und Metadosis – antike Vorstellungen von Ansteckung.” *Medizin, Gesellschaft und Geschichte* 11 (1992): 43–73.

Lombroso, Cesare, and Rodolfo Laschi. *Il delitto politico e le rivoluzioni* [...]. Torino: Fratelli Bocca, 1890.

Lucas, Prosper. *De l’imitation contagieuse ou De la propagation sympathique des névroses et des monomanies.* Paris: Didot le jeune, 1833.

Lund, Roger L. “Infectious Wit: Metaphor, Atheism, and the Plague in Eighteenth-Century London.” *Literature and Medicine* 22 (2003): 45–64.

Middendorf, Stefanie. *Massenkultur. Zur Wahrnehmung gesellschaftlicher Modernität in Frankreich.* Göttingen: Wallstein, 2009.

Moscovici, Serge. *L’âge des foules. Un traité historique de psychologie des masses.* Paris: Fayard, 1981.

Nutton, Vivian. “The Seeds of Disease: An Explanation of Contagion and Infection from the Greeks to the Renaissance.” *Medical History* 27 (1983): 1–34.

Nutton, Vivian. “The Reception of Fracastoro’s Theory of Contagion. The Seed That Fell among Thorns?” *Osiris* 6 (1990): 196–234.

Nutton, Vivian. “To Kill or Not to Kill? Caelius Aurelianus on contagion.” *Text and Tradition. Studies in Ancient Medicine and its Transmission. Presented to Jutta Kollesch.* Eds Klaus-Dietrich Fischer, Diethard Nickel, and Paul Potter. Leiden, Boston, Cologne: Brill, 1998. 233–242.

Nutton, Vivian. “Did the Greeks have a Word for it?” *Contagion. Perspectives from Pre-Modern Societies.* Eds Lawrence I. Conrad and Dominik Wujastyk. Aldershot, Burlington, Singapore: Ashgate, 2000. 137–162.

Nye, Robert A. *Crime, Madness, & Politics in Modern France. The Medical Concept of National Decline.* Princeton, NJ: Princeton University Press, 1984.

Rambosson, Jean. *Phénomènes nerveux, intellectuels et moraux, leur transmission par contagion.* Paris: Firmin-Didot, 1883.

Régnard, Paul. *Les maladies épidémiques de l’esprit* [...]. Paris: E. Plon, Nourrit et Cie, 1887.

Reichert, Ramón. *Der Diskurs der Seuche. Sozialpathologien 1700–1900.* Munich: Fink, 1997.

Roussin, Philippe. “Des liens humains (toucher, contagion, sympathie).” *La contagion.* Eds Jacques Cheyronnaud, Philippe Roussin, and Georges Vigarello. Paris: Édition du Seuil, 1998. 121–146 [*Communications* 66].

Sarasin, Philipp, Silvia Berger, Marianne Hänseler, and Miriam Spörri (Eds). *Bakteriologie und Moderne. Studien zur Biopolitik des Unsichtbaren 1870–1920.* Frankfurt a. M.: Suhrkamp, 2007.

Schaub, Mirjam, Nicola Suthor, and Erika Fischer-Lichte (Eds). *Ansteckung. Zur Körperlichkeit eines ästhetischen Prinzips.* Munich: Fink, 2005.

Sighele, Scipio. *La coppia criminale. Studio di psicologia morbosa.* Torino: Fratelli Bocca, 1893.
Sperber, Dan. *La contagion des idées. Théorie naturaliste de la culture.* Paris: Odile Jacob, 1996.
Stallmeister, Walter, and Helmut E. Lück (Eds). *Willy Hellpach: Beiträge zu Werk und Biographie.* Frankfurt a. M.: Lang, 1991.
Sticker, Georg. *Abhandlungen aus der Seuchengeschichte und Seuchenlehre.* Vol. I.1: *Die Geschichte der Pest.* Gießen: Alfred Töpelmann, 1908.
Strowick, Elisabeth. *Sprechende Körper – Poetik der Ansteckung. Performativa in Literatur und Rhetorik.* Munich: Fink, 2009.
Tarde, Gabriel. *Le lois de l'imitation. Étude sociologique.* Paris: Félix Alcan, 1890a.
Tarde, Gabriel. *La philosophie pénale.* Lyon: Storck, Paris: G. Masson, 1890b.

George Rousseau

The Overlap of Discourses of Contagion: Economic, Sexual, and Psychological

1 Frenzied Metaphors and Historical Contingency

The contagion that interests me is moral and metaphoric: specifically how homosexuals – gay persons – were historically configured as people who 'caught' their orientation from other homosexuals; an absurd position but not so for earlier masses. My focus is narrow, yet begs for comparison with the broad development of contagion discourse in Western culture. For example, recently the most glaring contagion discourse has permeated the banking sector, yet it did so a full decade *before* the current economic crisis exploded in 2007. The language of contagion became entrenched in the banking sphere by 1998, well before the credit crunch officially erupted (Glick and Rose 1998; Schoenmaker 1996; Woodward 1999). Can the parallel universes – sexual and economic – tell us anything from this lost decade's (1997–2007) discourse about 'contagious gays'?

The contagion described in the banking sphere of the 1990s was literal: removed from any metaphoric intention beyond that inherent in all language; its purpose internationally to alert policy makers to what was approaching on the horizon (Woodward 1999). In the late 1990s there was no frenzied rhetoric or wild metaphoric affirmation – these arose after 2007; after chaos and confusion set in, and when it became apparent that major economies were teetering owing to soaring national deficits. Heightened metaphoricity occurred *after* alarm bells sounded and panic set it. But if you scrutinize this discourse circa 1997–1998, a decade *before* the crisis erupted, it becomes clear that *rampant metaphoricity* is absent. If generalized the abstract principle suggests intense metaphoricity arises *after* the appearance of the phenomenon, no matter how confusing the original manifestation. Put otherwise, frenzied metaphors succeed less frenetic events, not vice versa. The duration of time lags varies depending on the event(s): bankers were troubled in 1997–1998 because they foresaw an oncoming economic crisis of unprecedented proportions and sought to describe what they identified as its potentially contagious elements (Glick and Rose 1998). Ten years later, in 2007, when the effects of the crisis became self-evident – too glaring to overlook – contagion's metaphoricity in the banking sphere swelled.

This recent metaphoric development contrasts with calmer historical moments. For example, post-Hobbesian philosophers discussed the contagion of benevolence, especially good works towards others; by the eighteenth century this 'contagion' spread to discourse about human sociability: the sense that humans are not merely sociable creatures, but that precisely by dint of being sociable we 'infect' others with a sense of what sociability entails. Shaftesbury, Hutcheson, and other early moralists acknowledged that shared sentiments could become dangerously contagious, disruptive forces; as Shaftesbury opined, "the disease [of doing good] is no sooner seen than caught" (Shaftesbury et al. 1999, 27). By the time Hume wrote his celebrated *Treatise of Human Nature* (1739) two decades later, the contagion of sociability was widely construed as the literal social connective tissue between humans:

> As in strings equally wound up, the motion of one communicates itself to the rest; so all the affections readily pass from one person to another, and beget correspondent movements in every human creature. (Hume 1978, 257–258)

Hume was less philosophically influenced by the Ancient notion of identification – especially Lucretius's arguments – than by recent Enlightenment challenges to the concept of selfhood articulated by Mandeville and the post-Hobbesians. But this metaphoricity differs from our banking version; generated, as it was, in philosophical discourse to persuade readers through the use of a few charged metaphors to adopt positions about unseen mechanisms in economic breakdown. No historical event or social outbreak – nothing financially ominous on the horizon, as it was in 1997–1998 – preceded the composition of Hume's *Treatise* of 1739–1740. He and his contemporary moralists would have articulated their theories of "contagious sociability" even if the post-Hobbesians had not endured into the eighteenth century. The alarms, however, in the banking sector since 2007 required something else.

It may be that human nature permits little alternative to the persistence – some will say tyranny – of the language of contagion (Bashford and Hooker 2001; Browning 1998). As a cultural and linguistic historian, I want to suggest how much steadier we are now in the domain of contagion metaphor than a century ago: not merely in the sexual sphere, which constitutes my main concern here, but others too. Stated pithily, levels of contagious discourse augur poorly for outcomes; the lower the level, the more rational and empirical the phenomena being described, as in 1998 versus 2007. Magisterial questions about the contagion of debt have been put, of course, to economists and policy makers since then, but few any longer invoke a reckless language of contagion without interrogation and reflection. Likewise, in philosophical and moral realms, as in my example from Enlightenment philosophy. Discourses of moral contagion may not be alien to us in the twenty-first century when every day, it seems, the news suggests the 'infection' of crime and violence; and when historians repeatedly document how we have survived waves of allegedly 'contagious violence' in which the *contagious component* is as noteworthy as the *criminality* of rioting and looting. Whether construed as copy-cat violence, imitative violence, or in other mimetic forms, the action is conceptualized through *contagion* as its overarching idea (Lynch 1996; Nuttin and Beckers 1975).

More locally, I have tried to understand the profile of the homosexual in history in the *longue durée* from the Ancients forward. Specifically, I have been preoccupied by the homosexual's symbolism and the mentalization of this sexual stereotype rather than the anatomical and pathological differences scientists and theorists have located (Rousseau 1991). Such retrieval is more fraught than meets the eye: anachronism is one of its supreme sins, and one reason we resist anachronism is that it compels us to think in odious ways. Yet perhaps even anachronism is less reprehensible than failure to ask *big* questions about the homosexual's configuration over time and space. A book devoting itself to contagion 1880–1933 has specific work to do and may be unable to devote time to the *longue durée*. Conversely, everything I have learned suggests that late nineteenth-century developments about the sodomite's presumed contagion arose within an ancient pedigree of precedence (Carlin 2005; Christensen 2005).

2 The Filthy Sodomite

The Ancients configured the sodomite along lines that included perceived filth. Alcibiades' boys apparently had dirty fingernails, and Juvenal's sodomites in the Roman world are often pictured as unbathed; the opposite of our modern, clean-cut, preppie gays obsessed with bodily pores sanitized by Dolce Gabbana. Did such body odors and earthy skins intensify desire; render these boys sexually more alluring? Juvenal is silent but his sodomitical youths are anything but physically clean (Davidson 2007). The Ancient world sets the stage for what follows.

Moral filth – as distinct from *literal* filth – had been intrinsic to most theories of contagion from its earliest days. Whether as miasma, pollution, or physical contagion, the moral imperative never strayed far from the tip of the imagination of doctors and patients, authors and readers, almost as if contagion itself were both a physical and *non*-physical category (Douglas 1966). What precisely is it about contagion that continues to lift it from its physical presence, and demand its moral dimension? Especially its moral dimension construed according to the local tenets of particular cultures (Aubry 1896)?

A potted history of homosexuality from the Greeks forward will, ruefully, not advance us much, yet some highlights are instructive for contagion's progress in relation to the sodomite. Albertus Magnus, the thirteenth century German Dominican friar and theologian, considered homosexuality a *contagious* disease, especially common among wealthy classes, and difficult to cure. In what sense *contagious?* Contagious, Magnus writes, within, or to, the individual body itself:

> If [man] fails to exercise restraint over his body, he opens the door to rapid weakening and deterioration, especially through the imagination and passions which accelerate the process of bodily corruption. (Magnus 1987, 64–65)

These physical and non-physical processes combine to produce the contagious disease, yet Magnus does not explain how. He is reasoning metaphorically.

Three centuries later Fracastoro noted in his 1546 *De contagione* that syphilis is transmitted through amorous ways and inquired: "Why should we think this late *Contagion* strange?" (Fracastoro 1930, 9) He uses the language of contagion – his word is *contagiosum* – and situates the cause of venereal disease specifically in contagious causes residing in human contact (*contactus*). In his earlier poem of 1530 about syphilis, Fracastoro had attributed venereal conditions to travel from country to country, hence the *contagium* of *contactus* as spreading geographically: the 'French disease' to Italy, where it becomes known as the 'Italian disease', the 'Italian disease' to Spain, where it becomes known as the 'Spanish disease,' and across national borders. The 'diseases' themselves are never designated by their local name in their home country; therefore the French disease is never called the French disease *within France*, only by that name in Italy and Spain, and so forth, immediately clarifying how contagious conditions historically contained built-in moral characteristics that were linguistically expressed from early modern times. But 'filthy diseases' were not the only contagious maladies in the Renaissance: supernatural illnesses, or at least conditions thought to have been brought about through supernatural means, also were, as when Robert Burton postulated in his *Anatomy of Melancholy* (Faulkner et al. 1989, 252) that supernatural illness was contagious. "Men if they see but another man tremble, giddy, or sick of some fearful disease, their apprehension and feare is so strong in this kinde, that they will have the same disease," contagious transmission made possible by the power of the imagination.

Then change occurred. During the Enlightenment, constructions of the sodomitical type never veered far from the image of an excessive masturbator. And vice versa too: the compulsive masturbator was routinely imagined as sodomitical.[1] Filth – literal and metaphoric – attached itself to this mental picture in the

1 Ironically, two hundred years later Freud wrote on 17 October 1899 to his confidante Fliess: "What would you think if masturbation were to reduce itself to homosexuality, and the latter,

form of 'filthy masturbators,' and the conjunction coagulated to form the main explanation for the stereotype within medical literature. Furthermore, from the early eighteenth century forward intuition about a "third-sex" arose: a gender physically "soft" and "flaccid" through the profligate waste of seed; a type ending in despair and madness (Rousseau 1991, 12; Herdt 1994). Widespread Enlightenment anti-onania campaigns not only disseminated fear that this excess would cause blindness, madness, depression, and suicide, but *also* a morally, and personally, polluted sodomite.[2] By the late eighteenth century the predominant explanation in Western Europe was that habitual self-abuse was also *catching:* if you associated with compulsive onanists you would join their ranks through uncharted contagious processes not so differently from the copy-cat contagion of political rioters, or the contagion of the failing Euro in Greece, Ireland, Portugal, and now Spain. Huge national debts in relation to Gross Domestic Product are doubtlessly onerous and economically catastrophic for individual countries. The two domains – economic and sexual – may appear disparate but their language thrives on remarkably similar metaphors; but *exactly how* does the failing Euro *spread* from country to country (Price-Smith 2009) and by what specific processes do copy-cat rioters enact their contagion? No one stipulates how, nor did the Enlightenment anti-onania doctors, but everyone invokes a rhetoric of contagion as if it were somehow clarificatory of the processes and adequate to explain the physics of the contagion.

In the era of Dr Samuel Tissot, the Swiss Enlightenment medical anthropologist, one theory aimed to delineate the physical pathway. This was the view that the *habit of onania* was not contagious *itself* – that is the consorting, or bearing contact with, other masturbators was not the culprit – but that physical blindness was. The visualized sequence was this: through repeated self-abuse masturbators grow blind; constantly wasted seed deprives their eyes of necessary, replenishing fluid; the anatomical fluid causing blindness in the eyes is the contagious material; contact with it also causes blindness, and subsequent madness, in others. The fluid itself is contagious. This flawed theory gained credence because it appeared logical, almost impossible then to refute: eyes obviously contained fluid. Why should that fluid not be contagious? Despite its appeal contemporary "mad doctors" – William Battie, the Monro brothers, William Perfect – resisted it in their belief about the nervous rather than contagious determinants of insanity. Yet the fluidists persisted, hammering in the idea that sodomites

that is male homosexuality (in both sexes) were the primitive form of sexual longing?" (Freud et al. 1985, 380).

2 These discourses invoked the terms catching, contagious, infectious, infected, and others indiscriminately; a lexical study of their appearances and sources would be useful.

shared anatomical characteristics that would be identified some day more specifically than the author of *Satan's Harvest Home* (1749) had been able. Michel Foucault derided these fluidists in his *Histoire de la Folie* for an unsubstantiated, assumed contagion whose agenda was moral rather than empirical. Foucault's specific indictment is that contagion is such a persuasive ideology it can seem self-evident, yet – as he argued – the whole history of science and medicine conspired in an opposite position. Sounder proof of contagion was needed.

3 Social Contagion

Lexical changes to the post-Enlightenment semantic roots of contagion also shed light. The young Edmund Burke, writing in his very first published work, the 1757 *Philosophical Enquiry into the Origin of our Ideas of the Sublime,* stipulates that "by the contagion of our passions, we catch a fire already kindled *in another,*" [emphasis mine] – that is, the "fire" of another *person* (Burke and Boulton 1987, 175–176). Laurence Sterne, Burke's contemporary and the author of *Tristram Shandy,* wrote that "to *read* is to lay oneself open to contagion," [emphasis mine] a puzzling position suggesting that words themselves are contagious, or at least contagious through psychological suggestion impinging on the body's senses and organs of perception (Loveridge 1982, 208). Philosopher-poet Coleridge observed that "[s]ensibility [...] proves little more than the coincidence or *contagion* of pleasurable sensations in different persons" [emphasis mine] (Coleridge et al. 1990, 4: 223). These examples from the period 1760–1820 aim to capture, however imperfectly, how human beings 'infect' each other with phenomena from "sensations" to emotions and even words. They also suggest how pervasive references to charged metaphors of contagion then were. The compilation of dozens of examples from this era would further demonstrate how the synergy of these uses converges in body-mind overlaps, whether in affects, emotions, or cognitive states. But – and this is the point – I find no similar specific pathways in the sodomitical condition except for the affirmation, made without any evidence whatever, that it is perfidiously contagious. Precisely how it is contagious, no one says.

The lexical heritage of *contagiosum,* both in Latin and English, further reveals how the sodomite's filth *increased* over the centuries. If the Enlightenment sodomite was morally repugnant and physiologically compromised, the Victorian and Bismarckian sodomitical body was imagined as *filthier:* exterior and interior body parts and guts. The homosexual has not yet been physically idealized as he will be – most of my observations derive from the male, the female having another historical trajectory – in the twentieth century. Costume and fashion disguise this bodily status, as in the early nineteenth-century effete British Dilletanti and Macaronis so often decked out in deceptive colourful frocks and tight trousers. But their nudities, if they could have been viewed, remained impure. Linguistically set the dials to c. 1800, or 1850, and filth has not yet entered the elevated metaphoric range it will inhabit later in the nineteenth century, in part to assist national campaigns to assert cleanliness over filth in developing British, French and other global empires. Purity and filth, in Mary Douglas's tropaic sense (1966), of course long antedated Enlightenment uses, yet the 'contagious sodomite' was also beginning (i.e., 1800 – 1860) to be configured along her axes.

Nineteenth-century additions to the configuration were racial, religious, even biogeographical after 1860, especially along lines of post-Darwinian degeneration and extinct species, but to a greater extent they were *contactual* through touch and infection (Christensen 2005). Contagion and infection differed: carriers could be contagious while not being infected. In the realms of sexual orientation the primary route for acquisition among the *not-yet-infected* was *social* contagion: the notion that when – what we call – straight and gay people 'interact' the gay person is somehow an active aggressor, the straight person a passive victim. Such a view is so abhorrent to our contemporary sensibility it appears offensive now to read; but anachronism is one of the gravest errors in retrievals of this variety and no matter how odious, the views of yesterday must be faithfully reconstructed if we are to understand them. In nineteenth-century constructions, the contagious pathway shows the passive party acquiescing to active advances, and by so doing immerses himself in 'catching contact.' For the passive victim, itself a loaded metaphor, the power of advance is too seductive to stave off, just as epidemical disease is too robust for immune systems to resist. By the 1890s, when Oscar Wilde is defending himself in court, the degree to which constructions of the post-Darwinian sodomite are thriving on metaphors of contagion is patent. A forlorn biographical example cries out for attention in the 1880s when Cambridge poet-scholar A. E. Housman, was living together with American-born Moses Jackson. After heterosexual Jackson rebuffed Housman and left England, the already reclusive Housman sequestered himself in a monastic existence at Trinity College Cambridge so he would not be – *infectious* to others. The notion of a 'contagious sodomitical Houseman' appears preposterous to us – too absurd to ponder and a further reason why we eschew anachronism – but was hardly so to the Edwardian mindset. Housman insisted his scout should leave his meals in front of his closed door for later collection.

Another nineteenth-century trend, concurrent with the rise of sexology during the 1870s, invoked the sodomite's defective blood and weak nerves, then believed to be constantly degenerating (Eder et al. 1999). Contaminated blood had long been ascribed as the source of other *morally* debilitating conditions ranging from antisocial behaviour to criminality. Weak nerves, especially those of males, had been much discussed since Werther's suicide a century earlier in Goethe's best-selling novel of that name (1774). The contagious capacity of both defects, blood and nerves, was mythical – a fiction; but speculation grew that even those who *associated* with such persons could themselves be contaminated, especially already nervous types bringing down the robust of health of others. Religions were implicated, Jews out for Christian blood, and Christians taking revenge by declaring their anatomic supremacy, further purified by the sacrament of the Eucharist (Bennett 2009). By the turn of the twentieth century, the Jew and sodomite are being yoked in this fantasy of impure sodomitical blood and corrupted, or debilitated, nervous systems, with Christians often declaring a need for reprisal (Gilman 1988). Time would expose it as a phantasmagoria thriving, above all, on heightened metaphoric language. Deplete these discourses of inferior blood and weakened nerves and the edifice crumbles.

A recent book by Canadian historian Guy Poirier, *L'homosexualitè dans l'imaginaire de la Renaissance* (1996), claims that the body of the sodomite in early modern European thought was anatomically constructed on the blueprint of the hermaphrodite. Physical contagion plays a part in Poirier's configuration: the hermaphrodite's *infectious melancholy.* Poirier demonstrates that the sodomite's repeatedly thwarted sexual desire historically predisposed him to chronic melancholy leading to insanity. It is an intriguing possibility. If indeed the hermaphrodite's tragedy had been perpetual melancholy – the gloom of unrelenting sexual frustration – it would have been recognizable to other melancholics. The contagion's pathway from melancholic to melancholic remained hidden but no great leap was necessary to grasp the enduring pathos of the sodomite's plight: desire forever aborting itself, eventually ending in Renaissance lunacy. This melancholy, Poirier believes, engendered a sense of the contagious hermaphrodite. Anachronism enters so prominently into Poirier's argument that we must turn ourselves, it seems, into near-magicians to disentangle it: first the hermaphrodite as ancestor of the homosexual – a difficult passage in its own right – followed by melancholy's bizarre contagion. When these various transhistorical tasks are accomplished, there is little difficulty granting that gloomy types preternaturally attract others to themselves – their sole pathway to a modicum of sociability.

Nineteenth-century French psychiatrist Esquirol, Professor of Medicine at the Salpêtrière in Paris, was an authority on the weak nerves of male patients. He had treated hundreds of soldiers suffering from nostalgia, then a physical disease – the chronic malady of longing for home presenting with symptoms as violent as less recondite ones – and reasoned that if nostalgia could be epidemic, so too might sodomy be among soldiers. The logic was unmapped but conditions ripe: male confinement, geographical removal from women, love for the soldier-brother in the trenches. But what was the dynamic progression of 'nostalgic sodomy'? Esquirol explained:

> When nostalgia prevails epidemically in an army; when mountaineers take up their abode in our cities; when monomania [that is, an *idée fixe* over sex usually accompanied by excessive masturbation mentioned earlier on grounds it will relieve the sexual *idée fixe*] is rife among a population, particularly superstitious monomania [the *idée fixe* that this over-arching preoccupation will never recede]; [...] then are suicides most frequent, and the *contagion* of mental illness manifests itself. [emphasis of "contagion" mine] (Esquirol 1965, 279–283)

The soldierly sodomy presumably becomes 'epidemical,' grows 'contagious,' by passing from brotherly soldier to soldier. Esquirol never defines the infection of sodomy, just its *epidemical potential*; he pronounces as a Catholic professor of medicine facing no contradiction between his religion and profession. Esquirolian epidemical mental illness is *au fond* a capability thriving on antecedent notions of medical contagion (Esquirol 1965, 275–294), and his view, originally published in 1823, was deeply influential.

4 Nervous Contagion

The Renaissance's melancholic sodomite shared features with Esquirol's nostalgic soldiers whose frayed nerves predisposed them – again contagiously – to sodomy. Similarly for the rise of neuroculture in the high Enlightenment, when it should have been predictable that the sodomite would be coupled to other weak-nerved, effeminate, and hypersensitive males. The homology among early nineteenth-century doctors – not all of them 'Romantic doctors' – becoming invested in the new neuroculture can have appeared logically ironclad:

- sensitive males have weak and flaccid nerves, like females
- their nerves are less taut than those of robust males
- sexuality is a nervous physiological activity determined by the condition of the nerves
- flaccid nerves lead to effeminate sexuality
- male nervous inferiority may be contagious even among robust males

If the nervous sodomitical paradigm was gender driven, its internal logic seemed irrefutable. As the nineteenth century unfolded the view was also generalized to other groups also stigmatized by weak nerves through a kind of Svengalian logic: Jews, gypsies, sodomites, lunatics, vagrants – all affirmed to be inexplicably nervous and morally defective (Pick 1989, 2000). The above syllogism appears crazed to us, but was then seriously entertained (Lucas 1847). The fewer the facts that can definitively be established about groups of people – for example sodomites, as they were still labeled in the early nineteenth century – the more numerous the myths circulating about them and more difficult to eradicate.

Moving forward chronologically, the possibility of nervous contagion paradoxically turns more cognitive and emotional. For example, James Mullingen was a Victorian British traveller whose two-volume compilation of medical curiosities published in 1837 attracted attention (Mullingen 1837). Modeled on Isaac Disraeli's best-selling *Curiosities of Literature* (1802–1812), his was a remarkably full compendium of early Victorian medical lore. Mullingen was vigilant to the cholera scares and other epidemical outbreaks of the 1830s, and fascinated by those who *consciously infect others* – that is, with the *conscious* intent of passing the disease on to *others*; as well as curious about those who have no intention to infect yet who themselves become infected by physical or mental conditions through *unexplained* processes. The unknown, unexplained component intrigued Mullingen. He had read Stendhal's account of his mystifying experience in 1817 in the Uffizi Gallery in Florence, which caused his heart to pound rapidly, caused dizziness, fainting, mental confusion and hallucinations. Stendhal had devoted a chapter of his own travel memoir, *Naples and Florence: A Journey from Milan to Reggio* (1817), to this episode, which he strove, unsuccessfully, to understand. Were his symptoms attributable, Stendhal wondered, to his hypersensitivity – itself a new category in 1817 and barely understood – or to some contagious phenomena he had 'caught' from the other traveller-admirers? He wrote:

> As I emerged from the porch of Santa Croce, I was seized with a fierce palpitation of the heart (that same symptom which, in Berlin, is referred to as an attack of the nerves); the well-spring of life dried up within me, and I walked in constant fear of falling to the ground. (Stendhal 1959, 72)

Stendhal's predicament repeatedly presented itself among other returning patients, until Italian psychiatrist Graziella Magherini labelled it the "Stendhal Syndrome" in 1979. Dr. Magherini had diagnosed similar psychosomatic conditions (racing heart beat, nausea, dizziness, delirium) amongst first-time visitors to Florence, especially those "catching the tears of others while watching paintings" (Elkins 2001, 3). Her explanation was *au fond* psychological despite the pronounced physical symptoms. The sight of so many other gazers immersed in overpowering religious art, she reasoned, overwhelms the mind. A century earlier Mullingen could have explained why: one visitor contracts it, another follows suit, tears are shared, others see them faint and reel, soon the whole group ails. Clearly mimesis – imitation – has generated disease as robustly as bacteria or other germs through group contagion.

Magherini wondered whether the groups were self-selecting. Were travelers to these places prone to copy-cat contagion? Set the dials back to the mid-Victorian period, and the sodomite, not yet the post-Darwinian homosexual, or – in the sexological language of the time – Urning, Arcadian, Uranian, Dorian, as he will variously be labeled after the 1860s, is also said to be engaging in another type of contagion based on mixed blood and compromised nerves. The contagious progression appears to be logically cogent but requires decoding for comprehension, especially insofar as heredity was not thought to play a role in transmission. For example: a Jewish male is attracted to a blond-and-blue eyed robust Christian partner possessing the right (i.e., pure) blood; the Jew is – as many Jews were then stereotyped – sensitive, talented, intelligent, and possesses other Semitic physical characteristics too: dark skin, big nose, hirsute body. Their consorting – so goes the sequence – corrupts the Christian boy's purity: bad blood infecting good, impure traits fraying the robust partner's nerves and morally incapacitating him. By the time classicist-poet A. E. Housman sought to explain his sexual "deviation" to himself in the 1890s, he too conceptualized the process as infection – as *infecting the other* – despite Housman's not being Jewish. Sodomitical contagion, whether physical or mental, was a fantasy posing as up-to-the-minute scientific theory. Little wonder that Housman, textual classicist *par excellence* of his epoch, resorted to lyrical poetry to idealize the uncorrupted asexual boys of his imagination as pure and uninfected "Shropshire lad[s]" (Housman 1906).

Darwinism altered the course of this "third sex" which had been configured for over a century before 1859, when Darwin's *Origin of Species* appeared. A generation later, by the 1880s, the "third sex" was embodied as an evolving, patently decaying, effete creature, successively "selected out," softening its physical constitution, and thereby rendering it vulnerable to contagion and susceptible to infection. Théophile Gautier, not himself a card-carrying member of the "third sex" but representative of the *literati* in Paris who spent much of their lives around them, commented that he had not the vaguest idea how such people *physically* became that way. He wondered whether they had been born normally but later became *infected* – contagion again. By the close of the nineteenth century, sexologists had constructed a vast phylogeny of these evolving third sexes, or, as utopian socialist Edward Carpenter named them, "Intermediate Types" (Carpenter 1914).

5 Criminal Contagion

Urnings and other "intermediate types" were commonly conceptualized as potential criminals: awaiting forensic classification and sentencing. They had been since the days of forensic doctor Paolo Zacchia in the sixteenth century

(Borris and Rousseau 2008, 75–81). "Agents of foul contagion," as one Renaissance legal philosopher called them (Borris and Rousseau 2008, 85), it was thought they could be identified by their rectal anatomy, especially the shape of their sphincters, folds of their *nates* and tears in their anal tissue through which infection had entered. Small surprise then that Edwardian author E. M. Forster wrote a postscript to his novel *Maurice* (composed in 1913–1914), the homosexual fiction he forbade publication before his death in 1970, accounting for the public loathing of post-Darwinian "Urnings" "not [because] they hate [homosexuality] itself but having to think about it" (Forster 1987, preface). Forster's was rhetorical ellipsis compounded by euphemism for the rectum. Polite Forster wrote to alert less-attuned readers to the *anatomic source* of their hatred: the forensic bum and buttock in the tawdry processes of contagion.

Marcel Proust, the great novelist, invokes the contagion trope with such jouissance at the beginning of the fourth volume of his novel *In Search of Lost Time* entitled *Sodom and Gomorrah* one could think he relishes it. The scene occurs when the narrator watches the Baron de Charlus engage in intercourse with the (male) tailor Jupien. Marcel is perched at the upper story of his parents' apartment in the Hôtel de Guermantes, watching for the Duc and Duchesse to return home. Eyeing a bee enter the courtyard, he descends the stairs to observe more exquisitely whether "the improbable insect would come to visit the tendered and forlorn pistil" of an orchid. Hidden behind a shutter, he remains unnoticed when the Baron enters to lunch at the apartment of Mme. de Villeparisis. Still waiting for the Guermantes and intrigued by the bee, the narrator watches Charlus return into the courtyard, "his half-closed eyes all of a sudden opened wide ... gazing with an extraordinary intentness at the former waistcoat-maker on the doorstep of his shop, while the latter, standing suddenly transfixed in front of M. de Charlus, rooted like a plant, was contemplating with an air of wonderment the ageing Baron's embonpoint [plumpness]" (Proust 1992, Vol. 4, 24; all passages in my discussion appear on pp. 24–32). Their sexual dance begins, Jupien invites Baron Charlus into his shop, the narrator follows them through a cellar passage into the room and hides behind partitions, where the voyeur (the narrator) savours their moans. "I might have thought," he comments, "that one person was slitting another's throat close beside me and that the murderer and his resuscitated victim were then taking a bath in order to erase their crime."

He glosses "their crime:" "I understood why [...] I had been able to think that M. de Charlus had the look of a woman: he was one!" Here lurks the subterranean contagion: André Gide admired Charlus's literary complexity yet complained bitterly to Proust that Charlus contributed to the habitual confusion between the homosexual and the invert, i. e., the identification of the homosexual-type with a man who has a woman trapped within him. Proust replied in the language of science: claiming that *both* types – homosexuals and inverts – are 'flowers' pollinating and infecting each other as ordained by Nature. When Charlus leaves the hotel after "infecting" Jupien with his own fluid, he deliciously crosses paths with the very same lingering bee the narrator had observed on its way to making "love" with the orchid. He astutely observes that the clinging of the two men is as "non-elective" as the bee's union with the orchid's pistil is hard-wired.

Proust's intuitive sexual contagion has modern parallels. In William Friedkin's film *Cruising* (1980), starring Al Pacino, young heterosexual detective Steve is assigned to catch a serial killer preying on the gay community by immersing himself in homosexual lifestyle. While cruising the leather bars, he becomes "infected" merely by exposure to this nether world. Without physical contact he suffers from night-sweats inducing him to think in alien ways. Prior, normative, missionary-position sex with his girlfriend ceases any longer to satisfy. He slowly is being converted to something else, "infected" too. Ultimately, his cat-and-mouse brush with the killer threatens to transform him into a murderer. Friedkin emphasizes psychological contagion over any other aspect, particularly Steve's psychosexual mimesis while being infected with the same murderous behaviour he putatively seeks to eradicate.

6 Psychic Contagion

One other crucial development after Darwin's *Origin* – the doctrine of psychic contagion – influenced the formation of the contagious sodomite. It occurred through the rise of suggestion psychology in the 1870s, and peaked during the last two decades of the nineteenth century. Suggestion as a means of influencing other persons had been ingrained in folk psychology for centuries; the difference now, in the 1870s, was its medicalization and pathologization. All sorts of doctors, especially the new psychiatrists, then turned away from other research to study its operations: Charcot in Paris, Ambroise-Auguste Liébeault and Hippolyte Bernheim in Nancy, Albert Moll in Germany, Vladimir Bekhterev in Russia, and others. Bekhterev brilliantly summed up suggestion in a single sentence in his book translated into English as *Suggestion and its Role in Social Life* (1897): "Suggestion is ... one of the ways of exerting influence of one person over another even under conditions of ordinary life" (Bekhterev 1995, 1).[3]

3 It first appeared in 1897 in Russian as a lecture, and was quickly translated into German in 1899 and French in 1910; Bekhterev then expanded it into a book of about two-hundred pages in 1903 and enlarged it again in 1908. The only English translation is the one cited in the References.

Discussions of "suggestion" usually occurred within contexts of hypnosis – another budding development in those two decades – and sought to explain how "psychic contact" developed. But these debates and discussions rarely evolved in neutral territory; the language invoked almost always depicted the "influenced person" as somehow infected or poisoned by the influence of the other. Bekhterev, for example, announced how this contagious dynamic spread throughout society in a book as culturally relevant as it was also then germane for the evolution of hypnotic therapies. He made no bones about the *contagious* aspects of the process:

> Psychic contact (*contagium psychicum*) ... which causes a psychic infection, whose microbes, although invisible with the microscope, nevertheless function here, there and everywhere, similarly to physical microbes, and are transferred through words, gestures, and movements of surrounding people, through books, newspapers, etc. in a word, wherever we are in the surrounding society, we are exposed to the action of psychic microbes and therefore we are in danger of being psychically, and contagiously infected. (Bekhterev 1995, 1)

No one had ever seen "psychic microbes" with the naked eye or with the assistance of microscopes, but the psychiatrists doubted not their existence. The *contagium psychicum* was specifically conceptualized as infection polluting body *and* mind. It was particularly effective through the pathway of sexual suggestion and rarely opposed by patients, especially nervous patients, as imaginative writers of the time continued to maintain. Psychic contagium had a social power, they thought, because the depressed contingent wished to belong more than they realized. Bekhterev generalized his theory of suggestion to human history, providing examples of mass contagion from events as far-flung as the 1720 South Sea Bubble in England, the early nineteenth-century Mississippi financial fiasco in America, and the German government's treatment of inflation during the 1920s, viewing these historical phenomena as high moments of the mass "*contagium psychicum*".

7 Dr. Radó and the Radoites

Whether as bee or Baron, whether as degenerating "third sex" or evolving "intermediate sex," these types were represented as more vulnerable than others to the diseases of contagion: venereal, syphilitic, consumptive, and eventually the malady par excellence of the 1890s, cholera. For decades cholera had transformed the realms of filth and elevated them to higher moral and metaphorical spheres (Briese 2003). It was precisely this medical milieu, whose ordinary daily language was charged with invading epidemics and their political undertones, into which Hungarian doctor Sándor Radó grew up. Born into a Jewish middle-class family in 1890 as the Austro-Hungarian empire was disintegrating, and intellectually maturing during the Freudian Era of Self-Discovery, Radó was medically educated in Budapest. When the empire finally collapsed he moved to Berlin, and became an entrenched member of the psychoanalytic community, migrating in 1931 to New York, before the Nazi menace threatened to destroy Jews like himself. In New York Radó spent a decade establishing the Psychoanalytic Institute, moving up the medical ladder at Columbia, and in 1944 accepted a professorship in psychiatry in its famed medical school (Radó et al. 1995). From that time to his death in 1972 he was the single most influential psychiatrist in America for the treatment of homosexuals, claiming to be capable of 'converting them' to heterosexuality (Radó 1956).

Radó's career can appear to be the success story of a Jewish immigrant physician in the new world, his pulse always in the right place at the right time. However, we wonder in amazement how anyone so theoretically defective, an exile himself who ought to have sympathized with other 'outsiders,' can have been so intolerant yet successful – such is the hazard and irony of anachronism (Mayer 1982). Yet Radó prevailed in wartime America, abetted by the political climate touting American patriotism enhanced by the virile bouillon of rugged masculinity. Although Radó was a classical Freudian who had been an assistant of Freud while still in Europe, he resisted Freud's aetiology of the male bisexual, arguing instead that all bisexual men were in actuality *homosexual men* in whose psychological soul was an 'unconscious fear of women' (Radó 1969, Ch. 4–6). Fear was the key signpost: fear of the female no less than the masses' fear that old-world sodomites could prove epidemical (Alcabes 2009); and Radó vigorously challenged Freud's position that homosexual men could *not* be cured. (He had no theory of lesbianism, which he did not see as a problem.) His model was grounded in the homosexual's unconscious terror of the invasive, castrating, predatory female mother; if not driven by a veritable Phaedre-complex then proximate to its tragic effects in the destruction of the son's integrity. As consequential for contagion, however, was Radó's reformulation of American psychiatrist Edward Kemp's prior theory of homosexual panic (Rosario 2002, 136–139).

According to Kemp homosexual panic is a temporary psychotic condition in which a heterosexual male acts violently – robs, steals, assaults, even murders – to stave off unwanted homosexual advances.[4] This is why homosexual panic could be a valid legal defence in America until the 1980s; the exonerated male who kills in self-defence in the state of psychotic panic. Biographically

4 For a recent case of homosexual panic resulting in brutal murder by an adolescent see http://www.bbc.co.uk/news/uk-scotland-20251281.

Radó had not heard of "Kemp's disease" (homosexual panic) in Europe during the 1920s, but he did after migrating to America in the 1930s, and amplified it to cover a broad base of what Radó termed "contagious homosexuality." Radó's formulation reduces to this syllogism:

- homosexual men crave sex more than anything else
- they seek sex primarily with straight men
- to enact it they cruise
- cruising involves interacting, suggesting, speaking, touching
- heterosexual men succumb to their advances and for inexplicable reasons continue to engage in this form of sexual contact
- Radó's solution: conversion

Each step of Radó's syllogism has been proved false, but its defects did not deter him from championing his solution: the "conversion" of homosexuals to heterosexuality. Given his premises his logic appeared irrefutable: especially in times of war during the 1940s America could not become a society of heterosexual men preyed upon by homosexuals who "converted" them. Radó's message was embraced during the MacCarthy Era of the 1950s while he reached his pinnacle at Columbia, which saluted his cultural message to the country (Berg and Allen 1958).

After President Roosevelt appointed Radó in the 1940s to the post of Psychiatric Consultant to the United States Army, Radó also championed the ban on gays in the military, on grounds that homosexuality was a contagious illness. Radó's simple solution? Eliminate homosexuals from the military: remove them, segregate them, and quarantine them on specific grounds of the "infection of cruising". The metaphor arrests: "cruising" is Radó's root cause. The homosexual was contagious precisely because he was compulsively promiscuous, a belief difficult to eradicate because then so religiously and psychologically entrenched in America. Radó's ban was his practical remedy, but on the psychoanalytical couch he touted "conversion from the contagion," claiming his conversion therapy was the only hope for homosexuals (Rousseau 1996). Every homosexual, he taught his medical students, could be "converted" if he merely refrained from cruising. Where were Proust and Gide now, who held such different positions just one generation earlier? Nowhere: for Radó they were deeply troubled "inverts" themselves who ought to have been converted by their doctors. Yet Radó's students historically became the most vocal psychiatrists of the MacCarthy era, espousing and touting the successes of their master – in the words of one, "homosexuality need not be your final destiny" (Radó et al. 1995, 74). Chief among these were three doctors – Edmund Bergler, Irving Bieber, and Charles Socarides. They had their moment of glory under the American sun until the Stonewall Riots, Gay Pride, and then

AIDS, exposed the fraud of their prejudice and vilified them (Bergler 1959; Bergler 1982; Bieber 1980; Bieber 1988).[5]

Radó's "conversion cure" amounted to monolithic elements set into a ruggedly patriotic context. Conversion was predicated on imitation: follow the therapist's example, who during Radó's four-decade reign was "straight" (women eluded the edict by suppressing their sexuality or keeping silent about it). Homosexual physicians were routinely denied entry to psychoanalytic institutes in America until the 1970s. Within psychotherapy the *gay patient* was deemed to demonstrate successful transference when he showed respect for, and idealized, the therapist's straight sexuality. The fee charged during the 1950–1960s was a sliding scale between 10 to 20 USA dollars per hour, converted to our buying power now approximately 200–300 dollars, or £140 per session. When homosexual playwright Tennessee Williams's southern doctor was unable to stem his alcoholism he sent him for "conversion" to New York psychiatrist, Lawrence Schlesinger Kubie, a Radoite. Williams was horrified at the mismatch: he did not want to be "converted," he wanted a boyfriend, and the price was too steep.

Williams has recounted this comic-tragic episode of his life. Kubie, he explained,

> "taught me much about my true nature but he offered me no solution except to break [with my lover] Merlo, a thing that was quite obviously untenable as a consideration, my life having been built around him." (Williams 1975, 173)

Williams was free-wheeling, drink-loving, and open-buttoned, the austere Kubie the opposite. Then in his sixties, Kubie was a bespectacled ivy-leaguer, starched member of the Harvard and Century Clubs in Manhattan, and by then – 1959 – an influential presence in the New York psychiatric establishment who had been trained by Radó. His textbook, *Theoretical Aspects of Psychoanalysis*, assured patients that the "homosexual neurosis could be cured" by converting from the love of men to women (Kubie 1950, Ch. 5).

Kubie told Williams he was "a violent man" (Williams 1975, 238), which Williams pensively took on board, and assumed "the Frenchman" – as Williams called him – meant verbally violent. But Kubie meant literally violent and persuaded Wil-

5 Despite attacks on them they carried on: Bergler died in 1962 before the attacks amounted to anything; Bieber continued to believe homosexuality an illness until his death in 1991; Socarides persisted until 2005, living into his eighties and maintaining until the end that his patients could be "cured of their illness" if they followed his conversion cure. Lawrence J. Hatterer was ancillary to these three, but campaigned that homosexuals were sick people in need of treatment and had to be changed (Hatterer 1970; Halberstam 1994).

liams that his alcoholism was ancillary to his homosexuality: convert to women and the drink will evaporate. But after eight months Williams quit, headed back south, began to drink again, and wrote more plays. When he again relapsed into heavy drink, his nephew, Jim Adams, set him up with another Radoite in New York, Dr. Ralph Harris (Williams 1975, 206). Williams perceived Harris as more "humane" than Kubie, but his message was identical: rid yourself of male lovers and convert to the love of women. Needless to say, Williams relapsed, the new emptiness he experienced drove him back to the bottle. Williams died 'uncoverted.'

8 Conversion Cures and Contagion

Two decades ago I tried to tell this story in greater detail; especially aimed to expose the confidence of its physician protagonists and their hypocrisies; to compile a biography of Radó on grounds he was the *fons et origo* of the American 'conversion movement' and teacher of the 'conversionists' who collectively did such damage to American psychological life. Any aspiration I had to provide a corrective to the history of psychiatry was secondary: too much havoc had already been done, too many lives ruined. After all, one of my own roommates at an American ivy-league university shot himself in the right temple at nineteen during his own "conversion therapy" with a Radoite treating him to learn *not* to cruise. Unable to imitate his straight therapist, this young collegian died thinking he had failed in the most important task of his newly adult life. When I sent his mother his remains they contained diaries documenting his sense of grief at failing to convert: "Mom, I have to cruise to live."[6]

Radó's biographical ending in 1972 was apparently not much happier. By then, the revolt against conversionism was making strides. Vietnam, 1968, the Free Speech Movement, Stonewall: all altered the political-sexual landscape; besides, the 'Marmorites' – New York psychologists and psychiatrists breaking with Radó who included Judd Marmor and Evelyn Hooker – denounced his conversion therapy and migrated to California to replace it with their own accepting heterodoxy. Sexual orientation, they proposed, was neurophysiological as well as psychological and genetically predetermined; nothing anyone could 'catch'. It could be a healthy way to live, precisely because it was *not* predicated on choice.

Moreover, by then American gays started to rebel against notions of their 'contagion' and beliefs about their existence in a state requiring 'conversion.' Martin Duberman (b. 1930), the distinguished historian and playwright, is a good exam-

6 The family does not permit to name the deceased or cite further than this from his rueful diary.

ple, although there are others. In his book *Cures* (1991) he recounts how desperately he searched to become 'straight.' A trained researcher, he knew how to use libraries, and tapped into the gay habit during those decades to trawl libraries "for cures." Having found nothing beyond conversion from cruising in books, Duberman consulted a string of psychiatrists on the American East Coast, Radoite conversionists Edmund Bergler, Sam Weintraub, Albert Igen, and Charles Socarides (1922–2005).[7] In *Cures* Duberman documents his treatment with "Karl," a medical fraud who may be based on Charles Socarides. Karl insisted that "to be cured" Duberman must convert to women. Eventually heroic Duberman walked out and redirected his energy to the Gay Movement. Redemption came in 1972 – the year of Radó's death – when a group of young anti-Radó psychiatrists at Columbia invited Duberman to debate "conversion therapy" with Irving Bieber. No less than Radó he touted conversionism and claimed he had never known "a homosexual man who had a loving, constructive father" (Duberman 1991, 268). At this point a Columbia undergraduate grabbed the microphone and declared he had just such a father. Bieber replied he placed no stock in "self-distorted evaluations" and offered to administer a proper battery of proper psychiatric tests if he would present himself at Bieber's waiting rooms. At this point, Duberman writes, "I [myself] grabbed the mike and in a tone that matched Bieber's unction, politely offered to test *him* for advanced symptoms of homophobia if he would trot round to my office" (Duberman 1991, 268).[8]

The Radoite position was pathetically sustained in the figure of the already mentioned Charles ("Karl") Socarides. For three decades after Radó's death in 1972, he continued to purport that homosexuals were as "sick" as they were psychologically contagious, yet by dint of his longevity Socarides did more damage than any of these psychoanalytic establishment figures except Radó (Socarides 1968, 1975, 1988, 1995; Socarides and Volkan 1990; Socarides and Loeb 2002). His homosexual patients, he believed, were not moral sinners but sick patients: psychologically ailing, developmentally diseased, and, not least, socially contagious.

Radó's demise a generation earlier had an opposite consequence: a fire in his house burned all his books and papers, rendering it impossible in that era before digital technology to compile a proper biography of his conversion ther-

---

7 An epitome of his work is found in his biographical entry on Wikipedia. http://en.wikipedia.org/wiki/Charles_Socarides (6 August 2012). It should be noted, however, that since Socarides' death in 2005 no one has attempted to redeem his monolithically negative profile.

8 Duberman sparred again with Bieber early in the 1970s in *The New York Times*, after Bieber derided him an amateur, "venturing into fields about which he knew nothing," and Duberman decried "the binary dualism theory of the binding mother/absent father" (Duberman 1991, 269–271).

apy set into its biographical and historical context.[9] When I tried, I was stymied by the lack of primary evidence. Books could be written about these immigrant and native American conversionists, but no painstaking study of the man himself who established conversion on American soil.

9 Conclusion: Contagion and Conversion

I cannot conclude without observing how hard old myths die. Although the homosexual predicament has made huge strides in our time, and conditions have never been more conciliatory for gays in the West, the contagionist position hangs on.

American Professor of Law Nancy J. Knauer has studied the so-called contagion model of sexual orientation and also believes it is far from dead:

> In the political arena, there are currently two central and competing views of homosexuality. Pro-family organizations, working from a contagion model of homosexuality, contend that homosexuality is an immoral, unhealthy, and freely chosen vice.[10]

Because homosexuality can so easily 'infect' so-called *normal people*, particularly children, any public image of homosexuality that is not negative (including simply the presence of an openly gay individual, such as an assistant scout master or a teacher), sends a dangerous message that must be forbidden, silenced, and repressed.

Knauer is right to focus on homosexuality's contagion model as one of its two predominant metaphors, abhorrent as the notion is in 2013. This forlorn state of affairs would be different if we were not now living in the midst of another crisis in contagion models: the economic one pertaining to banking. Homosexuality's contagion remains a psychologically vibrant rhetoric today, as has been all too apparent in the language recently dividing the worldwide Anglican church over the ordination of its bishops. But it was long ago disproved as having any scientific validity whatsoever. I have been arguing, in addition to the metaphorics and rhetorics of contagion, that these imbricated discourses – economic, sexual, psychological – should be viewed over the *longue durée* if we hope to understand how they have overlapped over time, and should be reconstructed with as little prejudice as possible against anachronism.

---

9 I owe this information to Dr John Truman (Professor of Paediatrics, Columbia University, Physician and Surgeons Hospital) and Dorothy Truman (Archivist, New York Academy of Medicine, New York).
10 Knauer, 403. Knauer's article on the "infectious rhetoric" of Radclyffe Hall's *Well of Loneliness* during the 1920s also demonstrates how the contagious model was then revived.

References

Alcabes, Philip. *Dread: How Fear and Fantasy Have Fueled Epidemics from the Black Death to Avian Flu*. New York: Public Affairs, 2009.
Aubry, Paul. *La contagion du meurtre: Étude d'anthropologie criminelle*. Paris: Félix Alcan, 1896.
Bashford, Alison, and Claire Hooker. *Contagion: Historical and Cultural Studies*. London: Routledge, 2001.
Bekhterev, Vladimir. *Suggestion and its Role in Social Life* (1897). Translated by Tzvetanka Dobreva-Martinova. New Brunswick, NJ: Transaction Publishers, 1995.
Bennett, Jeffrey A. *Banning Queer Blood: Rhetorics of Citizenship, Contagion, and Resistance*. Tuscaloosa: University of Alabama Press, 2009.
Berg, Charles, and Clifford Allen. *The Problem of Homosexuality*. New York, NY: Citadel Press, 1958.
Bergler, Edmund. *Homosexuality: Disease or Way of Life?* New York, NY: Hill and Wang, 1956.
Bergler, Edmund. *One Thousand Homosexuals: Conspiracy of Silence, or Curing and Deglamorizing Homosexuals?* Paterson, NJ: Pageant Books, 1959.
Bergler, Edmund. *Counterfeit-Sex: Homosexuality, Impotence, Frigidity*. New York: Grune & Stratton, 1982.
Bieber, Irving. *Cognitive Psychoanalysis*. New York, NY: Aronson, 1980.
Bieber, Irving. *Homosexuality: A Psychoanalytic Study*. Northvale, NJ: Aronson, 1988.
Borris, Kenneth, and George S. Rousseau. *The Sciences of Homosexuality in Early Modern Europe*. London: Routledge, 2008.
Briese, Olaf. *Angst in den Zeiten der Cholera*. 4 vols. Berlin: Akademie Verlag, 2003.
Browning, Barbara. *Infectious Rhythm: Metaphors of Contagion and the Spread of African Culture*. New York, NY: Routledge, 1998.
Burke, Edmund, and James T. Boulton. *A Philosophical Enquiry into the Origin of Our Ideas of the Sublime and Beautiful*. Rev. ed. Oxford: Basil Blackwell, 1987.
Carlin, Claire L. *Imagining Contagion in Early Modern Europe*. Basingstoke: Palgrave Macmillan, 2005.
Carpenter, Edward. *Intermediate Types among Primitive Folk: A Study in Social Evolution* London: Allen, 1914.
Christensen, Allan. *Nineteenth-Century Narratives of Contagion: Our Feverish Contact*. London: Routledge, 2005.
Coleridge, Samuel Taylor, George Whalley, and H. J. Jackson. *Marginalia*. 6 vols, Bollingen Foundation Collection. London, Princeton, N.J.: Routledge & Kegan Paul and Princeton University Press, 1980.
Conrad, Lawrence I., and Dominik Wujastyk (Eds). *Contagion: Perspectives from Pre-Modern Societies*. Aldershot: Ashgate, 2000.
Davidson, James. *The Greeks and Greek Love: A Radical Reappraisal of Homosexuality in Ancient Greece*. London: Weidenfeld and Nicholson, 2007.
Douglas, Mary. *Purity and Danger: An Analysis of Concepts of Pollution and Taboo*. London: Routledge & Kegan Paul, 1966.
Duberman, Martin B. *Cures: A Gay Man's Odyssey*. New York, NY: Dutton, 1991.
Eder, Franz, Lesley A. Hall, and Gert Hekma. *Sexual Cultures in Europe: National Histories*. Manchester: Manchester University Press, 1999.

Elkins, James. *Pictures & Tears: A History of People Who Have Cried in Front of Paintings.* New York, London: Routledge, 2001.
Esquirol, Jean Étienne Dominique. *Mental Maladies, a Treatise on Insanity, a Facsimile of the English Edition of 1845* History of Medicine Series. New York, London: Hafner, 1965.
Faulkner, Thomas C., Nicolas K. Kiessling and Rhonda L. Blair (Eds). *Robert Burton. The Anatomy of Melancholy.* Vol. I. Text. Oxford: Clarendon Press, 1989.
Forster, Edward Morgan. *Maurice: a Novel.* London: Guild Publishing, 1987 [1971].
Fracastoro, Girolamo. *Hieronymi Fracastorii De Contagione Et Contagiosis Morbis Et Eorum Curatione: Libri Iii.* New York, NY: Putnam, 1930.
Freud, Sigmund, J. Moussaieff Masson, and Wilhelm Fliess. *The Complete Letters of Sigmund Freud to Wilhelm Fliess, 1887–1904.* Cambridge, MA: Harvard University Press, 1985.
Gilman, Sander L. *Disease and Representation: Images of Illness from Madness to Aids.* Ithaca: Cornell University Press, 1988.
Glick, Reuven, and Andrew Rose. *Contagion and Trade: Why Are Currency Crises Regional.* London: Centre for Economic Policy Research, 1998.
Halberstam, David. *The Fifties.* New York, NY: Norton, 1994.
Hatterer, Lawrence J. *Changing Homosexuality in the Male; Treatment for Men Troubled by Homosexuality.* New York, NY: McGraw-Hill, 1970.
Herdt, Gilbert H. *Third Sex, Third Gender: Beyond Sexual Dimorphism in Culture and History.* New York, NY: Zone, 1994.
Housman, Alfred Edward. *A Shropshire Lad.* New York, London: J. Lane, 1906.
Hume, David, Peter H. Nidditch, and Lewis A. Selby-Bigge. *A Treatise of Human Nature.* 2nd ed. Oxford: Clarendon Press, 1978.
Knauer, Nancy J. "Homosexuality as Contagion: From the Well of Loneliness to the Boy Scouts." *Hofstra Law Review* 29,2 (2000): 401–501.
Kubie, Lawrence S. *Practical and Theoretical Aspects of Psychoanalysis.* New York, NY: International Universities Press, 1950.
Loveridge, Mark. *Laurence Sterne and the Argument About Design.* London: Macmillan, 1982.
Lucas, Prosper. *Traité philosophique et physiologique de l'hérédité naturelle dans les états de santé et de maladie du système nerveux.* 2 vols. Paris: Baillière, 1847–1850.
Lynch, Aaron. *Thought Contagion: How Belief Spreads through Society.* New York, NY: Basic Books, 1996.
Magnus, Albertus. *Man and the Beasts.* Translated by James J. Scanlan. Binghamton, NY: SUNY Press, 1987.
Mayer, Hans. *Outsiders: A Study in Life and Letters.* Cambridge, MA: MIT Press, 1982.
Mullingen, James. *Medical Curiosities.* 2 vols. London: Longman, 1837.
Nuttin, Jozef M., and Annie Beckers. *The Illusion of Attitude Change: Towards a Response Contagion Theory of Persuasion.* London: Academic Press, 1975.
Pick, Daniel. *Faces of Degeneration: A European Disorder, c.1848–c.1918.* Cambridge: Cambridge University Press, 1989.
Pick, Daniel. *Svengali's Web: The Alien Enchanter in Modern Culture.* New Haven, CT, London: Yale University Press, 2000.
Poirier, Guy. *L'homosexualité dans l'imaginaire de la Renaissance.* Paris: H. Champion, 1996.
Price-Smith, Andrew T. *Contagion and Chaos: Disease, Ecology, and National Security in the Era of Globalization.* Cambridge, MA: MIT Press, 2009.
Proust, Marcel. *In Search of Lost Time,* trans. C. K. Scott-Moncrieff, Terence Kilmartin and Andreas Mayor. 7 vols. New York, NY: The Modern Library, 1992.

Radó, Sándor. *Psychoanalysis of Behavior. Collected Papers*. New York, NY: Grune & Stratton, 1956.
Radó, Sándor. *Adaptational Psychodynamics: Motivation and Control*. New York, NY: Science House, 1969.
Radó, Sándor, Paul Roazen, and Bluma Swerdloff (Eds). *Heresy: Sándor Radó and the Psychoanalytic Movement*. Northvale, NJ: Aronson, 1995.
Rosario, Vernon A. *Homosexuality and Science: A Guide to the Debates*. Santa Barbara, CA: ABC-CLIO, 2002.
Rousseau, George S. *Perilous Enlightenment: Pre- and Postmodern Discourses: Sexual, Historical*. Manchester: Manchester University Press, 1991.
Rousseau, George S. "Queering the Pain: Diagnoses and Historiographies of Sexual Conversion." Unpublished conference paper delivered at the European Association for the History of Psychiatry, Geneva, Switzerland, 1996.
Schoenmaker, Dirk, and London School of Economics and Political Science. Financial Markets Group. *Contagion Risk in Banking*. London: LSE Financial Markets Group, 1996.
Shaftesbury, Anthony Ashley Cooper, and Lawrence Klein. *Characteristics of Men, Manners, Opinions, Times*. Cambridge: Cambridge University Press, 1999.
Socarides, Charles W. *The Overt Homosexual*. New York, NY: Grune & Stratton, 1968.
Socarides, Charles W. *Beyond Sexual Freedom*. New York, NY: Quadrangle, 1975.
Socarides, Charles W. *The Preoedipal Origin and Psychoanalytic Therapy of Sexual Perversions*. Madison, CT: International Universities Press, 1988.
Socarides, Charles W. *Homosexuality: A Freedom Too Far ... The Impact of the Gay Rights Movement on American Society*. Phoenix, AZ: Adam Margrave, 1995.
Socarides, Charles W., and Abraham Freedman. *Objects of Desire: The Sexual Deviations*. Madison, CT: International Universities Press, 2002.
Socarides, Charles W., and Loretta R. Loeb. *The Mind of the Paedophile: Psychoanalytic Perspectives*. London: Karnac, 2004.
Socarides, Charles W., and Vamik D. Volkan. *The Homosexualities: Reality, Fantasy, and the Arts*. Madison, CT: International Universities Press, 1990.
Stendhal. *Rome, Naples, and Florence*. London: J. Calder, 1959.
Williams, Tennessee. *Memoirs*. New York, NY: Doubleday, 1975.
Woodward, David, and Catholic Institute for International Relations. *Contagion and Cure: Tackling the Crisis in Global Finance*. London: Institute for International Relations, 1999.

Christoph Gradmann

Exoticism, Bacteriology and the Staging of the Dangerous

1 Dangerous Bacteria

Seen as an object of cultural practice, pathogenic microbes, when they entered laboratories, clinics and public discourse in the late 19th century, were strange fellows indeed: While few doctors and indeed none of their patients had seen them, everyone became increasingly aware of their presence and convinced of their dangerous character. While around 1860 doctors and the lay public would generally have considered the question of whether microbes were of specific relevance in relation to infectious diseases to be open and of limited importance, by a generation later, this had changed. By 1890, microbes had come to symbolise infectious disease to a degree that made it possible to treat the 'tubercle bacillus' as an embodiment of tuberculosis itself. Bacteria were now dangerous and they were almost equated with the diseases they caused: fighting tuberculosis and fighting the bacillus could easily have been seen as almost identical. Furthermore, when it came to understanding such bacteria, their raison d'être seemed confined to the attempted destruction of their host (Gradmann 2000; Hänseler 2009).

The history of how such a worldview gained acceptance has two different but entwined dimensions. First, bacteria were established as objects of scientific enquiry and medical practices. Second, bacteria acquired symbolic dimensions. They became popular embodiments of danger, thereby adding to the iconography of evilness as Elias Canetti has noted:

> The devils in their familiar shape are no longer to be found anywhere, their former large numbers not withstanding. But they have left traces [...]. They have now given up all the traits that might be reminiscent of human beings and have become even smaller. Much changed, therefore, and in even greater numbers, they have resurfaced in the nineteenth century as bacilli. Instead of the soul, they now attack the human body. And they can be quite dangerous to it. Very few people have ever looked into a microscope and actually seen them there. But everyone who has heard of them is always aware of their presence and tries not to come in contact with them, which is a somewhat vague endeavour, given their invisibility, their dangerousness and the concentration of outrageously large numbers of them in a very small space they have no doubt taken over from the devils. (Canetti 1984 [1960], 47, Italics in the original)

This paper is concerned with the trajectory of bacteria as embodiments of danger. It is particularly concerned with when and how bacteria were charged with these notions. On which other, perhaps more familiar notions of dangerousness did the idea of the dangerousness of bacteria reside? Was there a connection between the dangerousness of bacteria and the heroism of bacteriology? Based on the biography of the German physician Robert Koch (1843 – 1910), this paper will put forward the hypothesis that it was principally through travelling, and more specifically through presenting bacteriological hygiene as undertaken in exotic places, that bacteria were transformed from laboratory curiosities to public enemies.

The paper proceeds in three steps.[1] It begins with an introduction on the history of scientific research expeditions in the 19th century, bacteriological hygiene as a travelling discipline and Robert Koch as a traveller. In a second step we will take a closer look at Koch's cholera expedition of 1883/84 and more specifically at the issue of how that expedition gained publicity and which images of bacteriology and its research objects were created during the expedition. Finally, the paper will analyse the stability and impact of those images by looking at some of Koch's later travels.

2 Travelling Laboratories

Robert Koch liked travelling. Born into a petty bourgeois family where emigration was rather common, he had harboured dreams of emigration himself. He had originally aimed for a career as a travelling natural scientist, but for practical reasons settled for medicine. Yet, with the sole exception of his cholera expedition of 1883/84 travelling occurred during the later stages of his career after 1895 when he specialized in tropical medicine (Brock 1988). Thus, his passion for travelling was in several ways a fulfilment of youthful desires. The cholera expedition that this paper is going to look at played an important role in re-fashioning his youthful enthusiasm into a style of scientific work and also since it was widely reported in the press, in shaping the public image of medical bacteriology.

Bacteriological hygiene was one of the new laboratory-based disciplines that characterized medicine in the late 19th century (Bynum 1994; Cunningham, Williams 1992). It differed, however, in important respects from other disciplines, such as physiology, in that bacteriological hygienists had to reproduce the laboratory findings in the outside world. Whereas the physiologists were able to calculate such matters as the nerve conduction speed in the laboratory, the hygienists were always obliged to prove – in areas like the purification of drinking

1 In both material and argument the paper is based upon my own earlier work: Gradmann 2009, 171 – 229; Gradmann 2010. For a good introduction to Koch's biography also compare Brock 1988.

water, disinfection, or clinical diagnostics – that the relationships they had discovered in the laboratory could also be reproduced in the outside world. Turning the outside world into a laboratory was the objective and, as such, bacteriological hygiene became a science practised by travelling experts (Latour 1983). Such travelling also created privileged access to the public at home and could afford a laboratory scientist social prominence as a world traveller. The example of Alexander von Humboldt was well known to Koch and his contemporaries (Brenner 1990; Brenner 1991). To be sure, times had changed since Humboldt's great voyages, yet it was often still easier to gain public attention from the other side of the world – and also to guide it, given the absence of competition and the press.

As such, travelling was a traditional form of scientific work, but it increasingly changed in the nineteenth century. The place of the versatile discoverers, many of whom had travelled the world as amateurs in the eighteenth century, was gradually taken by specialized researchers who expanded their expert knowledge through their travels (Cittadino 1990; Osterhammel 1987). This development reflected the progressive specializations in medicine and the sciences as it was part and parcel of colonisation. While David Livingstone's "Dark Africa" turned more and more exotic in the contemporary imagination (Fisch 1989, 396), Africa was being physically colonised and equipped with infrastructure that supported research, such as the railways and the telegraph.

3 Cholera Wars

Let us now turn to what difference the cholera expedition meant in terms of the popularity of bacteria. What we need to keep in mind is that before 1884, when Koch returned from his expedition, medical bacteriology was not yet a public event. His identification of the tubercle bacillus had in 1882 achieved some recognition in scientific circles (Schlich 1996), but there is no indication that the event enthused the public to any extent. To be sure, it was on this occasion that Koch declared bacteria to be public enemies, noting that in relation to TB, medicine would no longer deal "with an undefined something, but with a concrete parasite, whose living conditions had been uncovered" [nicht mehr mit einem unbestimmten etwas sondern mit einem faßbaren Parasiten zu tun haben] (Koch 1912 [1882], 444). Earlier work, however, such as that on wound infections or bacteriological research methods, had been of an entirely technical nature. Looking at that work, however, presents us with an interesting aside to our investigations: the language of that early bacteriology contained comparatively little of that martial 'man against microbes' rhetoric that we associate with the field. This does not mean that it was void of pictorial language, but that expressions were drawn from everyday life, aiming to familiarize the observer with bacteria rather than to depict them as enemies (Hänseler 2009, 124–126).

The cholera expedition on which Koch and a small team of researchers embarked in August 1883, meant a departure from such lines of approach: bacteriologists were now investigating a disease that had an established reputation as an invader (Hamlin 2009).[2] Indeed the expedition itself had been made possible by an outbreak in the Middle East that seemed to threaten Europe. This had in turn triggered a response by European powers and several expeditions had set out from Britain, France and Germany. For the purpose of our investigation, a quick overview of the German expedition's travels is sufficient. In short, the team, after initial and unsuccessful investigations in Egypt, continued to Bengal where in February 1884 the bacterium that is today known as *Vibrio cholerae* was described. What is more interesting for us is that by travelling, Koch, his team and the bacteria they were aiming to investigate, acquired a degree of public recognition they had not received before.

The expedition made the front pages of German newspapers as early as September 1883, owing to circumstances that had little to do with cholera. More relevant in this instance was the competition with other research teams, particularly the French one, which had reached Egypt a few days before the German team (Coleman 1987, 318). As a rather unsavoury article in the *Berliner Tageblatt* of 26 September indicates, the press was eager to interpret the relation between the two research teams according to the pattern of Franco-German competition, with which the readers were familiar from the days of the 1881 Hygiene Congress at Geneva where Koch and Louis Pasteur had clashed in public (Gradmann 2009, 13 f.). Whereas the German team sought scientific truth, the article maintained, the French were only showing off:

> Within short order, rumour had it throughout town [Alexandria] that the German doctors had already achieved very good results. The French gentlemen pricked up their ears and of course, faithful to their national character, tried to wreck the Germans' parade with a giant cholera bacillus they claimed to have discovered. But with a few words of refutation from Geheimrath Koch they were sent back into their own narrow scientific backyard. [Binnen Kurzem kursierte in der Stadt [Alexandria] das Gerücht, die deutschen Aerzte hätten bereits sehr günstige Resultate aufzuweisen. Die Herren Franzosen spitzten die Ohren, suchten selbstredend ihrem Volkscharacter getreu, den Herren mit einem Riesenbacillus, den sie entdeckt haben wollten, in die Parade zu fahren, wurden indeß nach wenigen wiederlegenden Worten des Geheimraths Koch, in ihre engen wissenschaftlichen vier Pfähle zurückgewiesen.] (Anon. 1883)

2 On the cultural history of cholera in the German speaking countries, compare Briese 2003.

Note that the attention that the expedition received was organised rather than coincidental. To create publicity, Koch regularly sent reports to the Imperial Ministry of the Interior. These were – with one exception – lightly edited and published in periodicals such as the *Reichsanzeiger* or the *Deutsche Medizinische Wochenschrift* from where they could then find their way into other media.

Combining science and nationalism was one aspect of the public recognition that the cholera expedition gained, the fashion in which the work was presented another. In this respect the travel reports and their publication made a difference: the reports are interesting hybrids; partly scientific article, partly travel literature. Quite personal in tone, written as they were in the first person singular, they made use of eye-witness authority to report on scientific work. In reading descriptions of such things as the hygienic conditions in Damiette or in learning about the findings of an autopsy, the readers felt that they were participating in an adventure that touched on both the macro- and the microcosm. They purported to give the public authentic insights into Koch's scientific work that was of a kind that could not have been carried out in a laboratory at home. Such narratives could easily accommodate information that had not even been gained on the expedition. This was the case, for instance, on 17 September 1883, when Koch wove a short survey of the animal-experimental cholera studies by other scientists into the description of his own infection experiments. These travel accounts also accomplished something else. They depicted Egypt – no doubt accurately – as a country "very rich in parasitical and infectious diseases" [sehr reich an parasitischen und ansteckenden Krankheiten] (Koch 1912 [1883/1884], 5). In his reports Koch made considerable use of this *genius loci*, partly by way of emphasizing the dangerous character of the disease, and partly to stylize the scientific work directed against the epidemic as a heroic struggle. Instead of working, as they had done before, in modern and hygienic laboratories in Berlin, scientists now pursued epidemics in exotic and dangerous places and did their work under the most hazardous of conditions. Although the reports were not necessarily emotional in tone, they did cast the "Father of the Bacilli" (Koch) in the role of the crusader who, fighting the enemy in faraway lands, confronted him at the front lines.

It was on this next stage of his journey in Bengal that Koch included a significant extension to the air of exotic dangerousness that he had invested his bacteria with. In his final report he included a longer paragraph on the natural history of the disease under study. What this illustrates is that the rhetoric that touted bacteriological hygiene as a war against epidemics was particularly effective against the background of the exotic and dangerous places that were now presented as the home of disease. Koch provided a description of the Bengal jungle as the place of origin of the epidemic, leaving no doubt as to the dangerous character of the disease:

> Lush vegetation and a rich fauna have developed in this uninhabited area of the world, which, inaccessible to humans not only because of frequent flooding and the presence of many tigers, is above all avoided because of the pernicious fevers [...] It will be easy to understand that here microorganisms have a better chance to develop than almost anywhere else on earth [...] Under peculiar conditions a very peculiar fauna and flora is bound to develop, and in all probability the cholera bacillus is part of it. [Eine üppige Vegetation und ein reiches Thierleben hat sich in diesem unbewohnten Landstrich entwickelt, der für den Menschen nicht allein wegen der Ueberschwemmungen und wegen der zahlreichen Tiger unzugänglich ist, sondern hauptsächlich wegen der bösartigen Fieber gemieden wird (...). Man wird sich leicht vorstellen können, daß hier die Gelegenheit zur Entwicklung von Mikroorganismen geboten ist, wie kaum an einem anderen Platz auf der Erde. (...) Unter eigenthümlichen Verhältnissen muß sich in diesen eine ganz eigenartige Fauna und Flora entwickeln, der aller Wahrscheinlichkeit nach auch der Cholerabacillus angehört.] ('Valerius' 1884b)[3]

Unsurprisingly, such a description was received well in public reception. Consequently, it was with insignificant changes to the wording that it was reproduced by Germany's No. 1 popular magazine, *Die Gartenlaube*, which on that occasion also supplied a picture of the "much discussed and much feared comma bacillus in a faithful rendering" ('Valerius' 1884a). Koch's cholera expedition thus did a lot to create the image of the cholera bacillus as an invader and as the embodiment of that disease. In some sense this was a novel image of the disease, but at the same time it is obvious that Koch's cholera bacillus was also a re-enforcement of traditional ideas about cholera with which it swiftly combined. This disease had been considered an invader before and it might therefore just as well be argued that bacteriology equipped traditional ideas about the Asian scourge with scientific validation.

The notion that the outside world was where diseases breed was given a specific twist in Koch's speculation on the origin of cholera in Bengal. Tropical countries seemed the most likely places of origin for such dangers and the image of bacteriologists underwent changes as well; Koch had depicted Egypt, as it has been quoted above, as a country "very rich in parasitical and infectious diseases". He then made use of this *genius loci*, partly by way of emphasizing the dangerous character of the disease, and partly to stylize the scientific work directed against the epidemic as a heroic struggle. The cholera expedition, it can thus be argued, indicates the entry of Koch's bacteria to the public sphere and simulta-

---

3 Valerius cites Koch's account (Koch 1912 [1884], 36–37). Koch wrote of 'malignant fevers' which became 'pernicious fevers' in the *Gartenlaube*. Other than this the text was unchanged.

neously charged bacteria with the connotation of being public enemies. This became ever more obvious upon the expedition's return to Germany. The public echo was as widespread as it was specific: "Welcome, Victors!" [Willkommen, Ihr Sieger!] read the headline of the *Berliner Tageblatt* on 3 May (Anon. 1884), greeting the returning scientists in the "proudly armed New Germany" [waffenstolzen Neudeutschland]. The expedition headed by Koch was presented as a campaign of German science. Had not the scientists under their "commander" [Befehlshaber] Koch been dispatched to "discover the secret paths of one of the horrible pestilences that have plagued humanity for the last fifty years or more?" [um den Schleichwegen eines der furchtbarsten Plagegeister nachzugehen, von denen die (...) Menschheit seit nunmehr fünfzig Jahren und darüber heimgesucht wird.] Had they not pursued this "enemy all the way to his East-Indian lairs?" [Gegner bis in seine äußersten Ostindischen Schlupfwinkel].

On the occasion of a banquet honouring the returning scientists, the expedition was literally categorized as a victorious military campaign that could easily stand up to comparisons with the Franco-Prussian War:

> "Just as thirteen years ago the German people celebrated a glorious victory against the hereditary enemy of our nation, so does German Science today celebrate a brilliant triumph over one of humanity's most menacing enemies, one of the most dreaded and murderous epidemics of modern times: Cholera" [Wie vor 13 Jahren das deutsche Volk einen glorreichen Sieg über den alten Erzfeind unserer Nation feierte, so feiert heute die deutsche Wissenschaft einen glänzenden Triumph über einen der tückischen Feinde der ganzen Menschheit, über eine der gefürchtetsten und mörderischsten Volksseuchen der Neuzeit: Die Cholera] (Ibid.).[4]

The title page of the program for this banquet showed cartoon-like sketches of important elements of the travelling bacteriological laboratory and its public presentation. Special emphasis was placed on the exotic character of the countries visited. Thus nineteenth-century Egypt is simply portrayed as the land of the pharaohs; yet laboratory needs such as microscopes and experimental animals can also be found there. Also included are classic elements in the allegorical depiction of epidemics, such as the sick, grim reapers, and the angels of mercy. The latter are flanked by the members of the expedition in antique garb.

Officials in the Imperial Ministry of the Interior were quite aware of the image that was created and had in fact actively worked towards that particular aim: in spring they prepared a report for the Emperor. They proposed that the members of the expedition be given decorations. For Koch they envisaged the Imperial Crown Medal II Class – in fact a military decoration – and not without

4 On the notion of German Science, see Kollenbrock-Netz 1991.

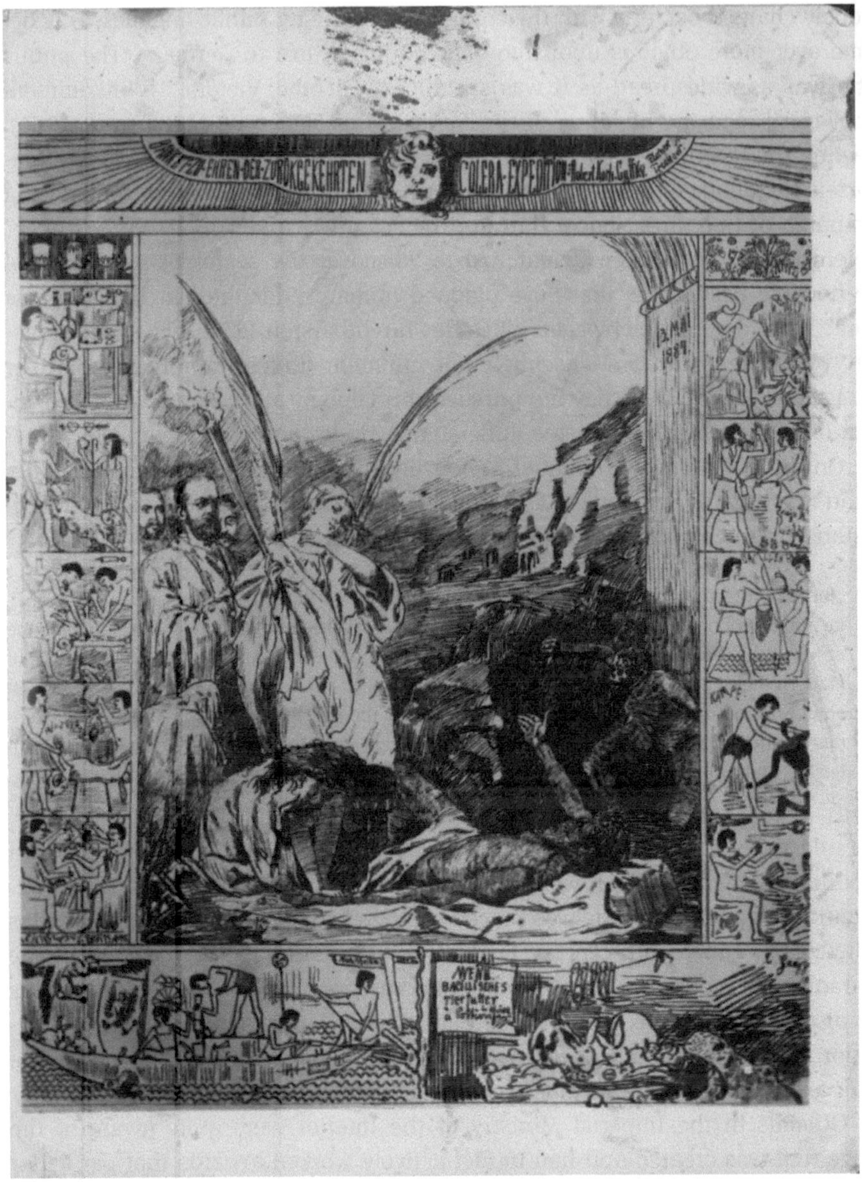

Fig. 1: Title page of the program for the banquet honouring the returning cholera expedition, 1884. Berlin. Robert Koch Institut, Koch Papers.

reason, according to Karl Köhler, the ministerial councillor and subsequent director of the Imperial Health Office who wrote the relevant memorandum:

> If there were a special reward for such accomplishments in the fight against the natural enemies of human life, analogous to the Iron Cross that is given for fighting the enemies of the Fatherland, I would suggest that in the present case that reward be included as well [Gäbe es für derartige Leistungen im Kampf mit den natürlichen Feinden des menschlichen Lebens eine besondere Auszeichnung, wie sie das eiserne Kreuz für den Kampf mit den Feinden des Vaterlandes bildet, so würde ich befürworten, im vorliegenden Falle, diese Auszeichung mitzuverleihen]. (Bundesarchiv Berlin. BA, R 1501 RMDI Nr. 11335)

When looking back on it, Koch himself particularly appreciated receiving the military decoration:

> My favourite decoration is my Imperial Crown Medal II Class, which our old Emperor personally bestowed on me after we returned from the cholera campaign to India. It is to be worn on a black-and-white ribbon, like a military decoration. And that is exactly what it was. [Mein Lieblingsorden ist mein Kronenorden II. Klasse, den mir unser alter Kaiser nach der Rückkehr von der Cholerakampagne in Indien persönlich überreicht hat. Er ist am schwarz-weißen Bande zu tragen, wie ein Kriegsorden. Er war ja auch schließlich einer.] (Quoted from Möllers 1950, 149)

4 Keeping the Enemy at a Distance

Bacteriology, when it became a popular science in the 1880s, was not just engaged in portraying disease as a bacterial invasion of the body, but also employed the notion that what applied to individual organisms could be assumed for larger entities such as towns, countries and indeed for the globe itself. Civilized countries, mostly with a cool climate, were threatened from the outside world that lacked either cool climate or civilisation or both. Upon inspecting the Hamburg cholera epidemic in 1892, Koch reportedly said "I forget that I am in Europe" (Evans 1987). The town, it seemed, had been hit by invaders. In a letter to his future wife Hedwig, Koch described his experience in graphic words: "It felt like walking on a battlefield. Everywhere are people who had been in best health just a few hours before, [...] now they lie side by side in long lines, killed by invisible projectiles" [Es war mir zu Muth, als wanderte ich über ein Schlachtfeld. Überall Menschen, die noch wenige Stunden vorher vor Gesundheit gestrotzt hatten (...) nun in langen Reihen dalagen von unsichtbaren Geschossen dahingestreckt, (...)] (Möllers 1950, 630). For Koch, there was no doubt about where that invader had come from: from the East, following the rivers. Consistent with this, it was later proposed to safeguard the German empire from such invaders by establishing a chain of bacteriological surveillance laboratories on its eastern frontier. Defending the human body and the nations' boundaries had both become a matter of applied hygiene (Berger 2009; Weindling 2000).

It is important at this stage to remind ourselves that what was called popular science was more than science for the public. Instead it can be argued that it provided a background for scientific work and in particular facilitated the assemblage of a multitude of facts into coherent pictures. Bacteriology thus became a science of microbial invaders for bacteriologists and the public alike in the 1880s. Marianne Hänseler has recently shown that it was in these years when Koch began to employ military metaphors in his public speeches (Hänseler 2009, 126–146). While often portraying the microbes as enemies, his use of pictorial language also tried to fuse bacteriological notions and older frames of reference. For example, in 1888, he talked about epidemics of war:

> Even in peacetime they slink about and sap the strength of armies, but when the torch of war is lit, they creep out of their hiding places, rear their heads to tremendous heights and destroy everything in their path. Proud armies have often been decimated, even destroyed by epidemics; wars, and with them the fate of nations, have been decided by them. [Schon im Frieden schleichen sie umher und zehren am Mark der Armee, aber wenn die Kriegsfackel lodert, dann kriechen sie hervor aus ihren Schlupfwinkeln, erheben das Haupt zu gewaltiger Höhe und vernichten alles, was ihnen im Weg steht. Stolze Armeen sind schon oft durch Seuchen dezimiert, selbst vernichtet; Kriege und damit das Geschick der Völker sind durch sie entschieden.] (Koch 1912 [1888], 277)

If one did not know otherwise, one would place the author of this and other texts in the pre-bacteriological era. To be sure, everyone knew that it was bacteria Koch spoke about. Yet, the actors in the text are the epidemics of war, not their pathogens. Koch speaks about typhus, not about the recently identified bacterium that causes it. Even if in the texts of the bacteriologists, and particularly in their popularizing accounts, bacteria appear as the embodiment of disease, it is striking to see that the bacteria do not dislodge the traditional image of epidemics, and that, particularly in public lectures, traditional and modern metaphors for epidemics combine swiftly. The bacteriological imagery of "man against the microbe", then, could easily accommodate the traditional representations of epidemics.

We can also find examples of how scientific thinking was invested with such imagination: When Koch designed a therapy for tuberculosis in 1890, its scientific rationale was based on a kind of scorched earth strategy that conceived of the human body as an active battlefield shared by bacteria and physicians (Gradmann 2009, 100). In a larger context, Paul Weindling and Silvia Berger have described how German bacteriological hygiene conceived of the country as a hygienic space to be defended from outside invasion, be it through bacteriological laboratories on the Eastern boarder before 1914 or through delousing protocols designed to keep war epidemics, such as typhoid fever, at bay during the Great War (Berger 2009; Weindling 2000). Defending the body could now easily be compared to a battle where the prime objective was to "keep the enemy at a distance" by means of a "full mobilisation" of the bodily defences (Dekker 1898, 13).[5]

5 Tropical Wars

When it comes to Koch himself, however, tropical medicine played an important role in all of this. It was a field that he entered in the 1890s for a host of reasons. One of those was to escape from colleagues and critics of whom he, as he saw it, had far too many in those days. Another, less obvious reason was to escape from the consequences of his own successes. Europe had, in his eyes, been fundamentally altered in its epidemiology to such an extent that the relationships between men and microbes were becoming increasingly hard to study in this place. Tropical countries, instead, represented a kind of natural state in the relationships between men and microbes. When in 1899 Koch studied malaria in New Guinea, his research was less on the aetiology of that condition than into understanding the rising and ebbing of epidemics. Studying these under conditions where they had not been influenced by medical intervention was, for Koch, particularly interesting. New Guinea possessed splendid qualities for becoming a veritable laboratory for the study of tropical infections:

> "The malaria expedition was given an opportunity in New Guinea that has become rare today: To study malaria under circumstances where it can develop totally undisturbed." [Die Malariaexpedition hat in Neuguinea die heutzutage wohl nicht mehr oft sich bietende Gelegenheit gehabt, die Malaria unter Verhältnissen kennen zu lernen, wo sie sich ganz ungestört entwickeln kann.] (Koch 1912 [1900], 422)

A few years later, when researching sleeping sickness in East Africa (Gradmann 2009, 201–225), Koch took some notes on the character of African nature in relation to the natural history of infectious diseases. Such note taking show that popular notions we would assume to be the result of such science were in fact also galvanising it. In August 1906, while officially being on an expedition to study sleeping sickness, Koch embarked on a boat trip on Lake Victoria. When it comes to its declared purpose of searching for patients who had been treated in Koch's camp earlier, the round trip was a failure and is of little interest to us.

5 The bodily defences are further specified as an 'army of leucocytes.' On martial metaphors of immunity see Kraut 1994.

Yet, there were also undeclared purposes, and these are more relevant to our argument. Koch, accompanied by a military sergeant and a team of oarsmen seemed to have been embarking on a hunting trip and in particular. focussed on killing as many crocodiles as they could. Having – erroneously – identified these animals as the reservoir of human trypanosomiasis, provided some justification for hunting them and trying out equipment for their extinction.[6] A reading of Koch's diary, however, gives the impression that hunting was far more random in terms of species targeted and that the scientific rationale, such as testing means for the mass-extermination of crocodiles was more a gloss over.[7] Koch and his companions basically shot at everything that moved from hippopotamuses to crocodiles, from herons to eagles. "Shot two pelicans" [zwei Pelikane geschossen] (Henneberg et al. 1997, 168), Koch noted on 8 August, "shot birds around the valley" [in der Umgebung vom Tale Vögel geschossen] (Henneberg et al. 1997, 169), on 9 September, and "shot a lot of other birds, among others a beautiful blue heron" [noch viele Vögel geschossen, darunter ein schöer Edelreiher] (Henneberg et al. 1997, 170), on 11 September. On 17 September he saw "a giant snake; we first demolished its vertebral column with a shot of pellets and then smashed its head with gunshot" [eine Riesenschlange, der mit einem Schrotschuß zuerst die Wirbelsäule zerschmettert und dann der Kopf zerschossen wurde] (Henneberg et al. 1997, 172). Many more entries of this kind could be cited. The diary also contains colourful descriptions of strenuous stalking:

> 12 September (...) Sat there for almost two hours, but the crocodile didn't come. Then we took off, crept along the edge of the island, suddenly saw between rocks and bushes the tail of a crocodile. The animal stayed on the spot because its rear was paralysed. Writhed and bucked in front and opened its jaws to catch our scent. Brought it down with a bullet to the head. [12/9 (...) Fast 2 Stunden gesessen, ohne daß das Crocodil kam. Dann aufgebrochen, am Rande der Insel hingeschlichen, plötzlich zwischen Steinen und Büschen ein Crocodilschwanz gesehen. Das Thier blieb auf dem Fleck, weil es hinten gelähmt war. Wälzte, krümmte sich vorn und riß witternd den Rachen auf. Durch Kopfschuß hingestreckt.] (Henneberg et al. 1997, 170)

---

6 Koch was initially unaware of the differences between those trypanosoma that cause human trypanosomiasis and those that can be found in crocodiles. Over the course of his expedition he became aware that there were more species than he had initially assumed (Gradmann 2009, 212f.).

7 The diary from which the following quotes are taken is reprinted in Henneberg et al. 1997, 166–181.

Even if some meat was needed to feed Koch's oarsmen, the number of animals killed was much too high for this purpose. Some of them, for instance the eagles, were hardly suitable food. At the same time, references to the scientific character of the undertaking are rather sparse. Occasionally the dispatched animals were photographed and autopsied, preparations for subsequent use were sometimes produced. Yet, it is often difficult to distinguish between the sporting and the scientific interest. Thus Koch noted on 27 September,

> Very soon come to a small clearing, where two crocodiles lie. One of them immediately flees, and at the same moment the other receives a shot through the vertebral column. It can't get away but snaps its jaws, hisses and growls. Is photographed when still alive, then killed and the head cut off. [Sehr bald an eine kleine Lichtung gekommen, wo zwei Krokodile liegen. Das eine flüchtet sofort, im selben Moment erhält das zweite einen Schuss durch die Wirbelsäule. Es kann nicht mehr fort, schnappt aber um sich und knurrt und faucht. Wird noch lebend photographirt, dann todtgeschossen und der Kopf abgeschnitten.] (Henneberg et al. 1997, 178)

A fixation on crocodiles in this expedition is unmistakable. It was not only a matter of shooting the animals, but also of finding their nests, counting their clutches, and then usually destroying them. It is therefore clear that Koch and Sacher engaged in an extermination campaign against crocodiles, which considering the number of crocodiles and the means at the hunters' disposal, definitively had something quixotic about it. However, judging by the diary entries, the undertaking gave Koch considerable pleasure, in part perhaps because the tangible results compensated for the disappointing outcome of the experimental treatment on Sese.[8]

"Under the beautiful cover sleeps doom" [unter der schönen Decke schlummert das Verderben],[9] the bacteriologist wrote in a letter from Lake Victoria. The hunting campaign provides insight into Koch's perception of nature and his understanding of disease, complementing what has been discussed earlier in this paper about his fascination with the Bengal jungles as the home of cholera. The scientist's enthusiasm for African nature was obviously symbiotic with an aggressive attitude, and to this extent is reminiscent of the contemporary clichés that depicted "Black Africa" as a fascinating and dangerous place. As a physician, Koch added specificity to this image. The characteristics of the Dark Continent that others viewed over the sights of a gun were also visible, albeit in a different form, through the lens of a microscope. In Koch's case, these were trivial images of a hidden and menacing nature.

---

8 After initially delivering promising results, this treatment turned out to be ineffective. In addition, serious side-effects became obvious, notably in patients loosing their eyesight.

9 Koch to Georg Gaffky, 30.7.1906, quoted in Möllers 1950, 312.

For all the beauty of nature, the bacteriologist uncovered innumerable dangers lurking under the surface:

> "Malaria, dysentery, recurrent fevers, all of this is amply present here as almost nowhere else. The place is swarming with anopheles; even on my mountain we have them almost in pure culture" [Malaria, Dysenterie, Recurrens, das ist hier so gründlich vertreten wie kaum anderswo. Alles wimmelt von Anopheles, selbst auf meinem Berg haben wir sie fast in Reinkultur.] (*ibid.*).

He wrote this from his camp, thereby providing a fine example of his perception of nature. An examination of his own rowers, "52 strong young men" [52 junge, kräftige Männer], yielded the results he had expected: "And by the way, of these 52 seemingly healthy young people, 47 had *Filaria perstans*, 26 had malaria parasites, and 2 recurrent fever spirilla in their blood. This is what the supposedly still healthy local population looks like." [Nebenbei bemerkt, hatten von diesen 52 anscheinend gesunden Leuten 47 Filaria perstans, 26 Malariaparasiten und 2 Recurrensspirillen im Blut. So sieht die noch für gesund geltende hiesige Bevölkerung aus] (*ibid.*).

6 The Nature of Infectious Disease

That nature is a source of dirt, danger, and above all disease was a fundamental conviction of Koch's. This attitude is revealed in his reflections on the natural history of cholera in the jungles of Bengal. We can conclude that for him, Africa was the apotheosis of dirt, danger and disease – a repulsive yet fascinating subject. The fundamentals of the orderly microscopic world, which the bacteriologist imagined, were mirrored in the macroscopic world of Africa or in the jungles of Bengal, where nature had not yet been tamed by civilization and hygiene. That Koch formulated very similar statements about nature as the source of dirt and infection over a timespan of several decades suggests that this was an intersection where science and ideology reinforced each other. Koch's concept of pathology was informed by the idea of lurking, minuscule, invisible dangers coming from without. These were characteristics he ascribed to bacteria as well as to nature as a whole. In the words of Ludwik Fleck, not the least important intention in creating such concrete and trivial images is to stabilize scientific thinking by relating it to everyday knowledge:

> "The concreteness of a body of knowledge has a special effect. First applied by the expert in order to make a thought understandable to others [...], this concreteness, initially a means, assumes the importance of a body of knowledge acquired. The image wins out over the specific proofs and often returns to the expert in this new guise" (Fleck 1988 [1935], 154 f.).

Robert Koch's imagined African nature, his ideas about the natural history of epidemics in Bengal and similar matters brought together ideology and scientific practice in a quite creative, if not necessarily sophisticated manner. His ideas expressed fundamental assumptions about the relationships between inside and outside, cleanliness and health, dirt and infection, that were as important to the scientific concept of infectious disease as they were for the popular ideas about cleanliness, hygiene, and the boundaries of the body.

There is, we realize, more than just an element of exoticism in the relationships between men and microbes as they were imagined by Koch and his audiences. Instead such relationships are portrayed against a backdrop of exotic nature and colonial politics. Tropical nature in particular is assumed to provide exemplary insights into the relationships of men and microbes, its images serving to amplify and guide the thought style of early bacteriology.

References

Anon. "Politische Tagesübersicht. Die deutsche Cholera-Kommission in Ägypten." *Berliner Tageblatt*, 26.9.1883.

Anon. "Willkommen, Ihr Sieger!" *Berliner Tageblatt*, 3.5.1884.

Berger, Silvia. *Bakterien in Krieg und Frieden. Eine Geschichte der medizinischen Bakteriologie in Deutschland 1890–1933*. Göttingen: Wallstein, 2009.

Brenner, Peter J. "Der Reisebericht in der deutschen Literatur. Ein Forschungsüberblick als Vorstudie zu einer Gattungsgeschichte." *Internationales Archiv für Sozialgeschichte der Literatur*, special issue 2. Tübingen: Niemeyer, 1990.

Brenner, Peter J. "Gefühl und Sachlichkeit. Humboldts Reisewerk zwischen Naturwissenschaft und Naturphilosophie." *Archiv für Kulturgeschichte* 73 (1991): 135–168.

Briese, Olaf. *Angst in den Zeiten der Cholera*. 4 vols. Berlin: Akademie Verlag, 2003.

Brock, Thomas D. *Robert Koch. A Life in Medicine and Bacteriology*. Madison, WI: Science Tech Publishers, 1988.

Bynum, William F. *Science and the Practice of Medicine in the Nineteenth Century*. Cambridge: Cambridge University Press, 1994.

Canetti, Elias. *Crowds and Power*. Translated by Carol Stewart. New York, NY: Farrar, Straus and Giroux, 1984 [1960].

Cittadino, Eugene. *Nature as Laboratory: Darwinian Plant Ecology in The German Empire 1880–1900*. Cambridge: Cambridge University Press, 1990.

Coleman, William. "Koch's Comma Bacillus. The First Year." *Bulletin of the History of Medicine* 61 (1987): 315–342.

Cunningham, Andrew, and Perry Williams (Eds). *The Laboratory Revolution in Medicine*. Cambridge: Cambridge University Press, 1992.

Dekker, Hermann. *Die Schutz- und Kampfmittel des Organismus gegen die Infektionskrankheiten*. Hamburg: Verlagsanstalt und Druckerei A.-G. [vormals J.F. Richter], 1898.

Evans, Richard J. *Death in Hamburg: Society and Politics in the Cholera Years 1830–1910*. Oxford: Clarendon, 1987.
Fisch, Stefan. "Forschungsreisen im 19. Jahrhundert." *Der Reisebericht. Die Entwicklung einer Gattung in der deutschen Literatur.* Ed. Peter J. Brenner. Frankfurt a. M.: Suhrkamp, 1989. 383–401.
Fleck, Ludwik. *Genesis and Development of a Scientific Fact.* Chicago: University of Chicago Press, 1988 [1935].
Gradmann, Christoph. "Invisible Enemies: Bacteriology and the Language of Politics in Imperial Germany." *Science in Context* 13 (2000): 9–30.
Gradmann, Christoph. *Laboratory Disease: Robert Koch's Medical Bacteriology.* Baltimore, MA: Johns Hopkins University Press, 2009.
Gradmann, Christoph. "Robert Koch and the Invention of the Carrier State: Tropical Medicine, Veterinary Infections and Epidemiology around 1900." *Studies in History and Philosophy of Biological and Biomedical Sciences* 41 (2010): 232–40.
Hänseler, Marianne. *Metaphern unter dem Mikroskop. Die epistemische Rolle von Metaphorik in den Wissenschaften und in Robert Kochs Bakteriologie.* Zurich: Chronos, 2009.
Hamlin, Christopher. *Cholera: The Biography.* Oxford: Oxford University Press, 2009.
Henneberg, Georg, Klaus Janitschke, Klaus Stürzbecher, and Rolf Winau (Eds). *Robert Koch II. Teil. Nach Fragmenten von Bruno Heymann.* Berlin: Robert Koch-Institut, 1997.
Koch, Robert. "Die Ätiologie der Tuberkulose." *Gesammelte Werke von Robert Koch.* Ed. Julius Schwalbe. 2 vols. Vol. 1. Leipzig: Thieme, 1912 [1882]. 428–445.
Koch, Robert. "Berichte über die Tätigkeit der zur Erforschung der Cholera im Jahre 1883 nach Ägypten und Indien entsandten Kommission." *Gesammelte Werke von Robert Koch.* Ed. Julius Schwalbe. 2 vols. Vol. 2,1. Leipzig: Thieme, 1912 [1883/1884]. 1–19.
Koch, Robert. "Erste Konferenz zur Erörterung der Cholerafrage." *Gesammelte Werke von Robert Koch.* Ed. Julius Schwalbe. 2 vols. Vol. 2,1. Leipzig: Thieme, 1912 [1884]. 20–60.
Koch, Robert. "Die Bekämpfung der Infektionskrankheiten, insbesondere der Kriegsseuchen." In *Gesammelte Werke von Robert Koch.* Ed. Julius Schwalbe. 2 vols. Vol. 2,1. Leipzig: Thieme, 1912 [1888]. 276–289.
Koch, Robert. "Zusammenfassende Darstellung der Ergebnisse der Malariaexpedition." *Gesammelte Werke von Robert Koch.* Ed. Julius Schwalbe. 2 vols. Vol. 2,1. Leipzig: Thieme, 1912 [1900]. 422–434.
Kollenbrock-Netz, Jutta. "Wissenschaft als nationaler Mythos. Anmerkungen zur Haeckel-Virchow Kontroverse auf der 50. Jahresversammlung der deutschen Naturforscher und Ärzte in München (1877)." *Nationale Mythen und Symbole in der zweiten Hälfte des 19. Jahrhunderts.* Eds Jürgen Link and Wulf Wülfling. Stuttgart: Klett-Cotta, 1991. 212–236.
Kraut, Alan M. *Silent Travellers: Germs, Genes, and the "Immigrant Menace".* Baltimore, MA, London: Johns Hopkins University Press, 1994.
Latour, Bruno. "Give Me a Laboratory and I will Raise the World." *Science Observed: Perspectives on the Social Study of Science.* Ed. Karin Knorr-Cetina and Michael Mulkay. London: Sage, 1983. 141–170.
Möllers, Bernhard. *Robert Koch. Persönlichkeit und Lebenswerk 1843–1910.* Hannover: Schmorl & von Seefeld, 1950.
Osterhammel, Jürgen. "Forschungsreise und Kolonialprogramm. Ferdinand von Richthofen und die Erschließung Chinas im 19. Jahrhundert." *Archiv für Kulturgeschichte* 69 (1987): 150–195.

Schlich, Thomas. "Ein Symbol medizinischer Fortschrittshoffnung. Robert Koch entdeckt den Erreger der Tuberkulose." *Meilensteine der Medizin.* Ed. Heinz Schott. Düsseldorf: Harenberg, 1996. 368–374.

Valerius (pseudonym). "Die Cholera-Gefahr." *Die Gartenlaube* 30 (1884a): 500–502.

Valerius (pseudonym). "Der Kommabacillus." *Die Gartenlaube* 32 (1884b): 598–599.

Weindling, Paul. *Epidemics and Genocide in Eastern Europe, 1890–1945.* Oxford: Oxford University Press, 2000.

Thomas Anz

Rousing Emotions in the Description of Contagious Diseases in Modernism

Contagious diseases pose problems in medicine and at the same time are a subject of cultural fascination with considerable emotional impact. In every cultural sphere, contagious diseases are very popular as metaphors for phenomena that have no medical significance. In the *Frankfurter Allgemeine Zeitung* of 19 July 2011 the lead story on the "Financial market" pages was entitled "Growing threat of contagion on the markets" [Wachsende Ansteckungsgefahr an den Märkten] (Braunberger, FAZ 19 July 2011, 17). The economic section in the same issue contained a commentary with the title "Threat of Contagion":

> On the financial markets in the last few days a word has been circulating that should send an alarm signal to all who still remember the serious crisis that followed the collapse of the American investment bank of Lehman Brothers in autumn 2008. In financial market jargon, that word is "contagion" [...]. It means that a crisis can suddenly jump from one market to another and thus spread without check. [An den Finanzmärkten kursiert in diesen Tagen ein Wort, das all jenen ein Alarmsignal senden sollte, die sich noch an die schwere Krise nach dem Zusammenbruch der amerikanischen Investmentbank Lehmann Brothers im Herbst 2008 erinnern. Das Wort heißt in der Sprache der Finanzmärkte "Contagion" (...). Damit ist gemeint, dass eine Krise plötzlich von einem Markt auf einen anderen überspringen und sich auf diese Weise unkontrolliert ausbreiten kann.] (Braunberger, FAZ 19 July 2011, 9)

'Contagion' as an "alarm signal": contagion scenarios are usually fear scenarios. People then talk about "the threat of contagion". This essay aims firstly to highlight the fact that talking or writing about contagious diseases has eminent emotion-arousing potential above and beyond the communication of certain cognitive concepts. Secondly, it aims, through examples of Literary Modernism and its criticism, to show that apart from fear, many other emotions can be associated with ideas about contagion scenarios. And in the process it will reconstruct some mechanisms and rules that enable these emotions to be aroused.

A look at texts of very different kinds reveals that contagion metaphors can even arouse positive emotions. For example, one of the latest developments in the advertising industry is called 'viral marketing management.' It is an attempt to get people to recommend certain products or services to others. A 'viral marketing manager' said recently: "I look for an idea that is worth passing on. Because it's only when the story is really worth telling that the viral snowball can start rolling." [Ich suche eine Idee, die es Wert ist, weiter erzählt zu werden. Denn nur wenn die Geschichte wirklich erzählenswert ist, kann der virale

Schneeball ins Rollen kommen.] (Pilgram, SZ 6–7 August 2011, 9). This form of advertising is called "viral" because, as the *Süddeutsche Zeitung* explained to its readers on 6/7 August 2011, "the message is to be passed on from person to person in a short time like a biological virus" [die Botschaft in kurzer Zeit wie ein biologischer Virus von Mensch zu Mensch weitergetragen werden soll] (*ibid.*). Such positive applications of the contagion metaphor, i.e. provoking joy, satisfaction or pleasure are not new and are also found in quite different cultural spheres. Stefan Zweig for example depicted Sigmund Freud's ideas in the nineteen-twenties as spreading like contagious bacteria, with no negative connotations at all. On the contrary: In just the same way, said Zweig in 1926 in a speech on the psychoanalyst's 70th birthday,

> the thoughts, the bold and often brilliant interpretations, with which Sigmund Freud has endowed and challenged our world today, [...] are alive and have created life. [...] Like bacteria, they have penetrated every organism of the intellectual world: everywhere, in poetry, in philosophy, in ethics, and even in everyday dealings and relations between the sexes there are clear signs of it. [So sind auch die Gedanken, die kühnen und oftmals genialen Deutungen, mit denen Sigmund Freud unsere Gegenwart beschenkt und herausgefordert hat, (...) lebendig und haben Leben gezeugt. (...) Sie sind wie Bazillen eingedrungen in alle Organismen der geistigen Welt: überall, in Dichtung, in Philosophie, in der Ethik, ja selbst in der Form gewöhnlichen Umganges und der Beziehung der Geschlechter ist ihre Spur deutlich zu erkennen.] (Zweig 1994, 232)

Similarly, albeit with a variety of connotations and emotions, disease metaphors have in fact now also entered the meta-language for discussing illness metaphors, when referring to their rapid and extensive propagation.

Despite, or perhaps precisely because of her warnings about the harmfulness of illness metaphors, Susan Sontag used the same type of metaphor when she criticised the popularity of cancer, AIDS and other diseases as metaphors (Sontag 1990). In 1987, Paula Treichler diagnosed an "epidemic of signification" in relation to the AIDS discourse (Treichler 1987). And Brigitte Weingart gave her investigation, published in 2002, of "Representations of AIDS" the title "Contagious Words" (Weingart 2002). The excellent introduction written by Weingart, together with the specialist in American studies Ruth Mayer, to the Symposium Proceedings which appeared in 2004 – *VIRUS! Mutationen einer Metapher* [VIRUS! Mutations of a Metaphor] (Mayer and Weingart 2004, 7–42) – makes several references to the fact that viruses, with their ability to lodge unnoticed in a host organism and change its code for their own purposes, are turning into metaphors that express and attempt to arouse positive emotions, especially in the intellectual environment of Postmodernism of the 1980s. It happens when they are used to illustrate processes in which existing orders, power structures and ideologies are destabilised, when established boundaries are dissolved. A subversive, deconstructive potential is then ascribed to viruses used as metaphors. We will see that this positive use of disease metaphors is widespread not just in the Postmodernist age, it already was in the epoch of Literary Modernism.

The expression and evocation of fear were and are still predominant in the metaphorical and narrative depiction of contagion scenarios. As such, contagion scenarios are instrumentalised for a wide variety of purposes. Literary Modernism around and after 1900 was affected in two ways. 1. The opponents of Literary Modernism tried repeatedly to stigmatise it as sick. 2. Literary Modernism intensified literature's interest in disease and integrated it into its anticlassical aesthetics and poetics. In both cases infectious diseases as well as contagion scenarios were of eminent significance.

1 Disease Metaphors in the War on Literary Modernism

1925 saw the publication of the first volume of a polemic, subsequently to be reprinted countless times, that used its rhetoric to criticise culture by employing excessively and militantly the 'healthy-sick' dichtotomy to vilify its opponents and impose its own moral values. The author of the text belonged, at least in age, to the 'Expressionist' generation. Here, an unsuccessful artist was attacking the more successful Modernist art, talking about "the sickly excrescences of lunatics or of degenerate people which since the turn of the century we have learned to know under the collective conception of cubism or dadaism" (Hitler 1941, 353), speaking of "excrescences", "intellectual degenerates" (*ibid.*, 359), "hallucinations of insane people or criminals" (*ibid.*, 360) and of the responsibility "of the government [...] to prevent a people from being driven into the arms of spiritual lunacy." (*ibid.*, 354)

For the cultural critic, the disease afflicting modern art since the turn of the century was of course the sign of a far more comprehensive malady of the epoch – like syphilis, on which the preceding passages of the book had declared war. It too was said to be only a symptom, "only the result of an illness of moral, social, and racial instincts." (*ibid.*, 349) Anyone who gives in to these afflictions has forfeited his right to exist. The present government has failed to control the disease:

> Towards syphilis especially one can describe the attitude of the national and State authority only with the words, complete capitulation. [...] The invention of a remedy of a questionable character as well as the commercial exploitation of the latter are able to help but little with this plague. [...] The cause, however, lies primarily in our prostitution of love. The Ju-

> daization of our spiritual life and the mammonization of our mating impulse sooner or later befouls our entire new generation. (*ibid.*, 337)

With printed emphasis, the author spelled out the consequences in traditional social-Darwinian terms: “When the energy for the fight for one’s own health is no longer present, the right of living in this world of strength begins gradually to withdraw” (*ibid.*, 351).

These sentences are in Adolf Hitler’s *Mein Kampf.* We know how Hitler acted on the threats associated with his diagnoses of disease. After the book burnings of May 1933, the ‘Degenerate Art’ exhibition of 1937 was a particularly spectacular event for the fight of the Nazis against Modernism, bearing out the pathologising verdicts of anti-Modernism. The pathologising concept of ‘degeneracy’ owed its career to the doctor and writer Max Nordau. In 1892/93 he published his two volume-text entitled *Degeneration* which was reprinted numerous times and translated into several languages. The book’s attack was aimed at the latest “fashions” in the top echelons of Paris society and their “imitators” in Germany, the “fin-de-siècle mood” that was spreading like an epidemic and its manifestations in the lifestyle and artistic tastes of a small but style-setting “minority” of “rich educated people” (Nordau 1895, 7). To him, Modernist art and literature are symptoms of diseases, which played a similarly prominent role in the psychopathology and cultural criticism of 1900 as ‘melancholy’ did in 1800 and ‘schizophrenia’ in the 20th century. Nordau diagnoses ‘degeneration’ and ‘hysteria’ with its weaker ‘neurasthenic’ forms. He mentions infectious diseases only in passing, when he makes various toxins responsible for the manifestations of degeneration he has diagnosed. The absorption of organic toxins caused by diseases such as syphilis and tuberculosis also creates degenerates in the subsequent generation who “[...] if they remain exposed to the same influences, rapidly descend to the lowest degrees of degeneracy, to idiocy, to dwarfishness, etc.” (*ibid.*, 34).

But in his descriptions of disease Nordau does not only highlight contagion phenomena in the metaphorical sense. The “formation of close groups or schools” of various kinds is said to be characteristic of all degenerates and hysterics. And according to Nordau’s observations, which in many ways had equivalents in the psychology and psychopathology of the time – and the psychoanalysis, with its concept of ’transference’ – , this is caused by contagious processes guided by an invisible hand.

> Criminals unite in bands, as Lombroso expressly establishes. Among pronounced lunatics it is the *folie à deux*, in which a deranged person completely forces his insane ideas on a companion; among the hysterical it assumes the form of close friendships, causing Charcot

> to repeat at every opportunity: "Persons of highly-strung nerves attract each other;" [...] and finally authors found schools. (*ibid.*, 30)

In this connection Nordau specifies what the chapter on the "symptoms" of the "fin-de-siècle mood" left unclear. Who are the sick subjects of this new fad: the painters, poets, composers and philosophers, in other words those actively producing culture, or those who like to enthuse about their works, a flock of critics, propagandists or passive hangers-on? The author suspects pathology at work in all of them.

> This is the natural history of the aesthetic schools. Under the influence of an obsession, a degenerate mind promulgates some doctrine or other – realism, pornography, mysticism, symbolism, diabolism. He does this with vehement penetrating eloquence, with eagerness and fiery heedlessness. Other degenerate, hysterical, neurasthenical minds flock around him, receive from his lips the new doctrine, and live thenceforth only to propagate it. (*ibid.*, 31)

The word "propagate" again points to the pathological aspect of this process, to its epidemic character. "Insane ideas" predominate among the active leaders and instigators of a school of aesthetics, weakness of will and a pathological hypersensitivity to suggestion, such as is especially typical of hysterics, predominate among "the associates, the disciples, the submissive part" (Nordau 1895, 31).

2 Pathophilic Modernism

Around and after 1900, Literary Modernism shared with its opponents the interest in pathological phenomena and excessive use of illness metaphors, but to a certain extent gave them new meaning. The scorn and anger Nordau directs at degenerates and which he tries to arouse in his readers along with a fear of the contagious spread of the symptoms of degeneration, did not exist in Modernist authors. On the contrary, Modernism was rather pathophilic. It imitated expressions of madness, identified with sick people and their social status as outsiders in contrast to the normality of the odious bourgeois, integrated physical diseases into its aesthetics of ugliness or saw illnesses as productive crises from which those affected were able to emerge cognitively, emotionally or psychologically stronger. Infectious diseases were also among the pathological phenomena which Modernism took a serious interest in and valorised to a certain extent.

As is well known, the disease motif is of central significance to all of Thomas Mann's writings. In 1904, Thomas Mann sketched out a plan that he used four decades later in his novel *Doktor Faustus:*

> Figure of the syphilitic artist: as Doctor Faustus and as one assigned to the devil. The poison has the same effects [on him] as intoxication, stimulant, inspiration; he may create wonderful works of genius in a state of enraptured enthusiasm; the devil himself guides his hand. In the end, however, *the devil comes for him:* paralysis. [Figur des syphilitischen Künstlers: als Doktor Faust und dem Teufel verschriebener. Das Gift wirkt als Rausch, Stimulans, Inspiration; er darf in entzückter Begeisterung geniale, wunderbare Werke schaffen, der Teufel selbst führt ihm die Hand. Schließlich aber *holt ihn der Teufel:* Paralyse.] (Mann 1992, 121 f.)

Since Paul Julius Möbius's pathography, *Über das Pathologische bei Nietzsche* [On the Pathological in Nietzsche], which appeared in 1902, syphilis had been closely associated with the notion of genius by German intellectuals. One Expressionist author swayed by this view of Nietzsche was Gustav Sack, whose fragment of a 1913 novel entitled *Paralyse* [Paralysis] presents syphilis as a stimulus for ecstatically unfettered thinking and fantasising. Anja Schonlau studied this in depth in her book on *Syphilis in der Literatur* [Syphilis in Literature] (Schonlau 2005, 381–399).

In the work of Thomas Mann, illnesses have a function in relation to the various messages the author intends to impart: as a component of an atmosphere of decay, as a form of remoteness from bourgeois society and the consequent suffering in isolation, as independence from society's constraints and as a necessary requirement for artistic genius. In Thomas Mann however, illness also not infrequently acquires a disillusioning function as the antithesis of 'healthy' greatness and superiority. The novella *Schwere Stunde*, 1905 [A Weary Hour] about Friedrich Schiller destroys a widely accepted portrait of the personality of the German Classical poet. The disease motif is employed here not without humoristic undertones, as it is later in the best-known of Expressionist poems, Jakob van Hoddis' *Weltende* [The End of the World], in which the apocalyptic fears evoked by the title are subverted *inter alia* by the verse: "Most people have a cold" [Die meisten Menschen haben einen Schnupfen]. Thomas Mann's narrative presented Schiller thus: "[...] coughing, drew together the folds of his dressing-gown [...] he snuffed hard through his nostrils to get a little air, for as usual he had a cold" (Mann 1936a, 290). Friedrich Schiller is presented to the reader as sick and completely exhausted. He owes his work to the "discipline and self-control" (Mann 1936a, 294) which enables him to cover up his weakness in a final agonising physical effort. In the novella *Der Tod in Venedig* [Death in Venice], which was published in 1912, it is the poet Gustav Aschenbach, initially extremely successful and exemplary in every way, who represents the ideals of his bourgeois audience. His moral strength and dignity are increasingly challenged in the course of the narrative and here, disease also acquires crucial significance. Cholera, that physically defeats the poet, is an image of psychic anarchic powers from which comes the defeat by this "enemy of the composed and dignified intellect" (Mann 1990, 260). The disease is part of a complex set of biological metaphors describing in a wide variety of ways Aschenbach's secret craving for the lowest reaches of intoxication, sensuality and beauty. At the beginning of the novella, Aschenbach is trapped in the vision of a rich, damp tropical swampland with "rank jungles of fern" and "hairy palm-trunks", and his heart throbbed with terror and mysterious longing" (*ibid.*, 200). The imagery is continued when Aschenbach hears the story of the spread of the plague. This is Indian cholera, produced by "the sultry morasses of the Ganges delta, rising with the mephitic exhalations of [...] that primitive island jungle shunned by man" (ibid., 256). The steps taken by the authorities of the affected countries to control and conceal the plague as outlined in the novella are given in this context the significance of a metaphor for the collective resistance and repression of sensual passion by conscience and morals – a repression which has been described in the second chapter as the reason for Aschenbach's success and greatness. The text repeatedly suggests the connection between disease and illicit libidinous behaviour. The infestation of the city is accompanied by a demoralisation "of the lower social levels", and the encouragement to "the dark and antisocial forces" (*ibid.*, 258). There was "intemperance, shameless licence and growing criminality" (*ibid.*, 258). Now enlightened about the disease-related events in Venice, Aschenbach has a dream during the night, the setting for which is "his own soul" (*ibid.*, 259). His resisting consciousness is overcome by the all-possessing, ecstatic, orgiastic followers of the god Dionysus. The panting bodies frenziedly dancing and yelling are surrounded by "an exhalation as of staling waters, with another smell, too, that was familiar: that of wounds and wandering disease" (*ibid.*, 260).

Aschenbach at one point alludes to "the profound instinctual fusion of discipline and licence" (*ibid.*, 240), on which the artist's nature and character rests. The existence of two opposing fields of psychic powers in the protagonist's character, like a split personality, forms the starting point for the issues addressed in the narrative.

In abstract terms, the handling of the narrative can be described as a shift from one field to the other; the sudden reversal is presented as terrifying. Towards the end, the condition of the already sick poet is described as follows: "He was being attacked by waves of dizziness, only half physical, and with them went an increasing sense of dread, a feeling of hopelessness and pointlessness, though he could not decide whether this referred to the external world or to his personal existence" (*ibid.*, 265). His fear relates to both: the disease-ridden outer world becomes increasingly sinister and frightening to him, as he also does to himself.

In a way very similar to several poems by the doctor and poet Gottfried Benn for example, disease in *Death in Venice*, related as it is to socially repressed aspects of human existence, has the function of destroying the prevailing ideas about human superiority and autonomy. But where Benn presents various diseases, including syphilis, with provocative ugliness, Thomas Mann is more closely bound by literary tradition in that he aestheticises Aschenbach's illness and suffering to quite a large extent both linguistically and thematically, even if the beautiful is often curiously mixed up with the ugly (the dirt and filth of Venice, the foul-smelling lagoons). Aschenbach the poet can distance himself from disease as little as he can from the sensual beauty of the sickly boy Tadzio. In that sense the novella identifies beauty and disease to a certain extent. The same is also very true of Aschenbach's death. It is a beautiful death, recounted in the refined vocabulary of a highly exalted style. This death has hardly anything terrifying about it.

A similar emotional ambivalence to that of Thomas Mann besets disease in Yvan Goll's little novel in an urban setting *Die Eurokokke* [The Eurococcus]. It appeared in 1927, in the same year as the German translation of *Ulysses*, Heidegger's *Sein und Zeit* [Being and Time] and also the second volume of Hitler's *Mein Kampf*. In many respects, the book is representative of those cultural crises, decadent fantasies and intense attempts at self-assertion that characterised both Literary Modernism and its opponents. In the Paris of the 1920s, Yvan Goll was one of the spokesmen of the Surrealist movement. The reflections of this Paris-based novel about fear and death recall Rilke's *Die Aufzeichnungen des Malte Laurids Brigge* [The Notebooks of Malte Laurids Brigge], the confrontation between a dying culture and the vitality of American civilisation could have been suggested by Alfred Kubin's apocalyptic novel *Die andere Seite* [The Other Side]. What the poet writes about the meaningless and simultaneously existence-illuminating disease of ennui can be read as an early existentialist equivalent of Sartre's novel *Nausea*, which appeared eleven years later. A number of things are very similar to Heidegger's critical verdicts on the 'forgetfulness of being' ['Seinsvergessenheit'] of Modernism or Spengler's speculations about the decline of the West. And behind it all are Nietzsche's analyses of nihilism and deconstructions of Western metaphysics.

The novel concentrates in a small space a rich diversity of impressions and stories about the metropolis. The Jewish author's interest and sympathy are devoted to the outsiders of society in particular: street girls, bohemians, beggars, the unemployed, criminals.

As in *Ulysses*, everything happens in one day. "I awoke from a dream that closed behind me like a gilded iron gate." [Ich bin aufgewacht aus einem Traum, der sich hinter mir schloß wie ein vergoldetes Gittertor.] (Goll 1988, 7). This is how the novel begins. The awakening is like being "expelled from paradise" [Vertreibung aus dem Paradies], from the blessed "slumber of numbness, of ignorance" [Schlummer der Taubheit, des Nichtwissens] into enforced awareness:

> I can sleep no longer, my eyelids have been snapped back. I must keep my eyes tightly, rigidly, directly focused on the truth, like dead people whose eyes no-one has closed. [Ich kann nicht

mehr schlafen, die Augenlider sind mir weggeschnitten. Ich muß die Augen hart, steif, gerade auf die Wahrheit richten, genau wie die Toten, denen niemand sie schloß.] (*ibid.*, 8)

The truth the narrator must see is that there is no longer any truth. The city is a polyphonic simultaneity of lies, facades, repressions and simulations, all hiding one thing: a paralysing, meaningless emptiness. Even nature is just "painted scenery, mise-en-scène, illusion" [Staffage, Kulisse, Täuschung] (ibid., 106). The title of the novel already supplies the surreal metaphor for that notion and it quickly becomes the focus for the whole text: a terrible disease has afflicted Europe and its agent is "the Eurococcus".

It is no accident that it has been discovered by an American scientist, representative of another, younger and more vital, culture than that of the old Europe. "The Eurococcus", he explains, "is the pathogen that is gobbling up European culture" [ist der Bazillus, der die europäische Kultur zerfrisst] and "some day will be responsible for the death of this continent" [einmal den Tod dieses Kontinents hervorrufen wird] (ibid.,74). It robs objects, animals and people of their inner substance, but leaves them externally intact. It does not kill; it sucks out their strength and their spirit. The American first found it on the towers of Notre Dame Cathedral. Notre Dame today is "just an imaginary building that no longer corresponds to reality because neither faith nor God live there: the Eurococcus has eaten them" [nur noch ein eingebildetes Gebäude, das der Realität nicht mehr dient, denn weder der Glaube noch Gott wohnen in ihm: die Eurokokke hat diese zerfressen] (*ibid.*, 74 f.).

A few years later he discovers the bacillus in an old book. It "was completely drained of all its spiritual content" [war seines geistigen Gehaltes vollkommen entleert] (*ibid.*, 75). And finally he also finds the Eurococcus in a human being, in a "decadent café." The narrator of the novel is sitting there. He has been attacked by the bacillus himself, by the "disease of emptiness, also known as ennui" [Krankheit der Leere, auch Langeweile genannt], and he is "the first European in whom the Eurococcus has visibly developed" [der erste Europäer, auf dem die Eurokokke sich in sichtbarem Zustand entwickelt hat]. No-one in fact had "sucked in the breath and torments of the city and the period as he had" [den Atem und die Qualen der Stadt und dieser Zeit in sich eingesogen] (*ibid.*, 82).

What the lonely and despairing hero still painfully perceives as a loss of Western values, other intellectuals are already starting to appreciate as the winning of an anarchic freedom. In the 'Bar de l'Ennui' and later in the 'Bar de la Mort', the narrator's friend preaches the ideal of a complete lack of ideals. "We take Western culture *ad absurdum*. We have declared it bankrupt." [Wir führen die okzidentale Kultur ad absurdum. Wir haben ihren Bankrott erklärt.] Only a complete lack of ideals, heroically rejecting every metaphysical prop, can give the people its greatest possession: “Absolute freedom is our first law and our last. The freedom of the ego takes precedence over morals, over friendship, over God. After all, we have nothing left to lose. [...] We have nothing left to fear, our story is behind us.” [Absolute Freiheit ist unser erstes und letztes Gesetz. Die Freiheit des Ich kommt vor der Moral, vor der Freundschaft, vor Gott. Wir haben ja nichts mehr zu verlieren. (...) Wir haben nichts mehr zu befürchten, wir haben unsere Geschichte hinter uns.] (*ibid.*, 110 f.).

In a discussion in 1929, Axel Eggebrecht called the book “the anthem of intellectual nihilism” [die Hymne des intellektuellen Nihilismus] (as in Goll 1988, 122). In the instructive postface to the new edition, published by Argon Verlag in 1988, Joachim Sartorius contradicted this. Yvan Goll, he said, is “more cautioning than nihilist” [mehr ein Mahner als ein Nihilist] (*ibid.*, 123), he is upholding a new (or old) faith against the agnosticism and triviality of his time. Both interpretations fail to understand what constitutes the aesthetic modernity of this novel: the perplexing absence of a clear standpoint on the part of a narrator who evades being unambiguously tied down by permanently changing his position and perspective. The postface by Barbara Glauert-Hesse in the facsimile edition which subsequently appeared provides details of Goll’s attempts to replace the first edition by a new one. For Goll, *The Eurococcus* was an incomplete, open work of art, a work, “which I’m always writing with all of my experience” [an dem ich mit meinem ganzen Erleben immer schreibe] (as in Glauert-Hesse 2002, 171).

In this realistic, and at the same time, fantastic novel, a huge placard is stretched over Paris, deeply confusing passersby who are only used to poster advertisements. In 28-meter high letters it says: “We do not know” [Wir wissen nicht]. It is directed at that imperious desire for knowledge, through which “everything is discovered and everything made technically possible” [alles entdeckt und alles technisch ermöglicht wird]. Renunciation of that desire would be “a new beginning *after* this culture” [ein neuer Anfang *nach* dieser Kultur] (Goll 1988, 30).

In its programmatic scepticism Goll’s novel is different from those critical verdicts of a degenerate and decadent culture that were always keen to offer terrifying diagnoses of disease and promising suggestions for treatment. The flawed and self-contradictory text distrusts therapeutic prescriptions and in its disillusion seeks refuge in old or new certainties. Its ending is left open, the last noun is: “mistake” [Irrtum] (*ibid.*, 116).

3 Rules of Emotionalisation in Literary Descriptions of Infectious Diseases

In the field of cultural studies, one of the most important recent publications on the history of infectious diseases is the volume *Bakteriologie und Moderne* [Bacteriology and Modernism], edited by Philipp Sarasin and others. This volume is symptomatic of current scholarly interest in the relations between the history of science, literature and art; it understands itself as a contribution to the 'history of knowledge' [Geschichte des Wissens] – referring to Michel Foucault among others. Crucial to this concept is the question of "transfer between different forms of science and the humanities on the one hand and non-academic forms of knowledge in modern societies on the other hand" [Austauschverhältnissen zwischen verschiedenen Wissenschaften einerseits und nichtwissenschaftlichen Formen des Wissens in modernen Gesellschaften andererseits] (Sarasin et al. 2007, 14).

The editors do mention, albeit incidentally, another important aspect of the public interest in bacteriology:

> [...] the entertainment value of the curious and exciting revelations from the realm of bacteria. Bacteria stories and epidemic narratives – Nancy Tomes calls them 'epidemic entertainment' – regularly led to high print runs of newspapers. Since bacteria and their sinister, life-threatening, secret activity could bring death and ruin to men at any time, they were also particularly suited to spark interest and arouse emotions in the public. [(...) Unterhaltungswert der seltsamen und aufregenden Mitteilungen aus dem Reich der Bakterien. Bakteriengeschichten und Seuchennarrative – von Nancy Tomes als 'Seuchenunterhaltung' bezeichnet – ließen die Auflagen der Zeitungshäuser regelmäßig in die Höhe schnellen. Da die Bakterien und ihre im Verborgenen stattfindende, unheimliche Tätigkeit jederzeit Tod und Verderben über die Menschen bringen konnten, waren sie auch besonders gut geeignet, beim Publikum Interesse und Emotionen auszulösen.] (*ibid.*, 35)

The editors add:

> While portraying bacteria and epidemics in an ominous way as 'invisible' and 'uncanny enemies' and as 'destroyers of mankind', popular articles play with skilful mastery on their readers' fears and arouse feelings of delightful and terrified horror. [Mit der nicht selten bedrohlichen Inszenierung von Bakterien und Seuchen als 'unsichtbare' und 'unheimliche Feinde' und als 'Zerstörer des Menschengeschlechts' spielten die populärwissenschaftlichen Artikel dabei sehr gekonnt auf der Klaviatur der Angst und förderten beim Publikum ein zugleich wohliges und Furcht einflößendes Grauen.] (*ibid.*, 35 f.)

This applies in a similar way to literary descriptions of infectious diseases.

Considering the relations between science and literature, one should generally assume that both are autonomous, distinct, self-generating and self-maintaining systems. For each of them, the other system is an exterior environment. Information and bodies of knowledge from the external environment are adapted to the internal order and functions of each system.

Despite all the affinities one can reconstruct historically between literature and science one should not underestimate their mutual boundaries and their autonomy. Creative writers do not only become influenced by certain scientific disciplines; they rather refer in their texts more or less playfully to academic or scientific works which they have read themselves, which they know from hearsay or which they assume are well-known among their readers. They integrate medical knowledge into their own order of knowledge and align it with the possibilities of literary representation.

In both cases, we have to assume the following: adaptions of knowledge from one system will be subordinated to the dominant functions of the other system. For example, the adaption of medical knowledge during the process of creative writing does not primarily serve the purpose of communicating certain insights. Instead, it creates suspense or other aesthetic effects, or it transmits certain ethical or aesthetic norms and values.

Poetry, wrote Robert Musil,

> is different from psychology, in the same way as poetry is different from science [...]. The distinction itself is simple: poetry does not transmit knowledge and insight. But: poetry *uses* knowledge and insight. [ist etwas anderes als Psychologie, so wie eben Dichtung etwas anderes als Wissenschaft ist (...). Die Unterscheidung selbst ist einfach: Dichtung vermittelt nicht Wissen und Erkenntnis. Aber: Dichtung benutzt Wissen und Erkenntnis.] (Musil 1978, 967)

Even if fictional stories about illness have absorbed the medical knowledge of their own era in a well-informed way in order to appear scientifically probable, their intentions are quite different from those of medical diagnosis and case studies; they integrate medical knowledge into their linguistic or cultural criticism or use it to communicate ethical and aesthetic convictions. And it is partly in this context that narrating illness aims to emotionalise the reader. It plays with his fears and hopes, arouses disgust, anger and various kinds of desire.

If we want to do justice to this process of emotionalisation, we must augment and modify current research on the relations between literature and science with its emphasis on history of knowledge and discourse and, increasingly, on narratology. We can do so by bringing in the most recent theories of emotion within the discipline of cultural studies.

To begin with, I would like to clarify some concepts. According to one of many psychological definitions, emotions are psycho-physical reactions through which an event from the exterior environment is perceived, processed, classified and interpreted; this process is accompanied by validation (Hülshoff 1999, 14).

In the act of reading, the literary text or a particular passage within the context of what has previously been read is the event from the exterior environment. But the literary text as external event must be distinguished from something like the sudden appearance of a snake – a frequently quoted example in research on emotions which goes back even to the time before Charles Darwin. Its sudden appearance causes emotional reactions in the subject which can be named as fear, terror, horror or panic. Texts on the other hand are artifacts and their artificial or, rather, artistic composition is intended to arouse certain emotions in the perceiving subject which he or she can decide to embrace or block out.

The definition I quoted which calls the emotional trigger an 'event from the exterior environment' is consistent with the assumption within psychology of emotions that emotions are not usually bound to the perception of an individual stimulus but rather to complex configurations of stimuli and scenarios.

Among the techniques of arousing emotions in literary texts is the evocation of imaginary scenarios that resemble real-life ones, and their emotional impact.

The phrase that, when reading, the literary text is the event from the external environment, can be enlarged on: the external event 'text' evokes among other things imaginations of various external events and scenarios to which the reader responds emotionally. Narratological and psychological interests intersect in the description of such scenarios.

Christiane Voss has developed a useful narratological concept of emotions in her monograph *Narrative Emotionen* [Narrative Emotions]. It makes reference to scenarios such as these and is attractive for our purposes insofar as narratological analysis belongs to the core competences of literary studies. The equivalent to the concept of 'scenario' in Voss' study is the concept of 'narrative.' 'Scenario' indicates an event while narrative means rather that an event is represented in a concrete way, from a certain perspective. Voss suggests the following: heterogeneous individual elements of complex emotions undergo a narrative synthesis in the emotional consciousness and experience of human subjects: that is, "through association and temporal relationships they are shaped into a meaningful chronological entity" [durch Assoziation und zeitliche Verknüpfung in ein chronologisches Sinnganzes gebracht] (Voss 2004, 186).

The poetics of illness stories in literary and scientific texts follow a pattern which is preserved as a narrative or as a script (if one wants to use the terminology of cognitive psychology) in the minds of authors and their readers – even if the texts do not present it in complete form. Incomplete, partial information about illness narratives are completed with the help of such 'scripts.' These narratives usually begin with a harmonic state of balance. This state is disturbed by some events or forces (compared in Yvan Goll's *Eurococcus* with the "expulsion from paradise") and transformed into a frequently threatening state of crisis. This crisis leads towards a situation in which the crisis will either be overcome in favour of the old or a new harmony; or where the crisis will turn into catastrophe.

This pattern and its narrative concretisation contain the potential to arouse emotions at all stages. The uncertainty whether the course of the illness will run happily or unhappily converges with narrative techniques of creating suspense. In traditional rhetorics, these techniques were already being defined as playing with the hopes and fears of the reader, namely "as a form of 'metabasis' that plays with spes and metus" [mit spes und metus spielende Ausprägung der 'Metabasis'] (Lausberg 1990, 950). Concerned is the transformation from good fortune to misfortune or from misfortune to good fortune. In the case of contagious diseases, fear often loses its connection to concrete sources of danger; it turns into a diffuse, uncertain 'angst' without an object which resembles the uncanniness of phantoms. Both novels *Death in Venice* and *The Eurococcus* contain many gothic elements. Thomas Mann's narrator compares cholera explicitly with a phantom and, in another section, Aschenbach is said to notice "uncanny developments in the outside world" (Mann 1900, 245).

With reference to the history of the gothic novel, Richard Alewyn articulated many years ago in an inspiring article the following hypothesis: fears can only arouse literary feelings of pleasure after they have in the main been mastered in reality and have disappeared (Alewyn 1965). Anja Schonlau picks up on this hypothesis in her book mentioned above. With some plausibility, she contradicts Susan Sontag's claim that illnesses lose their literary attractiveness as soon as they are medically understood and mastered. By contrast, Schonlau explains that in the case of syphilis, fears connected with the disease had to be reduced first by medical progress before they could be made 'enjoyable' in literature.

This claim is open to discussion; the most crucial aspect of Schonlau's theory is that the reader's 'pleasure in fear' requires a certain degree of safe distance from the horrors presented by a literary text. One component of the 'pleasure in fear' that accompanies the process of reading or the viewing of films is generally the feeling of relief: one is not acutely, or only to a much lesser degree than the fictitious characters, threatened by the dangers that are represented in the fictional mode.

However, apart from the aspect of 'pleasure in fear', illness narratives and the fears they conjure up frequently have a didactic function. The emotional effects of illness narratives intended by the texts, or rather by their authors, are accompanied by strategies to communicate certain norms or values. They concern mainly the evaluations of those involved in the illness scenarios: the causal agent of the illness; the one who is actually or potentially affected by the illness; those who can influence the course of the illness through their therapeutic or preventive abilities. With respect above all to the causal agent of the illness, it is frequently the case that illness narratives in literature are associated with the attribution of guilt. They include the appeal to avoid, eliminate or change what makes people ill. Illness appears as a sanction, arousing fear and disgust, for behaviour that does not conform to accepted or postulated norms. The fear of an illness is therefore not restricted to its potentially deadly consequences; it extends to the fear of things that are regarded as the cause of this particular disease. Theories on the causes of those illnesses that can be influenced by mankind bear implicit threats of sanctions. These threats prompt us to avoid the *negatively* and to pursue the *positively* evaluated forms of behaviour.

The enlightenment discourse on moralism tended to burden the sick person with a sense of guilt for behaviour that did not conform to accepted norms; the cause of the illness was sought in the victim itself. Social and cultural modernism, however, tends to absolve the diseased subject; the cause of the illness is attributed to social circumstances or to cultural norms and, therefore, rather the circumstances and norms are blamed than the sick person her- or himself. This 'modern' version of normative logic in discourses on health and illness no longer pursues the following sequence: 'Certain behavioural patterns make you ill, therefore avoid them!' This is transformed into a collective scheme – insofar as it is no longer the individual who is primarily made responsible for his own illness. Instead, certain forms of social existence and cultural norms are claimed to be responsible for an individual's illness and are presented as requiring change: 'Certain circumstances and living conditions make you ill, therefore they have to be changed!'. The fear which is evoked by illness narratives is no longer primarily the fear of behaviour that goes against the norm. It is rather a fear, mixed or alternating with indignation and disgust, of the social circumstances that make people ill. The emotional attitude towards the sick person tends to be dominated by compassion rather than schadenfreude, satisfaction, contempt or more aggressive forms of rejection.

In professional medical discourse all these aspects are related to 'aetiology', that is, the study of the causes of diseases and their normative implications. Yet it is not only ideas about what causes diseases that are full of normative claims. Equally normative are assumptions – frequently derived from aetiology – about things that prevent diseases, maintain health and cure those who are already ill; in medical discourse, these are above all the areas of dietetics, hygiene and therapeutics. Illness narratives are frequently dramatic and highly emotional scenarios of a struggle between powers that cause illness and powers that prevent or cure them. The novel *Death in Venice* contains many concepts and metaphors of battle, and to a lesser extent also Yvan Goll's novel *The Eurococcus.* "It felt as if there was an alien, hostile bacillus working in my blood" [Mir war, als arbeite ein fremder, feindlicher Bazillus in meinem Blut] (Goll 1988, 12), we are told there. But the sympathies and antipathies in the descriptions of various battles are much less clearly defined; in contrast to the militant critics of Literary Modernism their clear schemas of friend and foe are subverted.

The basic technique of literary emotionalisation through scenarios and narratives that typically evoke emotion frequently works as follows: the reader identifies with and develops empathy for fictional figures who are involved in a certain scenario and to whom certain emotions are often explicitly ascribed. Even if the reader has the distant perspective of an observer who follows events and even if his emotions are not identical with those of the fictional characters, his emotional involvement requires at least partial empathy with the figures in the text. The extent of this empathy depends on the extent to which the text represents its figures as objects of sympathy or antipathy. From this we can derive some fundamental rules of emotionalisation:

- Literary texts evoke compassion if those figures who suffer from an illness are represented in a sympathetic light.
- Literary texts evoke satisfaction if those figures who suffer from an illness are represented in an unsympathetic light
- Literary texts evoke indignation alongside compassion if those figures who suffer from an illness are represented in a sympathetic light and if those figures represented in an unsympathetic light seem to be responsible for the illness.

If one analyses techniques of literary emotionalisation and uses regularly concepts such as 'sympathetic' and 'unsympathetic light', then one needs additional concepts to explain literary techniques of regulating sympathy and antipathy. But going into detail on this point would go too far in the context of this paper.

Works of Literary Modernism on infectious diseases – such as the novels of Thomas Mann and Ivan Goll – deal with such rules in a much more subtle way than the discourses on illness within the movement of Anti-Modernism which focus on cultural criticism. In Goll's novel, an elite of artists and intellectuals meets in the 'Bar de la Mort.' The first person narrator thinks that the Eurococcus has had an especially negative effect upon these people. And he reflects: "Who knows, perhaps the bacillus was introduced by this elite!" [Und wer weiß, ob nicht von dieser Elite der Bazillus eingeschleppt worden war!] (Goll 1988, 114). This description definitely comes close to Max Nordau's verdict of 'degeneration.' Yet the spokesman in this milieu is not a detested adversary figure but rather a friend of the first person narrator. Infectious diseases are certainly also characterised as something threatening in the descriptions of Literary Modernism. However, time and again these descriptions also refer to certain benefits that come from disease; thus, they evoke substantial emotional ambivalence among their adressees.

One of the most sympathetic figures in the novel *Death in Venice* is, by the way, a young Englishman. At a travel agency, he tells the protagonist "in his straightforward comfortable language" (Mann 1990, 256) the truth about cholera that has been kept secret and denied by the Italian public authorities. Yet Aschenbach does not act on the Englishman's advice:

His thoughts dwelt upon

> [t]he image of the stricken disordered city, hovering wildly before his mind's eye, inflamed him with hopes that were beyond comprehension, beyond reason and full of monstrous sweetness. [...] What could art and virtue mean to him now, when he might reap the advantages of chaos? He said nothing, and stayed on. (*ibid.*, 259)

I cannot discuss here how we, as readers of that particular passage, react emotionally to Aschenbach's emotional state or how we are meant to react following the text's intentions; this would be the subject for another essay.

I would like to thank the translation company of Dagmar Förtsch in Glasgow, Martina King and Sheila Dickson for translating this essay which was originally written in German. They have also translated the quotes taken from the German publications. I would also like to thank Stefan Jäger and Vera Zimmermann (Marburg) for locating published translations of the German texts quoted and Thomas Rütten for further editorial assistance.

References

Alewyn, Richard: "Die literarische Angst." *Aspekte der Angst. Starnberger Gespräch 1964*. Ed. Hoimar von Ditfurth. Stuttgart: Thieme, 1965. 24–37.

Braunberger, Gerald: "Wachsende Ansteckungsgefahr an den Märkten". *Frankfurter Allgemeine Zeitung* (19.7.2011): 17.

Braunberger, Gerald: "Ansteckungsgefahr" (commentary). *Frankfurter Allgemeine Zeitung* (19.7.2011): 9.

Glauert-Hesse, Barbara: "Nachwort". Iwan Goll: *Die Eurokokke*. Ed. Barbara Glauert-Hesse. Mit neun Zeichnungen von Georges Annenkoff. Faksimile der im Martin Wasservogel Verlag, Berlin 1927, erschienenen Erstausgabe. Göttingen: Wallstein, 2002. 159–176.

Goll, Yvan. *Die Eurokokke*. Roman. Ed. Barbara Glauert-Hesse. Mit neun Zeichnungen von Georges Annenkoff und einem Nachwort von Joachim Sartorius. Berlin: Argon, 1988.

Hitler, Adolf. *Mein Kampf*. New York, NY: Reynal and Hitchcock, 1941.

Hülshoff, Thomas. *Emotionen. Eine Einführung für beratende, therapeutische, pädagogische und soziale Berufe.* Munich: Reinhardt, 1999.
Lausberg, Heinrich. *Handbuch der literarischen Rhetorik. Eine Grundlegung der Literaturwissenschaft.* 3rd ed. Stuttgart: Steiner, 1990.
Mann, Thomas. "A Weary Hour." *Stories of Three Decades.* Transl. from the German by H.T. Lowe-Porter. London: Martin Secker & Warburg Ltd., 1936a. 290–296.
Mann, Thomas. *Death in Venice and Other Stories.* Transl. and with an introduction by David Luke. London: Martin Secker & Warburg Ltd., 1990.
Mann, Thomas. *Notizbücher. Edition in zwei Bänden.* Ed. Hans Wysling. Vol. 2. Frankfurt a. M., 1992.
Mayer, Ruth, and Brigitte Weingart. "Viren zirkulieren. Eine Einführung." *VIRUS! Mutationen einer Metapher.* Ed. Ruth Mayer. Bielefeld: Transcript, 2004. 7–42.
Musil, Robert. "Fallengelassenes Vorwort zu Nachlaß bei Lebzeiten". *Gesammelte Werke.* Ed. Adolf Frisé. 9 Vols. Vol. 8. Reinbek: Rowohlt, 1978.
Nordau, Max. *Degeneration.* Transl. from the Second Edition of the German Work. New York, NY: D. Appleton and Company, 1895.
Pilgram, Jutta: "Ueberrraschung auf allen Kanälen". *Süddeutsche Zeitung* (insert ‚Beruf und Karriere') (6.–7.8.2011): 9.
Sarasin, Philipp, Silvia Berger, Marianne Hänseler, and Miriam Spörri. "Bakteriologie und Moderne". *Bakteriologie und Moderne. Studien zur Biopolitik des Unsichtbaren. 1870–1920.* Eds Philipp Sarasin, Silvia Berger, Marianne Hänseler, and Miriam Spörri. Frankfurt a. M.: Suhrkamp, 2007. 8–43.
Schonlau, Anja. *Syphilis in der Literatur. Über Ästhetik, Moral, Genie und Medizin (1880–2000).* Würzburg: Königshausen & Neumann, 2005.
Sontag, Susan. *Illness as metaphor* and *AIDS and its Metaphors.* New York, NY: Doubleday, 1990.
Tomes, Nancy. "Epidemic Entertainments: Disease and Popular Culture in Early-Twentieth-Century America." *American Literary History* 14.4 (2002): 625–652.
Treichler, Paula A. "AIDS, homophobia, and biomedical disourse: An epidemic of signification". *Cultural Studies* 1.3 (1987): 263–305.
Voss, Christiane. *Narrative Emotionen. Eine Untersuchung über Möglichkeiten und Grenzen philosophischer Emotionstheorien.* Berlin, New York, NY: de Gruyter, 2004.
Weingart, Brigitte. *Ansteckende Wörter. Repräsentationen von AIDS.* Frankfurt a. M.: Suhrkamp, 2002.
Zweig, Stefan. "Sigmund Freud – Zu seinem siebzigsten Geburtstage." *Über Sigmund Freud. Porträt. Briefwechsel. Gedenkworte.* Frankfurt a. M.: Fischer, 1994. 231–237.

Martina King

Anarchist and Aphrodite: On the Literary History of Germs[1]

1 Introduction – The Ambiguity of Germs

In the summer of 2011, Germany was attacked by a health hazard which was as unexpected as it was serious: the EHEC-bacteria epidemic. These microbes caused bloody diarrhoea, kidney failure, neurological impairment and death. But the EHEC bacilli not only led to panic among the public and disquiet amongst medical officials; they also became media stars – all major print and digital media offered daily EHEC entertainment with the features of a well-written crime story. The internet news magazine *t-online* reported on the "deadly strategy of the EHEC germs" [tödliche Strategie der EHEC-Keime] (http://nachrichten.t-online.de/forscher-entlarven-toedliche-strategie-der-ehec-keime/id_47063024/index), the *Süddeutsche Zeitung* on the bacteria "setting out on their deadly journey through Germany and Europe" [ihre todbringende Reise durch Deutschland und Europa antreten] and on "the world hunting for a phantom" [die Welt jagt ein Phantom] (www.sueddeutsche.de/wissen/ehec-erreger-die-jagd-auf-ein-phantom-1.1105849en.wikipedia.org/wiki/Totally_Gross_Germs,6.6.). And, apparently, germ horror is set to entertain media consumers every summer: "killer germs spread in the Baltic Sea" [Killer-Keime breiten sich in der Ostsee aus], *t-online* announced in July 2012 (http://nachrichten.t-online.de/killer-keime-breiten-sich-in-der-ostsee-aus/id_58117580/index).

So far so unsurprising – "Epidemic Entertainment" has been a long-standing tradition since the so-called 'golden age of bacteriology', well described by historian Nancy Tomes (Tomes 2002). Against this background, the bio-political rhetoric used by leading media seems rather familiar. Bacteria appear as sinister anthropomorphic creatures; as killers, foreign invaders, phantoms, whose clandestine strategy is fought tooth and claw by mankind. These tropes remind us of the metaphors of military interaction and invasion common in scientific and popular discourses after 1880 (see below). Cultural memory has preserved these metaphors, and perpetuated their wide currency.

1 My thanks to Samuel Cohn, Sheila Dickson, Richard King and Thomas Rütten for suggestions with English formulations.

But there is more to the recent EHEC media hype than just the familiar battle between mankind and microbe. There also seems to be an iconography of the beautiful germ. The pictures that accompany stories about anthropomorphic microbes on the attack are produced with a great deal of technical effort and focus on the sensual, aesthetic qualities of germs – representing them in soft organic, three-dimensional shapes, in an attractive contrast of colours, mostly green and pink, with a dramaturgy of brightness and shade. Clearly, there is a certain ambivalence: bacteria are represented as dangerous and beautiful, as killers and as aesthetic objects (http://www.physiowissen.de/thema-artikel4265-Klartext__EHEC___alle_Fakten.html).

This ambivalence has been touched upon by Olaf Briese, who claims that bacteria became "universal carriers of meaning" [universelle Bedeutungsträger] during the Koch era (Briese 2003, 385). It has furthermore been noted that Koch's microphotography of germs already follows certain aesthetic criteria; this tendency to aestheticise the bacterial microcosm becomes ever more evident during the development of microphotography in the 20th century (Stahl, Derenthal 2010, 25–30). Yet there has been no detailed historical reconstruction of this ambivalence of microbes, of their diverse iconic and metaphorical qualities. The question whether bacteria's polysemic significance is also rooted in the so-called 'golden age of bacteriology' remains unanswered so far. The historiography of bacteriology, dealing mostly with this period – the years between 1880 and 1900 in Germany and France – has hitherto focussed on the militaristic language of war, aggression and invasion that was common within scientific discourse and in popular media (Berger 2009; Sarasin et al. 2007; Sarasin 2004; Mendelsohn 1996; Gradmann 2000; Gradmann 1994) and seems generally centred on negative notions of contagionism, in particular on the infectious transmission of physical and moral corruption.

Scholars have revealed the intriguing connections between bacteriology and the politics of imperialism with respect to propagandistic language and practical action. Koch was widely supported by the Bismarck regime since his aetiological doctrine allowed for authoritarian state interventions and restrictions of free international trade, e.g. hampering British sea trade at the Suez Canal (Ogawa 2007). Against this background, the emerging scientific and popular discourse on microbes was profoundly affected by the imperialist climate in pre-war Germany. In order to make the abstract, minuscule object 'bacterium', which was inaccessible to sensual perception, accessible, anthropomorphism was widely used; the following terms came from the semantic repertoire of the militaristic, colonial state: "hostile intruder" [feindliche Eindringlinge], "immigration" [Einwanderung], "invasion" [Invasion], "battle" [Kampf], "extermination" [Vernichtung], "weapons" [Waffen], "the offensive" [Offensive] (Hänseler 2009, 119–145). Early medical bacteriology was obsessed with microbes, and therefore paid very limited attention to the host and its individual physical response (Gradmann 2005, 90–103). Bacteria were considered as necessary and sufficient cause for any infectious disease and therefore simplistically identified with the process of disease itself, and also with their carriers. The latter simplification proved to be a short circuit with long-term metaphorical and ethical implications: The equation 'bacteria are like their carriers' reached the level of a reciprocal normative identification of germs with political enemies or stigmatised human beings (Weindling 2007; Gradmann 2007, 344–346). The reactionary German philosopher Paul de Lagarde compared Jews with parasites in his infamous polemic *Juden und Indogermanen* [Jews and Indogermans] (1887) and recommended

> squashing this vermin. One does not debate with the trichina or the bacillus, one does not educate the trichina or the bacillus, one exterminates them as quickly as possible" [dieses Ungeziefer zu zertreten. Mit Trichinen und Bazillen wird nicht verhandelt, Trichinen und Bazillen werden auch nicht erzogen, sie werden so rasch und so gründlich wie möglich vernichtet]. (Bein 1965, 144)[2]

To sum up, scholarly work on the 'politics of bacteriology' has made it evident that the longstanding stereotype of the evil, menacing, invading, anthropomorphic germ in the 20th and 21st centuries originates around 1900.

But what about the other side, the visual beauty and narrative attractiveness that is apparently equally part of the cultural memory of microbes? Indeed, the career of microbe metaphors in the intellectual history of the 20th century is certainly not restricted to Koch's "enemies of mankind" [Feinden des Menschengeschlechts] (Koch 1912a [1890], 660), that is, to notions of contagionism, invasion, corruption and otherness, as could be assumed from previous scholarship (Sarasin et al. 2007). On the contrary, microbes were already circulating in various academic, popular and literary contexts around 1900 as ambivalent, even paradoxical objects of cultural knowledge between beauty, horror, wit and spirituality. This contribution to the debate will show that bacteria were perceived and constructed during the heyday of bacteriology both as bad, infectious threats and aesthetic, beautiful creatures, both as dangerous killers and our ancestors, both as alien and familiar, both as demonic and sacred. Sometimes their central connotation was one of evil contagion, sometimes they lost this entirely.

Encoding a variety of meanings, the living microbe reflects the paradoxes of modernism itself and likewise contributes to its paradoxical signature; it becomes, as will be argued, a collective symbol in the sense of Jürgen Link's dis-

---

2 On the links between German racism, extermination, bacteriological practice and language, as evidenced for example by the anti-typhus campaign in World War I, the practice of delousing and the identification of Jews with parasites, see Weindling 2000; 2007.

course theory (Link 1984, 1988, 1990). As an inter-discursive bridge between seemingly divergent cultural spaces it links together specialised discourses such as those of natural science, literature, art, philosophical scepticism and spirituality. It will be shown that these ambiguous metaphorical qualities of living microbes emerged within the field of medico-biological science, but that, however, popular scientific writings and especially literary texts played a crucial role in transforming Robert Koch's "enemies of mankind" into complex tropes which contributed to the intellectual history of Modernism.

2 Representation and Objectivity

The epistemological background for the striking ambiguity of microbes can be assumed as being the problem of 'mechanical objectivity.' The question how to represent scientific things in an objective manner, independent of the investigator and his subjective perception, judgement and interpretation became pressing from the mid-19th century onwards (Daston 2007, 115–190). In some respects, it culminated in the microscopic world and particularly in living microbes, which became more and more accessible after 1870. But what kind of accessibility was this, how did germs become working objects for scientists?[3] Microbes became scientific objects only through a series of sophisticated representational technologies, they underwent several media changes: pure culture, staining with Aniline pigments, examination under the microscope, microphotography, drawing, linguistic description (Schlich 1997; Sarasin 2004, 254–256). Thus the celebrated 'mechanical objectivity' of bacteria, achieved with advanced optical instruments and laboratory technologies, seems to be Janus-faced: the more the human subject disappears in the process of representation, the less one knows what kind of microscopic structures are actually displayed – living microbes, cells, staining artifacts (Daston 2007, 164–166)? The problem was already thorny in the heyday of early bacteriology. Koch, for example, complained that bodily fluids, as soon as they become stained with Aniline colours,

3 Bruno Latour has pushed the constructivist perspective on germs to the point of asking the provocative question "where were microbes before Pasteur?" (Latour 1999, 145). I think one does not necessarily have to go that far. It is certainly justified to distinguish epistemology and ontology here and to ascribe ontological reality to germs by taking epidemiological proof for current and historical disease causation into consideration, e.g. current standard microbiological diagnostics, epidemiological statistics or ancient DNA studies. One can assume that bacteria do cause disease and have historically done so, whether they have been identified or not.

> produce equally coloured precipitates which simulate bacteria by their granule-like or thread-like shape or which conceal existing bacteria by their voluminous mass. [Niederschläge geben, die ebenfalls gefärbt sind und entweder durch körnchen- oder fadenartige Gestaltung Bakterien vortäuschen oder durch ihre voluminösen Massen die vorhandenen Bakterien verdecken können.] (Koch 1912b [1881], 114)

Science was striving for the epistemological virtue of objectivity, yet the objectivity of its fanciest new topic, living bacteria, was apparently more than questionable. While Koch complained that pigments conceal bacteria, Koch's temporary competitor, Rudolf Virchow, who saw his own reputation and that of cellular pathology endangered by bacteriology, criticized the opposite in his essay *Der Kampf der Zellen und der Bakterien* [The Fight of Cells and of Bacteria]: the staining of bacteria conceals cells, makes them invisible. What Koch saw as objective truth is considered a flawed image of reality by Virchow (Virchow 1885). One can see that questions about the actuality and objectivity of microbes must remain unsolved, since the representational techniques of bacteriology seem to give only biased, selective images of the microcosm.

And this debate about the objectivity of invisible living germs reached beyond the restricted space of laboratory science, due to its general attractiveness for modernist ideas on perception, deception and contingency. Gerhart Hauptmann for example, former advocate of Zolaism, tells the story of a failed bacteriologist in his late novel *Atlantis*, who "instead of the anthrax bacillus, investigated [...] and described fibres in the staining pigment" [der statt des Milzbranderregers Fäserchen im Farbstoff untersucht und (...) beschrieben hat] (Hauptmann 1912, 420 f.). The flawed bacteriologist who struggles with the deceptive reality of germs becomes a symbol of Modernism in Hauptmann's narrative – his path becoming incoherent and leading paradigmatically from science to scepticism, poetry and erotic adventures.

In summary, we see that the series of representational techniques in the bacteriological laboratory leaves room for ambiguity and interpretation, accounts for contingency and invites literary adaptation. Contingency increases even more if one takes changes of medium into consideration. Pictures of germs require written comment; otherwise they remain abstract and incomprehensible. Thus germs are transformed from iconic – photographic or graphic – objects to linguistic objects and this process of conversion needs metaphorical tools: respectively anthropomorphisms or zoomorphisms. Germs – as opposed to geometrical viruses – do have round or curved organic shapes, their own metabolism, and sometimes even the capacity to move themselves; thus they inevitably trigger anthropomorphisms or zoomorphisms since they appeal to contemporaries as fascinating minuscule analogies to the macroscopic world of living beings.[4]

3 Microbes as Objects of Art Nouveau

Given these steps of representation, interpretation and increasing contingency, it is not surprising that the descriptive language for bacteria is diverse and differs widely according to the scientific field in question. If one looks for example at botany and medical bacteriology, which both draw upon microbes at almost the same point in time,[5] it seems that bacteria become different working objects for two divergent laboratory disciplines.[6] Marianne Hänseler has shown that Koch himself, in his early writings, refers to the ornamental language of botany but later on turns to the military rhetoric of the imperial power state (Hänseler 2009, 124–129). He then prefers the anthropomorphic talk of 'enemies', writing about being "at war with the smallest but most dangerous enemies of mankind" [im Kriege gegen die kleinsten, aber gefährlichsten Feinde des Menschengeschlechts], and "the microscopic and yet hitherto supremely powerful enemy within the human body" [des mikroskopischen, aber bis dahin übermächtigen Feindes im menschlichen Körper] (Koch 1912a [1890], 660). In botany however,

4 Interestingly, viruses do not only inherit the metaphorical qualities of bacteria as regards to positive or negative contagion, epidemic spread, etc. as pointed out by Thomas Anz in this volume. According to Brigitte Weingart (Weingart 1999, 214), viruses also become anthropomorphic hostile figures in popular scientific language of the 20th century, and the militaristic metaphors of classical bacteriology, such as 'killer', 'invasion', 'defence', reappear, e.g. in a popular book with the title *Viren. Die unsichtbaren Killer* [Viruses. The invisible Killers] (Willen 1995). Yet viruses are barely anything more than DNA/RNA without their own metabolism, on the threshold between live and inanimate nature; they just change the genetic programme of their host cell. Therefore, an additional semantic field is attached to the virus within postmodernist aesthetic and media theory and within science itself, covering concepts such as 'carriers of information', 'code', 'programmes of transcripition' or 'decoding', 'computer language', 'media' (Brandt 2004, Weingart 1999, 2003, Mayer/Weingart 2004). Given their rather formal than vital constitution, they seem to trigger a remarkably broad and vague set of functional analogies – communication, liminality, deconstruction etc.

5 Ferdinand Cohn started to work on bacteria in the late 1860s whereas Koch did so not earlier than 1873. Yet Cohn went on with his classificatory project during the 'golden years' of monocausal medical bacteriology in the 1880s.

6 Christoph Gradmann speaks of the heterogenous roots of medical bacteriology which give room for immanent contradictions and external competitions. See Gradmann 2005. This heterogeneity fits with the heterogenous narrative transformations of bacteriology's spectacular working object: the bacterium.

microbes appear as beautiful, ornamental zoomorphic creatures. The eminent botanist Ferdinand Cohn, one of Koch's teachers, uses an entirely different set of metaphors in his textbook *Über Bakterien, die kleinsten lebenden Wesen* [On Bacteria, the Smallest Living Beings]. It was firstly published in 1872 and was regarded as a programmatic text of early bacteriology:

> Most of the bacteria show extraordinarily vivid movements; and if they fill the drop of water in dense swarms, then the criss-crossing rods and spirals present a surprisingly exciting sight, comparable to a swarm of mosquitoes or an anthill. [...] they drift by in curving lines, sometimes slowly quivering and jiggling, sometimes shooting forwards with a sudden jump like a rocket, sometimes twisting across like a spinner [...]. The elongated filamentous bacteria bend their bodies while swimming, sometimes clumsily, sometimes swiftly and with agility, as if they were struggling to find their path through obstacles like a fish seeking its way through water plants. [Die meisten Bakterien zeigen ausserordentlich lebhafte Bewegungen; und wenn sie in dichtem Gewimmel den Wassertropfen füllen, bieten die nach allen Richtungen durch einander fahrenden Stäbchen und Schrauben einen überraschend fesselnden Anblick, den man mit einem Mückenschwarm oder einem Ameisenhaufen vergleichen kann. (...) sie ziehen in Bogenlinien dahin, bald langsam zitternd und wackelnd, jetzt in plötzlichem Sprunge raketenartig fortschiessend, bald der Quere nach gedreht wie ein Kreisel (...) Die längeren Fadenbakterien biegen ihren Körper beim Schwimmen, bald schwerfällig, bald rasch und gewandt, als bemühten sie sich, durch Hindernisse ihre Bahn zu finden, wie ein Fisch, der zwischen Wasserpflanzen seinen Weg sucht.] (Cohn 1889, 6)

Cohn was the first to classify bacteria systematically and claim that their distinct species are stable and consistent. His criteria were morphologic qualities such as 'spherical,' 'rod-like,' 'thread-like' or 'spiral' (Gradmann 2005, 60). Therefore it is hardly surprising that he did not focus on the central medical aspect, on the transmission of infectious disease that was already being debated in 1872, but on forms and shapes instead. However, his emphasis on fascinating beautiful motion, on the drifting in curved lines, the spinning twist, the swift and agile swimming is striking. As a matter of fact, few known bacteria actually propel themselves, but Cohn was a scientific storyteller and the abundance of zoomorphic metaphors and comparisons, even assonances, make this text clearly poetical. In the next passage, he describes "wave-like vibrios and corkscrew-like spirilli which turn rapidly around their own axis" [wellenförmige Vibrionen and schraubenförmige Spirillen (die) sich rasch um ihre Achse drehen] (Cohn 1889, 6). They seem as if they would "wriggle like an eel" [sich aalgleich schlängeln] or "jolt backwards and forwards like a meteor" [(...) zucken (...) meteorartig hin und her]. According to Cohn, bacteria quiver, "roll" [rollen], "move together in a circle" [bewegen sich mit den anderen im Kreise] and "glide slowly through the water" [schrauben sich langsam durch das Wasser] (*ibid.*, 6). All these remarkably visual images are very successful in turning the abstract object 'bacillus' into something concrete. But there is more to Cohn's account of microbe motion than just visualisation. It shows how germs are aestheticized, how they become objects of literature and art. With the wave-like vibrios, screw-like spirilli and their circular movements, bacteria are represented as decorative, beautiful, like the floral ornaments or floral female bodies in art-nouveau sceneries. Interestingly enough, a popular bacteriological textbook for housewives and servants with the title *Die Bakteriologie des täglichen Lebens* [The Bacteriology of Everyday Life] presents microbes not only as loathsome dangerous objects. In this book, the loathsome dangerous objects are also adorned – paradoxically – with bacterial beauty; that is, with art nouveau vignettes of bacilli garlands:

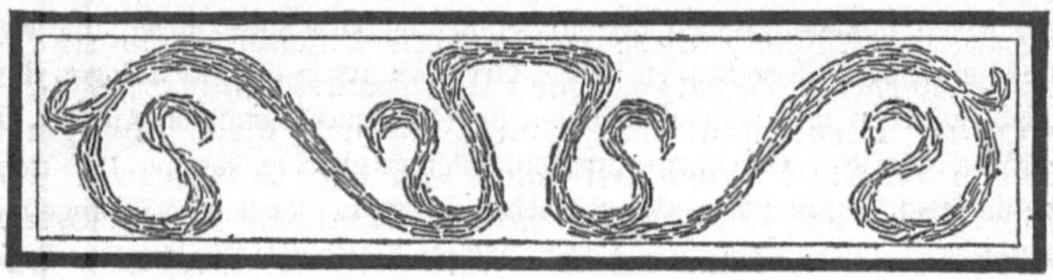

Fig. 2: Bacilli Vignettes from popular book *Die Bakteriologie des täglichen Lebens* (Jäger 1909, 302).

These ornaments clearly reference the art-nouveau floral and animal vignettes in popular scientific books such as Wilhelm Bölsche's famous work *Das Liebesleben in der Natur* [The Love Life in Nature] (1898/1901 [1906]) which was illustrated by art-nouveau artist Wilhelm Müller-Schönefeldt, and of course they cite Ernst Haeckel's paradigmatic book *Kunstformen der Natur* [Art Forms in Nature] (1998 [1904]). Only, the garlands of tendrils, leaves and blossoms, and Haeckel's symmetric arrangements of radiolares and medusae, are replaced by rod-shaped bacteria – which seem no less suitable for art-nouveau iconography.

And this is not the only aspect of convergence with art nouveau. The conception of vital, ornamental bodies and ornamental movement apparently applies to bacteria as well as to the contemporary discourse of free dance. Cohn's elastic bacterial gliding, drifting, spinning and body-bending sounds like a prelude to the movement of free-dance, represented by artists such as Loïe Fuller and Isadora Duncan. Both consider their performative art strictly naturalist: *The Serpentine Dance* (1891), the most famous choreography of Fuller, who regarded herself as embodiment of the art nouveau movement, is inspired by the ornamental movements of a snake and she compares it in her autobiography with a butterfly and an orchid (Fuller 1913, 31). Duncan, who admired Fuller greatly, likewise uses floral metaphors, describing an innovative programme as a "love movement, from the unfolding of which, like the petals of a flower, the dancer would stream as a perfume" (Duncan 1995 [1927], 59). The bending, gliding bacterial bodies of botany and the bending, gliding bodies of naturalist dancers Fuller and Duncan show how popular science and art shared the same obsession for exotic, spectacular, aesthetic subjects. 'Dancing microbes' seem to fulfil these purposes as they are exotic and spectacular, yet vital things. Given this neo-romantic proximity of art and nature, of artistic and organic movement, it is not surprising that Isadora Duncan came to know and admire Ernst Haeckel, the key figure of art-nouveau biology, who, conversely, interpreted Duncan's dance, so she says, as "an expression of monism, in that it came from one source and had one direction of evolution" (*ibid.*, 113 f.). 'Monism' meant for Haeckel the neo-pantheist unity of matter and spirit, nature and art, and above all of all living beings. The naturalist movement of artist Isadora fitted in with this complex belief system just as well as the artistic appearance of self-moving invisible natural beings – the kingdom of 'moners', with its most flamboyant exponents, bacteria. In his well-known work *Anthropogenie* [The Evolution of Man], Haeckel writes:

> The smallest of all moners are the famous bacteria (*bacillus*, *vibrio* etc.), the dreaded agents of many of the most dangerous diseases. These minuscule spherical or rod-like moners move by rotating, probably by means of a swinging flagellum; they proliferate very rapidly through division. [Die kleinsten von allen Moneren sind die berühmten Bacterien (Bacillus, vibrio u.s.w.), die gefürchteten Erreger von vielen der gefährlichsten Krankheiten. Diese winzigen kugeligen oder stäbchenförmigen Moneren bewegen sich rotirend (wahrscheinlich mittelst einer schwingenden Geißel) und vermehren sich sehr rasch durch Quertheilung.] (Haeckel 1891, 483)

This quotation highlights the beginnings of the ambiguity of bacteria and how they served Haeckel's aims as a propagandist of scientific culture: they are invisible and dangerous, famous and dreaded, killers and beautiful self-movers. Haeckel's "rotating motion, probably by means of a swinging flagellum" is particularly remarkable; as remarkable as Cohn's bending bacilli bodies. Non-medical biologists influenced by monism seem to be as obsessed with harmonious motion and versatile harmony as the free dancers who regarded themselves as plant- or animal-like; they all participate in the same hybrid project in which arts, storytelling, natural science and spirituality are united. This desire for unity, totality and wholeness can be taken as a regressive answer to the paradigms of cultural Modernism – differentiation, particularisation and scientific abstraction – which seem to cause the world to disintegrate into incomprehensible fragments.

The microbe writes intellectual history here, as it suits this synthetic project perfectly. It forms a link between the exoticism of free dance and art nouveau, philosophical neo-vitalism, and the gospel of evolution. Haeckel in particular is obsessed with the decorative flail, the flagella, which is part of the art-nouveau cosmos of ornamental flowers and animals – from Beardsley to Müller-Schönefeldt and to Haeckel's own *Art Forms of Nature*.[7] There, and also in his book *Natürliche Schöpfungsgeschichte* [The History of Creation] he depicts the species *flagellate*, which he translates as "flagellated swarmers" [Geißelschwärmer] (Haeckel 1904, plate 13; Haeckel 1902, 439). With the flail, Haeckel can show that even the most primitive beings such as bacteria are self-movers and therefore must have perception, feelings and soul (Haeckel 2009 [1918], 150 – 153). Given this status of the flail as core argument within neo-vitalism, we must not wonder that it appears with remarkable redundancy in Haeckel's work. He does not only speak about microbes which "move by means of a swinging flail". In another publication, he mentions "prehistoric plantlets whose shell of panelled cellulose adopt the most peculiar forms, move by means of a swinging flail" [Die Urpflänzchen, deren getäfelte Celluloseschale die seltsamsten Formen annimmt, bewegen sich mittelst einer schwingenden Geißel] (Haeckel 1901, 18); and in his famous work *The Riddle of the Universe* [Die Welträtsel] (1899) we learn that the "minute spermatozoa [...] are ciliated cells and swim about as freely in the sperm by means of their lashes or *cilia*, as the ordinary ciliated infusoria (the flagellata)" (Haeckel 1934 [1899], 111). The published translation "lashes or cilia" is flawed here insofar as it conceals the repetition of the phrase 'by means of a swinging flail'. The German original says that "[...] die sehr kleinen Samenkörperchen oder Spermien [...] sind Geißelzellen und bewegen sich mittelst ihrer schwingenden Geißel ebenso lebhaft schwimmend im Sperma umher wie die gewöhnlichen Geißelinfusorien (Flagellaten)" (Haeckel 2009 [1899], 179).

The flail as topic of biological art-nouveau apparently transforms minuscule living beings into serpentine dancers like Loïe Fuller. Correspondingly, the previously cited textbook *The Bacteriology of Everyday Life* also stylizes the flagellum into an art-nouveau ornament that has nothing to do with real microbial flagellas (Jäger 1910, 254).

To sum up: the invisible microbe, embodiment of scientific progress and specialisation, turns out equally to be a remedy against the horrors of scientification and specialisation. Notions of artistic beauty, theatrical self-motion and natural harmony amalgamate with the basic notion of scientific progress. Thus the microbe serves as an interdiscursive symbol for the pre-rational unity of science,

7 How relevant for Haeckel's art-nouveau cosmos flail-like organs for locomotion are becomes evident if one looks at the quite extraordinary jellyfish *desmonema annasethe* in table 8 (p. 88) in *Art Forms of Nature*.

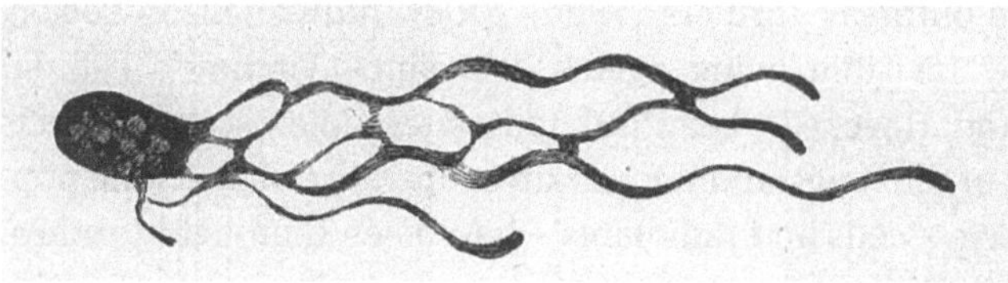

Fig. 3: Flagellated Bacillus from popular book *Die Bakteriologie des täglichen Lebens* (Jäger, 1909, 254).

art and natural philosophy; it represents an artistic counterworld of unbroken wholeness and totality. Later examples will demonstrate that microbe metaphors explicitly convey that criticism of culture, rationality and progress that was so typical for modernist intellectuals.

But first, we have to consider the genre in which these aestheticist connotations were attached to bacteria. With Cohn's and Haeckel's account, we can actually see how microbial entertainment, a popular mass spectacle for the educated public, came about. The authors were both eminent biologists who held chairs at Breslau and Jena, respectively. But, by contrast with Koch's rather dry, academic tone, both their styles are clearly popular; studies such as Cohn's *On Bacteria* and Haeckel's *Anthropogenie* represent a hybrid genre consisting of cutting-edge scientific contents and highly emotionalised language. Using a variety of poetic metaphors and rhetorical figures and transforming germ theory into thrilling narratives, they show how blurred the boundaries between science and popular storytelling were in the heyday of the laboratory revolution. They also show that bacteriology had a lot to offer for this new, partly-fictional genre of scientific storytelling. In *On Bacteria*, Cohn writes:

> In size, the smallest bacteria stand to human beings as a grain of sand does to Montblanc. [...] Our interest in bacteria increases in the light of the realisation that it is these most minute of creatures that are the most important, that they control with invisible yet irresistible power the most important processes in live and inanimate nature, that they even intervene in the existence of mankind in a mysterious and fateful way. [Die kleinsten Bakterien verhalten sich ihrer Grösse nach zum Menschen, etwa wie ein Sandkorn zum Montblanc. (...) (Es) steigert sich unser Interesse an denselben durch die Erkenntnis, dass gerade diese kleinsten Wesen von der allergrössten Bedeutung sind, dass sie mit unsichtbarer doch unwiderstehlicher Gewalt die wichtigsten Vorgänge der lebendigen und leblosen Natur beherrschen und selbst in das Dasein des Menschen zugleich geheimnis- und verhängnisvoll eingreifen]. (Cohn 1889, 4)

This language of extreme spacial contrasts makes use of the fascination of bourgeois society for microscopic worlds; it provokes not only fear and disgust but the irresistible mix of horror and curiosity that still provides high audience ratings for current disease-outbreak thrillers (Wald, 2008). Industrialized society has been fascinated by invisible living agents ever since Virchow's cellular state (Johach, 2008) and Haeckel's beautiful radiolares. Microscopic objects and metaphors are part of the longstanding narrative repertoire of scientific popularisers, and both objects – cells and radiolares – have been thoroughly anthropomorphised. Yet the mysterious bacteria show even more superior narrative qualities: they are decorative, autonomous, and, above all, self-moving, in contrast to the localized group-dependent and boringly round-shaped cells in Virchow's cellular state. They can thus be linked to contemporary neo-vitalism and to floral art nouveau. And in contrast to Haeckel's self-moving, decorative, but harmless radiolares with their swinging flagellum, they are dangerous killers with a swinging flagellum. They therefore also supply the thrill of a good detective story, and the ambivalence that is so significant for the whole epoch.

4 Aggression, Beauty and Cuteness: Ambiguous Microbe Narratives 1900–2000

Invisibility, beautiful self-motion and mysterious danger: these three core qualities attributed to microbes become ever more pronounced in the works of another key figure in German scientific storytelling, Wilhelm Bölsche. Being an autodidactic zoologist, an admirer of Darwin and Haeckel, a proponent of monist philosophy and a member of the famous *Friedrichshagener Dichterkreis* [Friedrichshagen Circle of Poets], Bölsche, more than anybody else, represents the interface between biology, literature, art and spirituality. His books transform Darwin's evolutionary theory into a hybrid mixture of fiction and natural philosophy; and he seems to be pretty knowledgeable about the entertaining qualities of bacteria as well, taking their ambiguity even further. In his work *Vom Bazillus zum Affenmenschen* [From the Bacillus to the Ape-Man], he refers in the traditional way to Koch's political and militaristic language: The bacillus appears as an "extreme individualist and anarchist" [extremer Individualist und Anarchist], bacilli are the "most consequent enemies of the state" [konsequenteste Staatsfeinde]. They attack the body with "mass invasion" [Masseninvasion] and "cannon of bacterial poison from an eternal ambush" [aus einem ewigen Hinterhalt die Kanonade mit Bazillengift] (Bölsche 1903 [1900], 5, 9, 38, 34). The bacillus as anthropomorphic yet alien invader is a well-known formula at the time. In the context of Bölsche's work, this formula reflects a rather aggressive type of social Darwinism common within popular anthropology and biology at the end of the century. It should be mentioned that Bölsche became a member of the *Deutsche Gesellschaft für Rassenhygiene* [German Society for Racial Hygiene] from 1905 onwards.

However, the invading enemy of the state and contagious anarchist is only one side of Bölsche's magic box of microbial images. At the same time as reproducing biopolitical stereotypes of early bacteriology, he emphasizes the issue of microbial harmony and decorative motion in another book, his previously mentioned text *Das Liebesleben in der Natur* [The Love Life in Nature], which is currently regarded as an exemplary work of German *fin de siècle* literature. Using numerous fictional elements, Bölsche contemplates among other things about cute microbial life on the prehistoric Cambrian beach; about "the damp primordial air where bacilli were swarming, or the primordial waters where they were wiggling, or the beach of primordial ooze where they were crawling" [die feuchte Urluft, in der die Bazillen schwärmten, – oder das Urwasser, in dem sie sich schlängelten, oder der Urschlammstrand, wo sie krochen] (Bölsche 1906 [1898], 99). The enemy of mankind with its cannon on the one hand, the swarming and wriggling movements of flailed minute dancers on the other – the scientific storyteller Bölsche apparently has no qualms about attributing to bacteria a kaleidoscope of meanings that has emerged from botany and medical bacteriology. In so doing he increasingly transforms them from scientific objects into objects of language and literature. For Bölsche then, bacteria serve not only as examples for decorative movement or evil contagionism; they are ideal candidates to enrich a hybrid genre that was very much in vogue among popularisers of science: the scientific fairy tale. Being minute, invisible, mysterious and traditionally anthropomorphic, they fulfil the criteria of liminal figures in a fairy cosmos, – figures such as dwarfs or trolls – , and further grotesque qualities can be attached to them. In a section about cell division which Bölsche explicitly entitles "a fairy tale" [ein Märchen] (*ibid.*, 130), microbes are depicted as "a clan of jolly little dwarfs" [ein Geschlecht lustiger kleiner Zwerge] (*ibid.*). They appear as "tiny dwarfs" [Zwergzwerglein] and "diminished rumplestiltskin" [Dezimierungsrumpelchen] (*ibid.*, 132, 133] who wear "pointed caps" [spitze Mützen] or as "grumpy hermits, who go fishing and hunting to their heart's content and, given the chance, will eat their belly full" [knurrige Einsiedler, (sie) jagten und fischten nach Herzenslust und assen sich bei guter Gelegenheit recht einen Ranzen an] (*ibid.*, 131).

The military language of medical bacteriology and of Bölsche's own book *From the Bacillus to the Ape-Man* is replaced by the infantile language of children's literature; the evil attacker of mankind is replaced by a funny little figure one can identify with. Such amazing catachreses illustrate how microbes can become multipurpose media stars on the one hand, and, on the other, collective symbols that reflect the paradoxical signature of modernism itself. It is noticeable that Bölsche's famous work of fact and fiction was widely read and became in fact the most successful work in popular biology of the early 20th century. For this reason it was highly likely to form literary traditions; at the very least it might help in explaining similar ensuing phenomena and apparent cultural heritage – such as bacteria becoming heroes of comic genres and children's literature.

Hilaire Belloc, Edwardian essayist, poet and collaborator of Chesterton, wrote a famous poem in his verse-book *More Beasts for Worse Children* (1897) with the title *The Microbe*. It was illustrated by his congenial friend Basil Temple Blackwood. Like Bölsche, Belloc depicts bacteria as imaginary creatures from a fantastic world, adding further topical and iconic elements from fairy tales to the narrative of funny germs. Rows of teeth, green eyebrows, seven tufted tails: in Blackwood's cute illustration the microbe is clearly represented as a fairy-tale figure, along the same lines as a troll – anthropomorphic and alien at the same time (Belloc, Blackwood 1897, 47, 48).

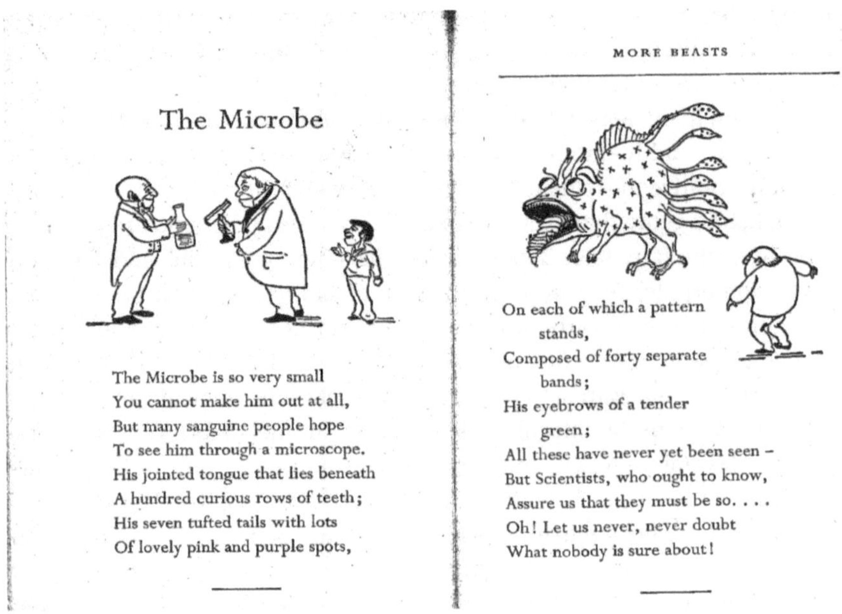

The Microbe

The Microbe is so very small
You cannot make him out at all,
But many sanguine people hope
To see him through a microscope.
His jointed tongue that lies beneath
A hundred curious rows of teeth;
His seven tufted tails with lots
Of lovely pink and purple spots,

MORE BEASTS

On each of which a pattern
stands,
Composed of forty separate
bands;
His eyebrows of a tender
green;
All these have never yet been seen –
But Scientists, who ought to know,
Assure us that they must be so. . . .
Oh! Let us never, never doubt
What nobody is sure about!

Fig. 4: Illustration by Basil Blackwood for Hilaire Belloc's poem *The Microbe*, 1897 (Belloc 1897, 130 f.).

Yet Belloc escalates the connotations 'comical' and 'entertaining' to the point of profound irony and scientific satire. In doing so he alludes to the doubtful reality of microbes and their apparently virtual, media-related existence, as did Robert Koch 18 years earlier. However, this virtual character of an object that has "never yet been seen" and is only *said* to exist by scientists, seems not to present any problems for the Edwardian poet. On the contrary, it is a chance to play the artistic game of meaning and meaninglessness, significance and absurdity. With Belloc's transformation of invisible microbes into linguistic objects of nonsense-poetry, we see how fruitful the questionable objectivity of bacteria has become; perhaps not for scientific clarity but certainly for aesthetic and symbolic purposes. Representational contingencies, as discussed above, initially seemed to facilitate the attachment of multiple, iridescent meanings such as evil, invading, beautiful, ornamental, self-moving, funny, twee, grotesque, and finally led to the purely autopoetic language-game.

It seems particularly remarkable how consistently the central connotation 'contagious' disappears – especially with Belloc, who combines the zoomorphic consistency and the sensual qualities emerging from botany, the wit and infantile tone introduced by Bölsche, and the general public fascination for spectacular invisible creatures into a cocktail of irony and contemporary scepticism. Instead of being conceived as murderous enemy, the microbe is made to seem absurd; a suitable protagonist for children's literature. And this phenomenon – bacteria as cute, witty, infantilized figures – becomes a *topos* in the literary history of germs from the late 19th to the 21st century. With Bölsche and Belloc, a kind of literary and iconic tradition is founded that has its next emulator in a famous picture book about dental hygiene and bacterial damage: *Karius and Bactus*, written and illustrated by Thorbjørn Egner, published initially in 1949 in Norway and followed by a puppet film in 1954. It was translated into German and subsequently became one of the most successful children's books ever published in Germany with no less than 42 editions by 2003. And yet, it can just as well be regarded as a historical failure. The original intention of *Karius and Bactus* was pedagogical – showing bad microbes in order to improve children's dental hygiene. But the opposite happened. Children identified with the friendly, seemingly familiar dwarfs and refused to brush their teeth in order to save the invisible inhabitants. Although psychological investigations and official warnings by dentists' associations exposed the process of identification incontrovertibly (Makuch 2006; Buschmann 2004), *Karius and Bactus* even had successors: 'Hicky' and 'Dicky', protagonists of the next dental picture book *Neues aus der Milchzahnstrasse* [News from Milk Tooth Street] (1993). It follows exactly the same narrative and iconic patterns.

It seems that the infantile, anthropomorphic, dwarf-like microbe has become just as much part of cultural memory as the bad alien invader-microbe. Generations of children considered nasty germs as their little friends, leading to a proper entertainment industry for children: in 1988, the popular UK comic *The Beano* introduced a weekly strip *Totally Gross Germs* by artists David Sutherland and

Vic Neill. Starring child-like, multicoloured germs named 'Ugly Jack Bacteria', 'Jeremy Germ' and 'Iris the Virus' who constantly annoy their host 'Ill Will', the strip became very successful. It ran for 12 years, from 1988 till 2000, and has been recently reprinted (en.wikipedia.org/wiki/Totally_Gross_Germs).[8] Germs currently even serve as cuddly toys, sold by the US company "Giantmicrobes, Inc". Their inventors transform deadly bugs such as *vibrio cholerae*, *yersinia pestis* and *salmonella typhi* into little sweeties of coloured plush with child-like physiognomies which are meant to sit on bed covers and sofa cushions (www.giantmicrobes.com/uk/).

In summary, one can assume that, in the long run, two distinct commercial narratives emerged from popular representations of bacteria around 1900 – ultimately grounded in contingencies arising from microbes' dubious objectivity. Based on contradictory metaphorical transformations in *fin de siècle* bacteriology, botany and popular science, these two commercial narratives can be traced as far as (post-) modern media culture; one could call them the dwarf-narrative and the outbreak-narrative, the latter following Priscilla Wald (Wald 2008). While the dwarf-narrative stresses qualities such as proximity, childishness, cuteness and humour and is successful in children's entertainment, the outbreak-narrative pursues the tradition of evil contagion and invasion that was so popular with medical bacteriology around 1890; it has been especially successful in the Hollywood film industry and in the commercial book market.[9] While the first is meant to arouse emotions such as comfort, closeness and identification, the latter evokes curiosity and the classical mix of fear and pleasure that grounds every successful detective story or crime thriller (see Anz's contribution in this volume). The process of commercialising a discursive figure that has evolved as a collective symbol in *fin de siècle* culture apparently involves a variety of linguistic and iconic media; it cannot be separated from media evolution and diversification – poetry, picture book, comic strip, film, internet. Yet there is one thing that all these best-selling representations have in common: they operate with the fascination for living things that are rooted in cultural memory as invisible and ambiguous.

It is significant that microbes, initially unconventional metaphors and narratives, apparently lose their suitability for high, artistic literature and remain restricted to the commercial sector – either in the toy or in the thriller industry – as soon as antibiotic treatments are firmly established. Indeed, some bacterial and

8 Thanks to Lucas and Kilian King who have drawn my attention to this source.

9 Of course the role of evil bacteria has been passed onto evil viruses or even evil mutant worms after the onset of the antibiotic era, but that does not change the patterns of the narrative, as is shown by thrillers such as *Outbreak* (Hollywood 1995), *Contagion* (Hollywood 2011), *Virus X., der Atem des Todes* [Virus X, the Breath of Death] (BRD 1997), *Deranged* (Korea 2012).

many viral epidemics cannot be cured nowadays and therefore still have the potential to evoke that curiosity and horror-pleasure that was already a best-selling recipe during the "late nineteenth century print revolution" (Tomes 2002, 629). However, microbe narratives were meanwhile losing other qualities – innovation, originality, opacity – which seem essential for autonomous artistic literature. Invisible parasites are no longer fascinatingly new, enigmatic and surprising; on the contrary, they are highly recognisable, which is, I think, a crucial criterion for longstanding commercialisation. They have undergone a predictable process of simplification and trivialisation that can be described with the conceptual instruments of discourse theorists. The microbe shows, for example, how a formerly strong collective symbol becomes conventional, a process described by Link referring to the balloon symbol in Jules Verne (Link 1984, 160, 161). One could equally speak about the emergence of a cultural stereotype in the sense of Sander Gilman (Gilman 1985, 15–37).

5 Microbes Metaphors and Criticism of Rationality around 1900

Things were, however, rather different around 1900 when microbes established themselves as strong symbols or even ciphers. That is not to say that there was not already a strong commercial aspect to the microbe mania after 1880, since it converged with the evolution of mass media (Gradmann 2000; Tomes 2002). However, microbes had been new and spectacular in those days, incomprehensible, surprising and controversial. These qualities make them as suitable for "protoscience journalism" (Tomes 2002, 630) in women's magazines as for modernist creativity and modernist ideas; the epoch is marked by a so-far unknown pluralism of controversial styles, ideologies, and aesthetic programmes. Microbes, instable working objects of an equally pluralistic scientific field but with a stable potential to attract attention, penetrate various aesthetic movements, epochs of style and discourses – such as monism, decadence, Avantgarde, philosophy of knowledge, mysticism, realistic storytelling.

Stanislaw Przybyszewski for example, a Berlin bohemian, partly shared Bölsche's intellectual environment. He was scientifically trained and propagated the metaphysical Darwinism of the later Friedrichshagen Circle. And he also used microbial metaphors: in 1893 he published his most famous short story *Totenmesse* [Requiem], which is regarded as a gospel of decadence. It is, however, rather an enigmatic reflexion on the evolutionary unity of all living beings and on the universal principle of sexuality, containing a profusion of organic and scientific metaphors. Among these are bacilli which, remarkably, become a metaphor for the soul and the intellect. For Przsybyszweski, soul and intellect had unfortunately and unproductively come to dominate over the principle of sexuality. Thus, rationality endangers and destroys the uninterrupted unity of life achieved in physical lust. This rather conventional opposition is described by means of an unconventional, surprising image: as a cannibalistic encounter of bacillus (soul) and leukocyte (sexual lust).

> The small bacillus devoured the leukocyte. In vain, the latter let all his lifeblood stream to the point where the bacillus sat and gorged, in vain, he threw his nucleus to his satanic bride in order to destroy her with the kernel of life. [...] The leucozyte dies. Agh! That was the wedding night, the incestuous wedding night of sexus and soul, the Song of Songs of the triumphant bacillus. [...] And thus, the soul must perish; thus, the triumphant bacillus must die of the leukocyte which it has resorbed. [Die kleine Bakterie frass den Leukozyten auf. Vergebens ließ er alle seine Lebenssäfte auf den Punkt zusammenströmen, wo die Bakterie saß und um sich fraß, vergebens warf er seinen Kern in seine satanische Braut, sie mit seiner Lebensachse zu zerstören (...). Der Leukozyt stirbt. Huh! Das war die Brautnacht, die blutschänderische Brautnacht des Geschlechtes mit der Seele, das Hohe Lied von der siegenden Bakterie. (...) Und so muß die Seele untergehen; so muß die siegende Bakterie an dem resorbierten Leukozyten sterben.] (Przybyszewski 1990 [1893], 12)

Again, microbes appear in connection with the regressive desire for unity and totality which is so typical for the *fin de siècle* climate, especially in monist circles. Such criticism of rationalism is a common pattern among intellectuals around 1900. More uncommon, however, is Przsybyszweski's metaphorical setting of bacillus against leukocyte in order to describe the conflict between cognition and sexuality. This shows how bacteriological motives are combined in the literature of the *fin de siècle* with seemingly incompatible intertextual elements such as the *Song of Songs* – producing catachreses, a characteristic sign of the literary epoch.

Equally remarkable is the way in which another famous critic of science close to the Friedrichshagen group made use of bacteria. They serve the philosopher Fritz Mauthner as an example for his sceptical perspectivism in his book *Beiträge zu einer Kritik der Sprache* [Contributions to a Critique of Language]. Mauthner argues in this work that we cannot have insight into the nature of things since we are unable to adopt perceptions other than our own and project this anthropomorphic perspective illegitimately on to other living beings – for example a so-called "bacterium photometricum":

> The most interesting case is that of the bacterium photometricum which is said only to react to infrared radiation [...]. This is certainly a subtle differentiation that even the human eye has not achieved. But is it legitimate to apply all these human concepts to protists? [Der interessanteste Fall ist der des Bacterium photometricum, welches nur auf ultrarote Strah-

len (...) reagieren soll. Gewiß eine feine Differenzierung wie sie nicht einmal das menschliche Auge erreicht hat. Wo aber nehmen wir das Recht her, alle diese Menschenbegriffe auf die Protisten anzuwenden?] (Mauthner 1901, 353)

Mauthner roughly follows Nietzsche's argumentation in *Ueber Wahrheit und Lüge im aussermoralischen Sinn* [On Truth and Lie in a Non-Moral Sense] (1873); but he radicalizes Nietzsche's position while replacing his example – the perspective of a bird – with something much more alien: a microbe.

Obviously, microbes come to serve more and more as the vehicles for distinctively modern ideas such as scepticism, perspectivism, parasitic dissociation, alienation, loss of coherence. The expressionist Avantgarde in particular is fascinated by germ metaphors; they serve their radical intentions to provoke and to destroy traditional values. In 1908, the Danish novelist Aage von Kohl, who worked with the *Sturm*-circle in Berlin, published a trilogy on the Russian-Japanese sea war with the programmatic title *Im Palaste der Mikroben* [In the Palace of Microbes]. Parasitic dissociation – of human morals, identity, narrative coherence – becomes the leading motive, microbes become the leading metaphor – for example when the hero warns his comrades on a war vessel about the fundamental ethical decline accompanying war:

> We are, admittedly, all bacteria together. [...] The poor people, says God: see, they have become microbes without exception. They have, respectively, become rod-like bacilli, microbes of corruption, or bacilli of murder, all together. [...] All together, we are our mutual, blameless and impenitent microbes – in the whole armada! [Wir sind, offen gestanden, Bakterien alle miteinander! (...) Die Armen, sagt Gott: siehe, sie sind alle ohne Ausnahme Mikroben geworden! (...) Sie sind respective zu Stabbazillen, Fäulnismikroben oder Mordbakterien geworden, alle zusammen! (...) Alle zusammen sind wir unsere gegenseitigen, unverschuldeten und reuelosen Mikroben – auf der ganzen Flotte!] (Kohl 1909, vol. 2, 163, 164)

While Kohl uses bacillus metaphors to indicate the 'infectious' spread of negative decomposition – similar to Yvan Goll in his novels *Die Eurokokke* [The Eurococcus] (1927) and *Der Goldbazillus* [The Gold-Bacillus] (1927) – another figure of the European Avantgarde movement, Filippo Tommaso Marinetti, turns this classical connotation upside down and suggests the opposite: productive decomposition. In his text *Die futuristische Literatur. Technisches Manifest* [Technical Manifesto of Futurist Literature], Marinetti proclaimed the following:

> Art means the desire to destroy and disperse oneself, in that they, like a giant watering-can, flood the country with heroism. The microbes, do not forget that, are necessary for blood and for art, for the extension of the forest of our blood vessels that expands outside our body in the infinity of space and time. [Die Kunst bedeutet das Bedürfnis, sich zu zerstören und zu zerstreuen, indem sie, eine riesige Gießkanne, das Land mit Heldentum überschwemmt. Die Mikroben, vergesst es nicht, sind notwendig für das Blut und für die

> Kunst, für die Verlängerung des Waldes unserer Adern, der sich außerhalb unseres Körpers ins Unendliche des Raumes und der Zeit ausdehnt.] (Marinetti 1912, 195)

This not entirely consistent image of positive, productive bacterial dissociation stands for the fundamental destruction of any aesthetic and epistemological tradition, the rational subject, even meaning and syntax – a utopian programme promulgated by the European Avantgarde. This 'positive dissociation' was meant to release a new artistic language and a new type of artistic self without limits and beyond any conventions, marked by the image of a microbially contaminated "forest of our blood vessels" growing beyond the boundaries of the body.

By this point it should be clear that the microbe was not only subject of art and literature, but also a constitutive element of the intellectual history of Modernism. Popular books on biology and works of literature transform it into a "collective symbol" in the sense of Jürgen Link; that is a representational and explanatory pattern shared by a whole society in a distinct epoch. For Link, a collective symbol is a complex trope where the literal side, in our case the microbe, contains various concepts, such as 'invisible object', 'laboratory', 'triumph of science', 'infectious disease' – like a semantic field. This complex set of concepts does not correspond with only one meaning, bad and alien, but with various, sometimes contradictory meanings, in our case horror and beauty, alien and familiar, wit and threat, soul and sensual perception, negative and positive dissociation, finally the loss of coherence, meaning and sense. Link uses the terminology of emblematics, *pictura* and *subscriptio*; one *pictura* has several *subscriptiones* and this emerges from a collective, anonymous process of "creative writing" – by journalists, critics, philosophers and poets (Link 1984, 150 – 157). This is exactly what happened with bacteria: a collective process of creative writing, by popular Darwinians, creative writers, theorists of Modernism. Thus, the microbe integrates seemingly remote discursive fields and provides descriptive schemes for collective experiences – which is the functional purpose of any collective symbol within Link's conception (Link 1988, 297–301).

6 Microbes and the Modern Religion of Art

One of the core experiences at the turn of the century was the loss of religious beliefs, of an all-encompassing, satisfactory explanation of the world. With Darwinian biology, mankind counted no longer as an image of God, but as a contingent product of evolution, nothing that would be categorically different from any other natural being. To overcome this metaphysical crisis, the German monist movement replaced former transcendental models with a new immanentist spirituality. Its core belief was the concept of life and the eternal unity of all living beings – granted no longer by a transcendental authority but by the idea of evolution itself. In order to guarantee the absolute harmony required by this new pantheistic, natural religion, aggressive elements such as the "struggle for existence" had to be pushed aside by monist thinkers in favour of the teleological principle of continuous, uninterrupted progress. Everything was connected with everything, an uninterrupted chain of beings united in cosmic harmony, generated by speculation rather than by scientific proof (Sprengel 2004).

There was only one problem left. After removing the creator, one ends up in infinite regress and a new principle of origin is therefore needed, the origin of life. Here, bacteria seem an ideal solution; they are so primitive, so small, so simple, they must be the first form of life emerging spontaneously from unanimated matter. They can even embody the cosmic principle of life as such in this new religion of faith – if one leaves aside connotations of otherness, evil invasion and threat. And this is exactly what one of the leading monist propagators of metaphysical Darwinism, Wilhelm Bölsche, speculates in his *Love Life in Nature* publication mentioned above. Microbes come into being by spontaneous generation from unanimated matter; at least they must have done so in prehistoric times when there was still no life on earth:

> For these bacilli [the first bacilli of the earth], something has to be assumed that distinguishes them fundamentally from all their offspring up to you yourself [...]. Imagine [...] the first bacillus at the borderline of water, air, and soil, so on the ocean's beach, for example, suddenly emerging from 'dead' matter, from any unorganic mixture [...]. [Für diese Bazillen wäre etwas anzunehmen, was sie von allen ihren Nachkommen bis zu dir herauf fundamental unterschiede. (...) Denke dir (...) den ersten Bazillus an der Grenze von Wasser, Luft und Erde, also am Meeresstrande etwa, aus 'totem' Stoff, irgend einer anorganischen Mischung plötzlich erwachsen (...)]. (Bölsche 1906 [1898], 106)

Bölsche seems not to care at all that this speculation is anachronistic by 1900; laboratory science had ended the longstanding discussion about bacterial spontaneous generation and permanent transformation with a clear verdict against this superstition.[10] Yet Bölsche is clearly not interested in scientific questions such as classification, distinct species and their stability. Discussing distinct species such as *vibrio cholerae* or tubercle bacilli would weaken his narrative composition around primordial spontaneous generation, insofar as spontaneous generation is linked to transformation and pleomorphism theories for contempo-

10 Cohn, Pasteur, and of course Koch, argued against the transformation hypothesis, whereas the botanist Naegeli pursued it (Gradmann 2005, 48–50, Berger 2009, 36), followed by Haeckel and Boelsche.

raries, not to species stability. What Bölsche accordingly cares about is the microbe as such, as holistic phenomenon. This almost magical object[11] can connect the unanimated and the animated world, the monocellular organism and the human being, microcosm and macrocosm. It serves Bölsche as the first and therefore seminal principle of everything, since the first prehistoric bacillus is said to "have fallen from God's hand through a mystical act" – evidently an object of religious dignity (ibid., 98). Accordingly, microbes are portrayed in *Love Life in Nature* not only as decorative wriggling dancers on a prehistoric beach or as child-like dwarfs, not only as liminal figures, but also as our own and the innermost part of us. Thus, they can fill the last gap in the gospel of descendance and embody the unity of all living beings:

> The unorganic matter could become bacillus. Therefore, it had to contain in itself the preconditions in the same sense as the bacillus could never have become human if it had not contained in itself something genuinely connatural to mankind, something leading towards mankind. [Das Anorganische konnte Bazillus werden. Es musste also die Bedingungen dazu schon in sich tragen, genau so, wie der Bazillus niemals hätte Mensch werden können, wenn er nicht etwas innerlich diesem Menschen Verwandtes, etwas auf diesen Menschen Hinleitendes schon in sich trüge.] (*ibid.*, 109)

This rather pre-scientific idea of pre-formation allows for the universal unity 'All-Einheit' monists believe in because one can skip the disruptive thought of selection, and it clearly shows Bölsche's strategy – identity replaces otherness – which is the narrative principle in *From the Bacillus to the Ape-Man.* There, germs appear as the utmost foreign, evil principle and illustrate the violent struggle for existence. Here, they appear as progenitor, even as the sacred origin of everything. The 'scientific novelist' apparently combines germs in two different books with two different sorts of Darwinism, namely with the aggressive social Darwinism of the naturalist generation and with the metaphysical Darwinism of monist philosophers.[12] Within the latter belief system, the first ancient bacillus appears as "the Adam of life" [Adam des Lebens] who "could create his own Eve through the curious process of self-division" [(der) durch den merkwürdigen Pro-

---

11 Nancy Tomes points out that microorganisms have longstanding magical connotations: inexplicable, unknown, therefore demonic in the pre-bacteriological era; an object of superstition for the non-scientific layman and housewife in the 'post-bacteriological era' of the 20th century, due to excessive advertising and popularization (Tomes 1998, 7 f.).

12 German bacteriologists in general shied away from Darwinism – apart from Cohn and Hueppe, see Berger 2009, 68–71. Bölsche's insistent and careless linking of Darwinism and germ theory again points to his idiosyncratic position between science, creative writing and natural philosophy (King 2012).

zess der Selbstteilung sich selber seine Eva schaffen konnte] (*ibid.*, 106). Allegorizing contagious germs to the biblical progenitor of *Genesis* – we see the modern process of secularization and its flip-side, the sacralisation of science emerging. According to the principle of pre-formation, not only mankind but also his most advanced works of art and culture are already present in prehistoric forms. Thus, microbes found not only a new religion, but also the religion of art:

> The first bacillus was the Adam of life – and, at the same time, Aphrodite. [...] Aphrodite, who emerges from the foam by the grace of a holy hour in her naked human beauty. [Dieser erste Bazillus war Adam des Lebens zugleich – und Aphrodite. (...) Aphrodite, die unter der Gunst einer heiligen Stunde in ihrer nackten Menschenschöne dem Schaum entsteigt.] (*ibid.*, 106)

Telling the tale of an all-encompassing unity and communion of living beings, of organic and non-organic nature, nature and culture, Bölsche transforms bacteria into various language objects: into human ancestors, into the principle of origin, into mythological figures of Christian-Jewish and Greek tradition, that is to say into an allegory of the beautiful arts. Bacteria are no longer alien, they no longer symbolise otherness, which was the shared basis of all metaphors created by medical bacteriology. Instead, they symbolise identity, harmony, unity, coherence and the communion of all things – either unanimated, animated or artificial; they serve as an immanentist principle of creation and as the core figure of this new synthetic religion of art and nature. Needless to say Bölsche carefully avoids any notion of contagion in his prehistoric reverie of microbial origin.

All in all, microbes might be stable species for laboratory science – at least after the initial representational difficulties had been resolved with more sophisticated techniques. But they are certainly not stable objects of language or stable carriers of meaning. Instead, we see how, at a time when they were new, striking, confusing, they become almost soluble symbols with a broad variety of paradoxical meanings: decorative self-movers within the context of the biological art nouveau; enemies of mankind within the bio-political propaganda of the German power-state; grotesque and friendly objects of nonsense poetry; metaphors for contemporary criticism of rationalism and knowledge; symbols for the contemporary crisis of the subject; articles of religious faith and, last but not least, an allegory of the fine arts and of the religion of art.

Consisting of *pictura* and diverse *subscriptiones* and emerging from an anonymous process of collective writing, it is evident that the microbe turns into a strong, new and striking collective symbol between 1890 and 1930; it provides descriptive schemes for the non-homogenous, disruptive experiences of a whole society. The interdiscursive language object 'microbe', which connects the incongruent and manifold and which builds affinities, is also a remedy against contemporary suffering from pluralism and fragmentation. It combines the thrilling but daunting experience of rapid progress and differentiation with the regressive and ubiquitous desire for unity and coherence.

Given this enormous range of cultural meaning, it seems anything but surprising that this soluble symbol became topical; not only within commercial Hollywood narratives but also in canonical fiction of the 20th century. Thomas Mann's *Doktor Faustus* – a novel whose first draft dates from 1904, when germs still had the striking newness and opacity discussed in this article – forms the culmination point of paradoxical microbe metaphors between deadly contagiousness and sacred beauty. In the central chapter, the tertiary narrator, here the devil himself, speaks about anthropomorphic germs and belittles them, in a similar way to Bölsche, and with an irony that we have come to know from Belloc. Syphilis microbes are repeatedly portrayed as "our small folk" (Mann 1997, 247–249), and as "our dear guests from the Indies" (ibid., 247). The intertextual similarities with Bölsche are indeed striking and encompass art-nouveau-beauty as well as sacredness and the religion of art. In Bölsches *Love Life in Nature*, microbes appeared as "funny little dwarfs", who show love and passion (Bölsche 1906 [1898], 99, 105, 106) and "swarm in the primordial air". In Mann's *Faustus*, microbes are portrayed as "the small folk", who, with "a passion for the uppermost [...] would swarm ardently thither" (Mann 1997, 249). Even the allegory of the ancient goddess of beauty occurs once again. The devil introduces the syphilis germ *spirochaeta pallida* as "our pale Venus [...] that is the true sort" (ibid., 247) – the Greek goddess is merely replaced by the Roman version.

What else belonged to the configuration of bacteria within the discourses of monism and art-nouveau? Like Ernst Haeckel, Thomas Mann is obsessed with self-motion, specifically with the flail. The devil speaks about the "living corkscrews" (*ibid.*, 247) and insists, at least in the German version, on the compound noun "Geißelschwärmer" (Mann 2007, 338). The latter has been translated as "flagellants" (Mann 1997, 251) in the English version, but Haeckel's concept "flagellating swarmers" would be more appropriate. For Mann's devil distinctly talks about "flagellating swarmers" *and* "flagellants", referring to modern microscopic creatures and medieval self-punishers. The crucial point is that in German there is just one word for scourge and flagella: Geißel. Thus, the devil joyfully plays with assonances and intertextual allusions and thereby forms an intricate play on words:

> As if I spoke of the vagabonding guild of penitents, scourging their backs for their own and all mankind's sins. But I mean the flagellates, the tiny imperceptible sort, which have flails, like our pale Venus. (ibid., 247)

Of course the devil means both, the flagellants and the flagellates, medieval mystics and modern medicine, the whipping scourge of the penitents and the decorative flail of the microbes – this is Thomas Mann's inventive art of montage. However, behind this originality the long shadow of biological art nouveau and monism becomes visible; it has been shown what eminent role the flail played there as an argument for the self-motion of microscopic beings and thus for an implicit neo-vitalism. Thomas Mann was familiar with this kind of metaphysical Darwinism. He definitely possessed Haeckel's *Art Forms of Nature*, where he could have found the picture of the 'flagellated swarmer'; motifs of evolutionary monism have been shown to be manifold in his novels, above all in *Felix Krull* and *Doktor Faustus* (Herwig 2004, 26–32, 143–266). All in all, it becomes obvious that Mann's *spirochaeta* semantics have not only a medical but also a monist signature. They point back to the *fin de siècle*, when the first draft of the novel was written and when Ernst Haeckel and Wilhelm Bölsche celebrated spectacular invisible parasites as the new gospel of life – as embodiment of vitality, universal unity and immanent spirituality.

To conclude: microbes, instable objects of a pluralised scientific field, become part of cultural memory around and after 1900. They are perceived as spectacular, enigmatic living beings and arouse a predictably high level of interest and attention within late bourgeois societies. Integral to this process of reception are the transformations of microbes into ambiguous iconic and language objects by scientists, popularisers, creative writers, philosophers – from Koch's and Cohn's classical textbooks to the artistic tales of popular Darwinism, the fictions of decadence and expressionism and finally to Mann's famous Faust-saga. In these multifaceted texts, reflecting the pluralism of intellectual modernism, microbes appear as attractive self-movers and contagious attackers, as the origin of life and an allegory of sacred beauty, as the object of natural science and creativity myths.[13] From Robert Koch's 'vicious enemies', writers and intellectuals created a highly artificial metaphorical product, light-years from the one-dimensional military language of the medical laboratory; aesthetic microbes became fundamental building blocks of the intellectual history of the epoch. They linked questions of knowledge and consciousness, of communication and secular religion, and are therefore suitable to express the extreme contradictions of the epoch itself.

Given this substantial role in the history of consciousness and mentalities, it becomes evident that notions of 'microbes' cannot simply be equated with notions of 'contagion.' One should clearly distinguish both concepts and not assume unques-

---

13 Thomas Anz' article in this volume supplements my claim insofar as it emphasises the "substantial emotional ambivalence" that is evoked by narratives of infectious diseases.

tioningly that 'microbe' necessarily falls under 'contagion', especially if one investigates historical or current phenomena of literal or metaphorical infection. Both concepts have their own history and semantic field which overlap only up to a certain point; 'contagion' of course has been on the cultural stage for a much longer time than the more recently occurring 'microbe.'[14] But whereas the former has rather circumscribed connotations of good or bad transmission, communication, circulation of 'illness,' the semantic field of the latter is, as has been shown in this article, unexpectedly multifaceted and paradoxical.

References

Bein, Alexander. "Der jüdische Parasit. Bemerkungen zur Semantik der Judenfrage." *Vierteljahrshefte für Zeitgeschichte* 13 (1965): 121–149.

Belloc, Hilaire, and Basil Temple Blackwood. "The Microbe." *More Beasts for Worse Children.* Eds Hilaire Belloc [verse] and Basil Temple Blackwood [illustrations]. London: Duckworth, 1897. 47 f.

Berger, Silvia. *Bakterien in Krieg und Frieden. Eine Geschichte der medizinischen Bakteriologie in Deutschland 1890–1933.* Göttingen: Wallstein, 2009.

Bölsche, Wilhelm. *Das Liebesleben in der Natur. Eine Entwickelungsgeschichte der Liebe mit Buchschmuck von Müller-Schönefeldt.* Vol. 1. 3rd ed. Jena: Diederichs, 1906 [1898].

Bölsche Wilhelm. *Vom Bazillus zum Affenmenschen. Naturwissenschaftliche Plaudereien.* Leipzig: Diederichs, 1903 [1900].

Brandt, Christina. *Metapher und Experiment. Von der Virusforschung zum genetischen Code.* Göttingen: Wallstein, 2004.

Briese, Olaf. *Angst in den Zeiten der Cholera.* 4 vols. Vol. 1: *Über kulturelle Ursprünge des Bakteriums.* Berlin: Akademie Verlag, 2003.

Buschmann, Cordula. "Rote Karte für Imagekiller von Zahnpflege und Zahnärzten. Karius und Baktus/ Neues aus der Milchzahnstraße." *Mitteilung des Arbeitskreises Jugendzahnpflege.* Ed. Landesarbeitsgemeinschaft Jugendzahnpflege in Hessen (LAGH), 2004. [www.jugendzahnpflege.hzn.de/.../2012_Rote_Karte_Imagekiller.pdf]

Cohn, Ferdinand. *Über Bacterien, die kleinsten Lebewesen.* New York, NY: Henry Holt and Company, 1889 [1872].

Daston, Lorraine, and Peter Galison. *Objectivity.* New York, NY: Zone Books, 2007.

Duncan, Isadora. *My Life.* New York, NY, London: Liveright, 1995 [1927].

Egner, Thorbjørn. *Karius und Baktus.* 42nd ed. Munich: C. Bertelsmann, 2003 [1954].

Fuller, Loïe. *Fifteen Years of a Dancer's Life with some Account of her Distinguished Friends.* Boston: Small, Maynard and Company, 1913.

Gilman, Sander. *Difference and Pathology: Stereotypes of Sexuality, Race, and Madness.* Ithaca, NY: Cornell University Press, 1985.

Gradmann, Christoph. "'Auf Collegen, zum fröhlichen Krieg'. Popularisierte Bakteriologie im Wilhelminischen Zeitalter." *Medizin, Gesellschaft und Geschichte* 13 (1994): 35–55.

14 See the introduction and Olaf Briese's article in this volume.

Gradmann, Christoph. "Invisible Enemies: Bacteriology and the Language of Politics in Imperial Germany." *Science in Context* 13 (2000): 9–30.
Gradmann, Christoph. *Krankheit im Labor. Robert Koch und die medizinische Bakteriologie.* Göttingen: Wallstein, 2005.
Gradmann, Christoph. "Unsichtbare Feinde. Bakteriologie und politische Sprache im deutschen Kaiserreich." *Bakteriologie und Moderne. Studien zur Propädeutik des Unsichtbaren 1870–1920.* Eds. Philipp Sarasin, Silvia Berger, Marianne Hänseler, and Myriam Spörri. Frankfurt a.M.: Suhrkamp, 2007. 327–353.
Haeckel, Ernst. *Anthropogenie oder Entwicklungsgeschichte: Gemeinverständliche wissenschaftliche Vorträge. Teil 2: Stammesgeschichte des Menschen. Wissenschaftliche Vorträge über die Grundzüge der menschlichen Phylogenie.* 4th rev. and augm. ed. Leipzig: Engelmann, 1891.
Haeckel, Ernst. *Aus Insulinde. Malayische Reisebriefe.* Bonn: Emil Strauss, 1901.
Haeckel, Ernst. *Natürliche Schöpfungsgeschichte. Gemeinverständliche wissenschaftliche Vorträge über die Entwickelungs-Lehre.* Second part: *Allgemeine Stammes-Geschichte.* 10th ed. Berlin: Reimer, 1902.
Haeckel, Ernst. *The Riddle of the Universe.* Transl. by Joseph McCabe. London: Watts & Co., 1934.
Haeckel, Ernst. *Kunstformen der Natur.* Reprint. Munich, New York, NY: Prestel, 1998 [Leipzig, Wien, 1904].
Haeckel, Ernst. *Die Welträtsel.* Reprint of the 11th ed. (Jena 1918). Hamburg: Nikol, 2009 [1899].
Hänseler, Marianne. *Metaphern unter dem Mikroskop. Die epistemische Rolle von Metaphorik in den Wissenschaften und in Robert Kochs Bakteriologie.* Zurich: Chronos, 2009.
Hauptmann, Gerhart. *Atlantis.* Berlin: Fischer, 1912.
Herwig, Malte. *Bildungsbürger auf Abwegen. Naturwissenschaft im Werk Thomas Manns.* Frankfurt a.M.: Klostermann, 2004.
Jaeger, Heinrich. *Die Bakteriologie des täglichen Lebens in achtzehn gemeinverständlichen Vorträgen.* Hamburg, Leipzig: Voss, 1909.
Johach, Eva. *Krebszelle und Zellenstaat. Zur medizinischen und politischen Metaphorik in Rudolf Virchows Zellularpathologie.* Freiburg, Berlin, Wien: Rombach, 2008.
King, Martina. "Staatsfeind und Schönheitsgöttin. Bakteriologisches Wissen in Wilhelm Bölsches populärdarwinistischen Schriften." *'Was wir im Verstande ausjäten, kommt im Traume wieder.' Wilhelm Bölsche 1861–1939.* Eds Gerd-Hermann Susen and Edith Wack. Würzburg: Königshausen & Neumann, 2012. 287–319.
Koch, Robert. "Über bakteriologische Forschung (1890)." *Gesammelte Werke von Robert Koch.* Ed. Julius Schwalbe. 2 vols. Vol. 1. Leipzig: Thieme, 1912a [1890]. 650–660.
Koch, Robert. "Zur Untersuchung von pathogenen Organismen (1881)." *Gesammelte Werke von Robert Koch.* Ed. Julius Schwalbe. 2 vols. Vol. 1. Leipzig: Thieme, 1912b [1881]. 112–163.
Kohl, Aage Hermann von. *Im Palaste der Mikroben.* Vol. 1–3. Transl. by Mathilde Mann. Leipzig: Haupt & Hammon, 1909.
Latour, Bruno. "The Historicity of Things. Where Were Microbes before Pasteur?" Bruno Latour. *Pandora's Hope: Essays on the Reality of Science Studies.* Cambridge, MA: Harvard University Press 1999. 145–174.
Link, Jürgen. "'Einfluss des Fliegens! – Auf den Stil selbst!' Diskursanalyse des Ballonsymbols." *Bewegung und Stillstand in Metaphern und Mythen.* Ed. Jürgen Link, and Wulf Wülfing. Stuttgart: Klett-Cotta, 1984. 149–165.

Link, Jürgen. "Literaturanalyse als Interdiskursanalyse am Beispiel des Ursprungs literarischer Symbolik in der Kollektivsymbolik." *Diskurstheorien und Literaturwissenschaft.* Eds Jürgen Fohrmann and Harro Müller. Frankfurt a.M.: Suhrkamp, 1988. 284–307.

Link, Jürgen, and Ursula Link-Heer. "Diskurs/Interdiskurs und Literaturanalyse." *Zeitschrift für Linguistik und Literaturwissenschaft (LiLi)* 77 (1990): 88–99.

Makuch, Almut et al. "Die Eignung von Kinderbilderbüchern zur Zahngesundheitserziehung in Kindergärten." *Oralprophylaxe & Kinderzahnheilkunde* 28.3 (2006): 124–130.

Mann, Thomas. *Doctor Faustus: The Life of the German Composer Adrian Leverkühn As Told by a Friend.* Transl. by John E. Woods. New York, NY: Vintage, 1997.

Mann, Thomas. *Doktor Faustus. Das Leben des deutschen Tonsetzers Adrian Leverkühn, erzählt von einem Freunde.* Eds Ruprecht Wimmer and Stephan Stachorski. Frankfurt a. M.: Fischer 2007.

Marinetti, Filippo Tommaso. "Die futuristische Literatur. Technisches Manifest." *Der Sturm* 3.133 (October 1912): 194 f.

Mauthner, Fritz. *Beiträge zu einer Kritik der Sprache.* Vol. 1. Stuttgart: Cotta, 1901.

Mayer, Ruth, and Brigitte Weingart (Eds). *Virus! Mutationen einer Metapher.* Bielefeld: Transcript, 2004.

Mendelsohn, John Andrew. *Cultures of Bacteriology: Formation and Transformation of a Science in France and Germany, 1870–1914.* Princeton, NJ: Princeton University Press, 1996.

Ogawa, Mariko. "Die Cholera und der Suezkanal. Die britische Debatte über Robert Kochs Theorie des Cholera-Bazillus." *Bakteriologie und Moderne. Studien zur Biopolitik des Unsichtbaren 1870–1920.* Eds Philipp Sarasin, Silvia Berger, Marianne Hänseler, and Myriam Spörri. Frankfurt a. M.: Suhrkamp, 2007. 285–327.

Przybyszewski, Stanislaus. *Werke, Aufzeichnungen und ausgewählte Briefe.* Complete ed. by Michael M. Schardt and Hartmut Vollmer. 8 vols. Vol. 1: *De profundis und andere Erzählungen.* Paderborn, Oldenburg: Igel, 1990 [1893].

Sarasin, Philipp. "Die Visualisierung des Feindes. Über metaphorische Technologien der frühen Bakteriologie." *Geschichte und Gesellschaft* 30 (2004): 250–276.

Sarasin, Philipp, Silvia Berger, Marianne Hänseler, and Myriam Spörri (Eds). *Bakteriologie und Moderne. Studien zur Biopolitik des Unsichtbaren 1870–1920.* Frankfurt a. M.: Suhrkamp, 2007.

Schlich, Thomas. "Repräsentationen von Krankheitserregern. Wie Robert Koch Bakterien als Krankheitsursache dargestellt hat." *Räume des Wissens. Repräsentation – Codierung – Spur.* Eds Hans-Jörg Rheinberger et al. Berlin: Akademie Verlag, 1997. 165–190.

Sprengel, Peter. "'Vom Ursprung der Arten' zum 'Liebesleben in der Natur.' Metaphysischer Darwinismus in der Literatur des frühen 20. Jahrhunderts." *'Scientia poetica.' Literatur und Naturwissenschaft.* Eds Norbert Elsner and Werner Frick. Göttingen: Wallstein 2004. 293–315.

Stahl, Christiane, and Ludger Derenthal (Eds). *Mikrofotografie. Schönheit jenseits des Sichtbaren.* Ausstellungskatalog Sammlung Fotografie der Kunstbibliothek, Staatliche Museen zu Berlin, Preußischer Kulturbesitz und Alfred Ehrhardt Stiftung, 01.10.2010–09.01.2011. Ostfilden: Hatje Cantz, 2010.

Tomes, Nancy. *The Gospel of Germs: Men, Women and the Microbe in American Life.* Cambridge, MA: Harvard University Press, 1998.

Tomes, Nancy. "Epidemic Entertainments: Disease and Popular Culture in Early-Twentieth Century America." *American Literary History* 14.4 (2002): 625–652.

Virchow, Rudolf. “Der Kampf der Zellen und der Bakterien.” *Archiv für pathologische Anatomie und Physiologie und für klinische Medizin* 101 (1885): 1–13.
Wald, Priscilla. *Contagious: Cultures, Carriers, and the Outbreak Narrative.* Durham, NC: Duke University Press, 2008.
Weindling, Paul. *Epidemics and Genocide in Eastern Europe, 1890–1945.* Oxford: Oxford University Press, 2000.
Weindling, Paul. “Ansteckungsherde. Die deutsche Bakteriologie als wissenschaftlicher Rassismus 1890–1920.” *Bakteriologie und Moderne. Studien zur Biopolitik des Unsichtbaren 1870–1920.* Eds Philipp Sarasin, Silvia Berger, Marianne Hänseler, and Myriam Spörri. Frankfurt a. M.: Suhrkamp, 2007. 354–374.
Weingart, Brigitte. “Parasitäre Praktiken. Zur Topik des Viralen.” *Über Grenzen. Limitation und Transgression in Literatur und Ästhetik.* Eds Claudia Benthien and Irmela Marei Krüger-Fürhoff. Stuttgart: Metzler, 1999. 207–230.
Weingart, Brigitte. *Ansteckende Wörter. Repräsentationen von AIDS.* Frankfurt a. M.: Suhrkamp 2003.
Willen, Karin. *Viren. Die unsichtbaren Killer.* Munich: Heyne, 1995.
Webpages:
www.giantmicrobes.com/uk/
http://nachrichten.t-online.de/forscher-entlarven-toedliche-strategie-der-ehec-keime/id_47063024/index
http://nachrichten.t-online.de/killer-keime-breiten-sich-in-der-ostsee-aus/id_58117580/index
http://www.physiowissen.de/thema-artikel4265-Klartext__EHEC___alle_Fakten.html
www.sueddeutsche.de/wissen/ehec-erreger-die-jagd-auf-ein-phantom-1.1105849en.wikipedia.org/wiki/Totally_Gross_Germs

Nicholas Saul

"[...] an entirely new form of bacteria for them": Contagionism and its Consequences in Laßwitz and Wells

In this essay I want to say something about the symbolic function of bacteria in two remarkable science fiction novels, both produced just before the turn of the nineteenth century: Kurd Laßwitz's *On Two Planets* [Auf zwei Planeten] (1897) and H. G. Wells's *The War of the Worlds* (1898). Wells's novel has established canonic status, and not just in the SF genre. The Laßwitz, perhaps because of its great length (900 pages in the modern edition), perhaps because of its markedly philosophical tone as a novel of ideas, is less well known even in Germanophone lands. Yet there has been something of a renaissance of Laßwitz scholarship in the last twenty years, pioneered by Arno Schmidt (who counted Laßwitz among his favourite unrecognised greats), and led by Rudi Schweikert, who produced the standard Zweitausendeins annotated edition, and William B. Fischer, who produced the first lengthy study (Fischer 1976; Schweikert 1979, esp. 902–1113).[1] More recently there have been weighty studies by Götz Müller, Hans Esselborn and Karl Guthke (Guthke 1983; Müller 1989; Esselborn 1992). Most recently, in the work of Esselborn, Ingo Cornils and Patricia Kerslake (Cornils 2003; Kerslake 2007) there has formed itself a tradition of comparing the two novels, which are wholly independently written and as different as can be, except of course insofar as they were probably both inspired in respect of their main motif by Schiaparelli's observations and maps in the 1870s of what appeared to be canals on Mars (Schiaparelli 1888), and Percival Lowell's ideas in the mid-1890s (Lowell 1896, 201–212), which used these observations as evidence for postulating the existence of advanced life on Mars. Both, then, share the conceit of the Earth's invasion by Martians. Mars in itself is the occasion, not the main cognitive interest of these works. That, rather, is the possibility of life on Mars and exploration of its relation to humanity. Both novels, then, are fundamentally Darwinian novels, choosing a scientific theme in the era characterised by Werner von Siemens as the "age of science" and when, as Paul Weindling and others have noted (Weindling 1989), Darwinism was the dominant cultural discourse and the life sciences were beginning their rise to the dominance they today enjoy. Evolutionism, in short, in the dual context of Earth and Martian otherness, is their originary aesthetic impulse.

1 On the Arno Schmidt reception see Schweikert 1979, 954–964.

We can list the commonalities to start. Both presume that life will arise spontaneously where appropriate conditions are met, and that life will evolve according to the universal Darwinian principles of the struggle for existence and adaptation through natural and other forms of selection. Both, like Lowell, know that Mars is an older planet and so postulate that Martian life is much more highly developed than that of Earth, and both therefore, in accordance with the observational evidence, postulate that Martian life is in the autumn or winter of its evolutionary cycle. Both show the Martians as being driven by lack of planetary resource to explore and ultimately exploit Earth. There, however, the parallels diverge. Wells's Martians are of course wonderful Victorian Gothic monsters: physiologically and psychologically repellent, aggressive, destructive, wholly non-communicative and single-minded colonisers, indeed would-be farmers of humans seen as mere food. Laßwitz's Martians are humanoid, indeed often ethereally beautiful in the classical aesthetic tradition of German idealism. They are also conciliatory, tentative, highly self-conscious and with high ethical ideals in their committed attempts to communicate with their less sophisticated Earth brethren. They end up as colonisers, of course, but before that happens they reveal themselves to be winningly inexperienced and cautious in first contact, despite their sophistication clumsy and uncertain in their own understanding of self and other, at worst believers in a sort of Kiplingesque interplanetary White Man's Burden, keen to propagate what they believe to be universal ethical and political ideals. As the names of their planet, "Nu", themselves, "Nume", and their spiritual ideal, "numenosity" [Numenheit] (Laßwitz 1979, 57), indeed even of the originator of their ideals, the great philosopher Imm (*ibid.*), suggest, all this is transparently coded by Laßwitz as allusions to Immanuel Kant's distinction of *noumenon* and *phainomenon*, the spiritual world and the world of appearance.

Yet from both of these contrary starting points the authors lead their races to war on Earth. Wells has his Earthlings crushed and defeated with shaming rapidity, until (with heavy irony) evolution emerges as the *deus ex machina* of his narrative strategy and rescues humanity. Famously, "our microscopic allies", terran "putrefactive and disease bacteria" (Wells 2005, 168), contained in the human blood which is the highly-evolved vampiric monsters' sole food, and against which humans are immune (a privilege acknowledged to have been bought by the Darwinian sacrifice in past æons of untold human lives) infect and consume the Martians alive. Wells's ending is markedly dystopian and pessimistic, a frightening extrapolation of unending Darwinian conflict following victory in what may only be the first battle (Wells 2005, 178). In the Laßwitz, by contrast, we have a sort of intercultural parable of the dialectic of Enlightenment. The first Martian attempts are not to colonise but to communicate with the less sophisticated species. These attempts are however frustrated by fear and clumsiness on both sides (of which more anon). This quickly leads to war with the leading jingoistic colonial power of the nineteenth century, England. Crushed, albeit with minimal loss of life, England serves as an example to the other, scarcely more appealing, nineteenth-century Great Powers, and they are forced to acquiesce in the establishment of a Protectorate of the Earth, only half-willed by the Martians. The Martians take control everywhere, but possession only of the North and South Poles, to draw off the resources they require. They attempt to appease their Kantian conscience by setting up faintly sinister "Institutes of Further Education" [Fortbildungsinstitute] (Laßwitz 1979, 621), attendance at which is compulsory and designed to educate the Earthlings into true freedom, complemented by the even more sinister "Psychological" or "Psychophysical Laboratory" [Psychologisches Laboratorium, psychophysisches Laboratorium] (*ibid.*), a kind of brainwashing institute where they send those who refuse to attend the "Further Education". At last, and not least with the aid of more understanding Martians, the Earthlings acquire Martian weapons, this fundamentally ambiguous regime is overturned, and peace and freedom are, at a price, re-established. First contact is thus a learning process for both sides. And this is certainly a utopian (if bruised) ending.

Now those who compare these two, almost exactly contemporaneous works tend to make broadly similar points, evident I hope already from my summaries. Both novels, like much SF, are a reflection of the present in the future. Both are highly critical meditations on the characteristically nineteenth-century phenomenon of racially motivated colonialism. Rather like Stoker's co-eval *Dracula* (with which there are many parallels), they are allegories of reverse colonialism, of colonisers with poetic justice colonised, attempts to raise Victorian and Wilhelmine consciousness of the problematic relation of self and cultural or racial other. The Wells is perhaps somewhat one-dimensional in its treatment of the theme. His Martians are intellectually not very fascinating. Wells clearly relishes more than Laßwitz (and is more skilled at) the telling of adventures. The Laßwitz is an elaborate and often slightly ponderous reflection on the difficulties of intercultural communication between superiors and inferiors, advanced and less advanced, whereby both parties oscillate unpredictably between comprehension and misprision, between (as it were) cosmopolitanism and nationalism, civilisation and barbarism, progress and atavism. Violence and totalitarianism are spawned precisely by this highly foregrounded miscommunication.

However there is one thing missing from the trend of helpful comment by the comparatists on the Wells and the Laßwitz in their remarks on the Laßwitz: bacteria. Bacterial contagion, we recall, is the Nemesis of Wells's Martians. That bacterial contagion should be thus emphasised in comment on the Wells is no surprise. It is, rightly, a commonplace of scholarship that in Robert Koch's writings and elsewhere, pre-existing aggressive, nationalist, colonialist and racist mentalities offered themselves as metaphors of scientific cognition for the description of the relation between humans and bacteria, and conversely, that such metaphors, once as it were naturalised in the scientific domain, were transferred out once more to contaminate with their pathological and parasitic connotations the political and social discourse of the age (Gradmann 2005; Weindling 2000, 3–108, Weindling 2007; Sarasin et al. 2007; King 2008 and 2010).[2] This lack of substantive comment is perhaps conditioned by the different scientific backgrounds of the two writers. Wells, we know, was a trained chemist and biologist.[3] Laßwitz, by contrast, possessed a physics doctorate in fluid dynamics, but was also a trained philosopher, friend and colleague of Dilthey (no less), and although he never got a philosophy Chair, he was one of the editors of the (still current) historical-critical Akademie-Ausgabe of Kant's complete works. Yet of course there *are* bacteria in Laßwitz's *On Two Planets*, even if those who do attend to them make little of them, as if they were a blind motif (Rottensteiner 1971, 293; Fischer 1971, 170; Cornils 2003, 37; Kerslake 2007, 102f.). Wells tells us – oddly to modern and even nineteenth-century ears (for there was a popular theory propounded by Helmholtz and Lord Kelvin that life originated as single-celled organisms transmitted from space to Earth by comets) – that there are no bacteria on Mars (Wells 2005, 168, 176). Perhaps this is a narrative strategy to ensure that the Martians can possess no evolutionary defence mechanism – even if one then wonders how life on Mars will have evolved at all for Wells, if not from such single-celled primitive organisms. But Laßwitz in fact offers us both terran and Martian bacteria. It is my contention in this paper that Laßwitz's depiction of bacterial contagion *does* make a significant contribution to the intended meaning of his novel.

In what follows I shall reconstruct the narrative path of Laßwitz's bacillus motif and then comment on its semantic achievement, before finally placing this briefly in the context of medicine and literature around 1900.

"Gragra," as Laßwitz calls it, is a bacillus which reverses Wells's figure in two ways: it is Martian, and so, although Martians seem to be immune, threatens both Martians and Earthlings (even if the consequences for Martians are realised only later) (Laßwitz 1979, 883). Now on present-day Mars gragra, rather like measles, has been reduced to a children's illness (*ibid.*, 675), to which adult Martians have been immune for thousands of years (*ibid.*, 677). Martian children display symptoms of tiredness and a mild rash, and the thing passes in a few days.

2 The metaphorisation of aggression dominated scholarly discourse also, compare Virchow 1870 and Virchow 1885.

3 Or mainly so. See Wells 2005, viii.

But that was not always so. In Mars's agrarian cultural epoch, some 18,000 Martian years ago (*ibid.*, 427), the bacillus was cruel and lethal – Laßwitz's narrator compares it with tuberculosis (*ibid.*, 675). A "terrifying plague," a "dreadful pestilence" [entsetzliche Plage; furchtbare Pest] (*ibid.*), gragra, when it was able to deploy its entire life cycle unhindered by the host's immunity, would depopulate entire regions. This took not an acute form but (again like tuberculosis) that of "chronic [...] poisoning" [chronische (...) Vergiftung] (*ibid.*), destroying the host in unspecified ways over a period of years. On the cusp of a shift from the agrarian into the industrial epoch – an age characterised by the worst internecine political conflict and wars in Martian history – Martians of course developed "inoculations" [Impfungen] (*ibid.*). However further measures seem to have been necessary, chiefly the general transition – also around this time – from vegetable nourishment to artificial food chemically derived from mineral rocks (*ibid.*, 412, 427, 677 f.). The bacillus (like anthrax) perhaps resides invisibly in vegetable hosts during the early part of its life cyle, and enters the body through ingestion and/or other unspecified forms of incorporation. Now, however, as Dr Hil, the Martian expert physician in the novel, explains to Ell, the so-called "Kultor" or chief governor of the German-speaking lands, the Martian bacillus, brought in by the colonisers themselves and "an entirely new form of bacteria for them" [eine für sie ganz neue Form von Bakterien] (*ibid.*, 676), has rediscovered favourable growth conditions. Clearly Laßwitz sees an analogy between water- and vegetation-covered Earth, in its current stage of cultural evolution just post-dating the industrial revolution, and not the arid Mars of the present, but the damper and more fertile Mars 18,000 Mars (or 36,000 Earth) years since. The once-tamed chronic form is now, in its new environment, resurgent – not, for the moment, in Martian hosts, but in humans, who possess no natural or acquired immunity, and who are, as Hil anxiously concludes, exposed to the "old, pernicious form" [alte perniciöse Form] (*ibid.*). In a few years, if nothing is done, "devastations" [Verheerungen] (*ibid.*) of the human race are to be expected. Laßwitz's analogy here is less that of western travellers unwittingly importing something like the cholera bacillus from the exotic Orient, more that of American colonists unwittingly importing pathogens such as smallpox into the unprotected native Red Indian population of the New World. This complex is explicitly encoded into the novel. One of the chief Earthling characters, Saltner, repeatedly compares his race's relation to the Martians with those of Red Indians to white men, failing to comprehend what (White Man's) "medicine" might be (*ibid.*, 148, 497). The threat, then, is to the invaded, not the invaders.

Now at this stage it should be noted that Laßwitz, like the evolutionary palaeobiologist Simon Conway Morris today and his contemporary Wilhelm Bölsche (Conway Morris 2003; Bölsche 1906a, 310 f.), and unlike even Martian enthusiasts such as Lowell and Wells himself (and Conway Morris's contemporary opponent Stephen Jay Gould) (Lowell 1896, 210–212; Lowell 1906, 376; Gould 1991),[4] must have held the concept of convergent evolution. Whereas for Gould, following his studies of the Burgess Shale fossils, the tape of evolution can never be replayed, and evolution, following an inherent law of punctuated equlibrium, will always pursue divergent developmental paths, Conway Morris (and before him Bölsche) claim that even under divergent conditions certain basic organs (the eye, the brain) and even certain basic body plans (limb dispisitions) will be independently and homologously evolved to a point of convergent similarity across species. Thus Mars, just like Earth, turns out for Laßwitz not to generate monsters or at any rate radical aliens, but sameness in difference, to possess charmingly varied Martian equivalents of many familiar creatures from the terran orders: insects, arachnids, flowers and trees, and, at the apex of the evolutionary process, humanoids. And bacteria. There seem to be no significant physiological differences between Martian and Earth people. Interbreeding is possible. The central figure, Ell, is himself the offspring of a Martian explorer (stranded on Earth) and a German mother (and hence at home, or homeless, on two planets). Martian heads (no doubt because of their brain evolution) and eyes are slightly larger by proportion, but not unpleasingly so, and sexual dimorphism and gender role play are closely similar to those on Earth. Martians are (as in Wells) somewhat handicapped by the Earth's greater gravity and denser barometric pressure, in particular also by the humid and windy climate of Earth. Thus not only can and do Martians fall in love with and marry Earthlings, they can, like the Earthlings with gragra, also be infected with earthly germs. In particular they suffer under cold and humid conditions from "Earth fever", which they unsuccessfully try to treat with a remedy called "Anthygrin" [Erdkoller] (Laßwitz 1979, 668 f.) – notably Hil himself and the man who later emerges as the villain of the piece, Space Captain Oß. As with Earthlings, physiological indispositions can also prompt nervous conditions (*ibid.*, 668). It therefore goes without saying that Martian doctors can and do treat Earth patients (Isma). Thus Laßwitz founds his medical symbolism in an interpretation of evolutionism diametrically opposed to that of Wells, but equally grounded in one school of contemporary scientific authority. To return to gragra: So close is the analogy with tuberculosis that Hil – who also treats Earthlings – notes that the incipient outbreak of the pernicious form of the disease is currently able to be detected only by Martian technology, "through our special radiation methods" [durch unsere besonde-

4 By contrast Henri Bergson (Bergson 1912, 75, 85, 90, 105–107) sees the evolution of life as an equilibrium of essentially explosive and tendentially divergent *élan vital* and tendentially convergent constraining functional-adaptive tendencies.

ren Strahlungsmethoden] (*ibid.*, 678). This obviously suggests something like the use of X-ray machines to reveal infection in bodily organs much as described in *Der Zauberberg* [The Magic Mountain] (Mann 1999, 201–217).

Precisely this leads to the traditional relative neglect of Laßwitz's gragra, namely, that it seems after this promising introduction not to be an issue at all in the rest of the novel, and this despite its prominent coding in the spirit of the age as the familiar signifier of colonial invasive threat, leading to domination and/or destruction. In what follows Ell, the hybrid Earthling-Martian, despite being immune thanks to his Martian ancestry, and despite having recently returned from Mars, is revealed to his relief not to be a "carrier" [Ansteckungsherd] (*ibid.*, 679).[5] He has, moreover, even back on Earth, fortunately converted to Martian synthetic food (*ibid.*, 678), which he finds he prefers. Relying on their theory of convergent evolution, the Martians realise that Earthlings need immediately to be vaccinated en masse, that physical contact and/or proximity between Martians and Earthlings must be avoided, and that Earthlings in their own interest be weaned off organic food and turned on to its chemical alternative (*ibid.*, 677) – the latter are attempting to do this anyway, but even they realise that this change is unlikely to occur in the near future (*ibid.*, 658, 679). And this is just what they do. The epidemic thus never comes, or at least not in biological form. But this is *not* the end of the story. What happens instead – and this is one chief narrative-strategic function of the gragra motif – is that the prophylactic measures to save the Earthlings reveal the key tragic weakness of the Martian colonisation plan. For in addition to accepting the necessity of mass vaccination, the Martians also realise that they, from the standpoint of communication and informativity, are fatally compromising their project of Kantian Enlightenment (*ibid.*, 658, 684–687). They realise that, having established their would-be benevolent dominion on Earth, with its concomitant control apparatus of "institutes of further education" and so forth, one thing they cannot do is reveal to Earthlings that they bring to Earth anything other than blessings, trustworthy promises of ultimate utopia (*ibid.*, 677); furthermore, that they should not exercise compulsion (*ibid.*, 677 f.). All this would undermine their Kantian ethic, to treat humans not as ends in themselves, but as instruments or objects, and in any case tend to produce the opposite of the intended effect (indeed, Martians are in principle at least psychologically incapable of exercising compulsion upon any other being who demonstrates true ethical autonomy, and even spiritual love is understood among them as unable to compromise the highest value of personal autonomy [*ibid.*, 214.]) But these are precisely the things that they actually do. The Martian

5 On this concept Gradmann 2007, 28; Weindling 2007, 358.

powers that be overrule Ell's reservations of principle, take the view that relations between Martians and Earthlings are one area of legislation which by definition does not require the assent of Earth legislatures, and pass a compulsory mass immunisation decree (*ibid.*, 695 f.). Thus Earthlings of all ages are compelled non-consensually to submit in each "Province" [Bezirk] (*ibid.*) to what amounts to a self-evidently unethical experiment on fellow human beings – inoculation by a Martian physician. Until this has been universally carried through, Earthlings are to maintain a certain physical distance from their colonisers, to refrain from entering dwellings or rooms used by Martians or any form of transport used by them on pain of "severe penalties" [strenge Strafen] (*ibid.*, 696). Worse, no explanation is given as to why, merely an obfustication: "a general indication that it would improve the state of health" [einen allgemeinen Hinweis auf Besserung des Gesundheitszustandes] (*ibid*). The majority of Martians, it seems, has recognised frankly the need for despotic compulsion (*ibid.*). The gragra episode, then, occasions the first step on the road which leads from reason to totalitarianism and crass instrumentalisation of human life.

This in itself, even though it involves an immediate self-contradiction of means and end, may not seem an ethically *very* terrible action to inflict upon the Earth population. Even if clinically dubious and therapeutically risky it is motivated by genuine therapeutic interest of a kind. However Laßwitz takes the move to its logical conclusion, which is perhaps not quite so innocuous. At this point in the multistranded plot, attention shifts to the figure of Josef Salten, colleague of Ell, one of the first to encounter the Martians at their North Pole base. In this capacity Salten has been accorded the status and privileges of Martian citizenship, and indeed, as a visitor to Mars, been routinely vaccinated against gragra. Interestingly, there is no Ellis Island on Mars, and the Martians, despite their expertise in bacteriology, welcome Earthlings literally with open arms: "there were no barriers" [Absperrungen gab es nicht] (*ibid.*, 403). On arrival in his home province of Bozen, Salten however sees with displeasure that here the Provincial has made the prophylactic decree much stricter than elsewhere. Not only do the uninoculated need to keep a much greater distance from their Martian betters (an absurdly increased six paces [*ibid.*, 698]), the punishments for non-compliance are also much more severe (500 Gulden or compulsory re-education in the psychophysical laboratory [*ibid.*]). The Nume have furthermore claimed the right to use the force of their anti-gravity revolvers to move the Earthlings away (*ibid.*). But worst of all is the official stigmatisation: Those Earthlings who have been inoculated are henceforth compelled to display on their headgear for the benefit of Martians the token issued by the Martian medical authorities as proof of harmlessness (*ibid.*, 697 f.) (although the carrier issue is not adumbrated). There thus duly ensues conflict between Salten, who naturally wears no token, and his draconian Provincial, none other than former Space

Captain Oß (which we need not pursue here). What matters is the token. Laßwitz's analogy is doubtless with the rattles used by lepers to signal their presence in advance, although he stigmatises those without the outward mark rather than those with. But the chilling anticipation of an age when outcasts as allegedly contagious carriers of imputed infection were required to wear a yellow star or pink triangle is clear enough. The bacterial motif has been extended metonymically to the human subjects. It is equally remarkable to note here that what is in fact a threat to the health of Earthlings has mysteriously been transmuted into a threat to power of Martians, and perhaps indeed also to the well-being of the hitherto seemingly immune Martians. This strand of the gragra plot code at last extends to encompass the end of the novel. It transpires that Provincial Oß ultimately becomes the leader of the anti-Earth faction on Mars, in a parliament equally divided between factions pro- and anti-Earth. Oß loses the election called to decide how to prosecute the crisis between Earth and Mars. He loses, because his opponent – Ell – has discovered and published Oß's secret plans for prosecuting the conflict should he win. They contain, as one might perhaps guess in this prophetic novel, designs for genocide. One plan involves deployment of Martian anti-gravity technology to stop the rotation of the Earth (which would fry or freeze the inhabitants depending on their position [*ibid.*, 881 f.]). The other, however, involves the de facto weaponisation of gragra, apparently even at the risk of endangering Martians (*ibid.*, 883 f.). In this Laßwitz would appear once more to preempt Wells, in this case his "Stolen Bacillus" story (Wells 1904).

In the last part of my paper I shall link the gragra motif more closely with the intercultural communication theme, and develop Hans Esselborn's arguments a little. Esselborn has rightly emphasised how the novel can be used as a didactic tool to teach intercultural communication. Him apart, it has rarely been noted just how far *On Two Planets* is in some ways not a science fiction novel at all, but a novel about communication in which communication of all kinds is repeatedly thematised. This is another curious parallel with *Dracula*. In that novel there is an inverse parallelism between the atavistic world of vampire contagion and the modern world of high-tech Victorian information-gathering and dissemination. Friedrich Kittler noted how the infectious blood-sucking of the parasitic vampire was strangely mirrored by the way in which the latest in modern technology (from Mina's Remington traveller's typewriter to Seward's wax-coated phonograph cylinder) relentlessly swallowed information and then transformed it, before passing it on to the next carrier (Kittler 1997). In Laßwitz, we find a similar parallel fascination with the possibilities of new information and communication technologies. Quite apart from the telephone, the radio-telephone and the kinematograph, we find mechanical books with pages which turn automatically and self-convert into spoken form (Laßwitz 1979, 62–64), laser-style light-information technology for instant communication under correct alignment between Mars and Earth of a "telephotic report" [telephotischer Bericht] (*ibid.*, 403) and, almost as amusing, the electronic visualiser, which provides Google Earth-style colossal magnifications of the planet surface from space (*ibid.*, 223–225). Best of all is the "Retrospektiv". This device uses Martian anti-gravitational technology to exploit the alleged fact (in this age before Einstein) that gravitational waves travel much faster even than light. A machine constructed on this principle is thus able to capture light waves, and the images they contain, long after they have moved away from Earth, and then to reproduce them in the present. If the correct spatio-temporal co-ordinates are available, then, historical events can be captured and reviewed in real time (*ibid.*, 434–436, 498–500, 510–512) – thus apparently transcending the distorting mediations of conventional historiography.

Beyond this however *On Two Planets* also reveals itself to be a decidedly modern, indeed proto-modernist, novel in the number of self-reflections it contains about the communicative act itself. Misprisions and misunderstandings dominate here, from the low-level "gossip" [Stadtklatsch] in Ell's provincial home town which links him romantically (and falsely) with Isma, a colleague's wife (*ibid.*, 315 f., 519, 582, 618, 693), to newspapers on both Mars and Earth which skew the presentation of information in the cause of one or other pro- or anti-alien Earth or Martian party and sway public opinion erratically (*ibid.*, 351–353, 484–486, 567, 582, 632, 822 f.), to, most seriously, the falsified ethnographical representations of the Martian Museum of the Earth. In this anthropological museum, clearly Laßwitz's critical reflection on the newly flourishing museum and exhibition culture of the colonial epoch (Brecht/Nikolow 2000; Penny 2002), we find not only comic contrasts between Martian populist representations of Earthlings and their real counterparts, but also a representation of the first encounter between the Martians and the English on an Arctic island – a key encounter, because it led to the first conflict, the destruction of English military power (Laßwitz 1979, 359–361, 453–455), and ultimately the subjection of Earth. This disastrous encounter is occasioned by a genuine misprision. English sailors are injured and then die in a fall. Their bodies are recovered by the Martians, who are then however surprised by another English party, which assumes the worst, and things go on uncommunicatively from there. The museum authorises and perpetuates this misprision in the form of a crude and emphatic diorama version of the Martian side of the tale which, on its first viewing, and in the presence of Earthlings, culminates in an outbreak of frenetic Martian nationalism and what Laßwitz frankly calls "incitement to hatred of humans" [Menschenhetze] (*ibid.*, 455). This cascades infectiously through the newspapers (*ibid.*, 456), and war ensues. The use of the "Retrospektiv", which establishes the true facts, comes tragically too late (*ibid.*, 511–513). Laßwitz has a very modern lesson for us here: Technological means do establish redemptive objective truth beyond subjective mediation. But the processes of mass-communication outstrip and nullify the dynamic of Enlightenment. Thus, in negative form, Laßwitz elaborates his main argument: that violence done to information ultimately generates real violence.

The positivisation of this negatively-couched argument is the final, quasi-religious tableau of the novel, in which the central figure of the hybrid Earthling-Martian Ell, at the outset a being who is at home on neither planet, finally makes himself at home, in a sense, on both: through a self-sacrificial act of perfect intercultural communication. This ultimate communicative situation is precisely positioned in the extreme contact zone between two cultures: an American airship at the zenith of its range in the frozen and almost airless upper atmosphere; a Martian spaceship at the uttermost limit of its range just above the atmosphere in the ether, but in immediate vicinity; both races encased in technology. The conflict is at tipping point: A new outbreak of war and technological disaster threatens. The message of peace from Ell's new government must be transmitted to Earthlings. But the technology fails. Worse, the American captain is dubious, trigger-happy, and misunderstands (*ibid.*, 890) the good intention. In desperation Ell moves to the external bridge of the spaceship, removes his oxygen mask, and just manages to call the redemptive message across the ether before he collapses and dies, blood – his gragra-immune blood – trickling from his mouth (*ibid.*, 890 f.), his intercultural mission accomplished at the price of his life, his hybrid dual voice surpassing *in extremis* the capability of all other forms of technological and cultural mediation. Ultimately, then, the novel abandons its fascination with frankly glamorised utopian technology to propagate a visceral and body-centred, yet also theological concept of communication (Fischer 1971, 136).

This, then, in addition to the motif of the sharing of bacteria-immune blood, makes a further link between the bacillus contagion theme and the central theme of communication. When Oß, the would-be genocidal manipulator of gragra, is publicly exposed by Ell for what he is, the general Martian reaction is "universal outrage" [allgemeine Entrüstung] (Laßwitz 1979, 883) and the entire phenomenon of information and communication abuse is diagnosed as the symptom of mass regression in political culture. Just this shock leads cathartically to its overcoming:

> Indeed the whole method of secret plots and machinations, which seemed to the Martians a worrying symptom of political regression, and worse still the decay of mentality, the contempt for the morally good and the noble outraged the consciousness of those who for a time had allowed themselves to be turned into enemies of humanity, and awoke in them the sense of their dignity as Nume. [Schon die ganze Methode geheimer Pläne und Machinationen, die den Martiern als ein bedenkliches Zeichen politischer Rückschritte erschien, noch mehr aber der Verfall der Gesinnung, die Mißachtung des sittlich Guten und Edlen

> empörte auch das Gemüt derer, die sich eine Zeit lang hatten zu Menschenfeinden machen lassen, und erweckten sie zum Bewußtsein ihrer Würde als Nume.] (*ibid.*, 883 f.)

In short: As the resurgance of the gragra bacillus is symptomatic of the atavistic past *physiologically* revisiting the present in the encounter of alien cultures under new evolutionary conditions, so the rise of Oß and his abuse of power mark the *cultural* degeneration of the Martian race under those same conditions. Indeed, it becomes clear that the intellectual perspective of the villainous Oß has been clouded all along by his exposure to physical conditions to which he cannot adapt, hence to an extreme case of infection with the otherwise less elaborated "Earth fever" infection, and finally to psychosis proper (*ibid.*, 671, 699–701, 822, 858; compare Esselborn 1992, 98) – as Dr Hil had warned when he identified the Earth bacillus:

> [...] there is a danger, an ethical danger, which will compel you to exercise particular care in your selection of officials. I have noticed a general phenomenon: that our Instructors, after several months, no longer possess the tranquillity of mind and equanimity which we customarily observe in the Nume. Intercourse with humans, at least in the context of the autocratic position they assume, has – if you forgive my expression – a rather coarsening effect on them. And that manifests itself first in their way of speaking, in the neglect of aesthetic form, second in the overestimation of their own importance, and finally in a domineering mentality which exceeds the morally acceptable. Indeed, I have observed cases in which one can speak plainly of psychosis. I call it "Earth fever". [Es ist (...) eine Gefahr da, eine moralische, die Ihnen in der Auswahl der Beamten ganz besondere Vorsicht auferlegen wird. Es ist mir im allgemeinen aufgefallen, daß die Instruktoren nach einigen Monaten nicht mehr die Ruhe und das heitere Gleichmaß der Gesinnung haben, die wir an den Numen gewohnt sind. Der Umgang mit den Menschen, wenigstens in der autokratischen Stellung, die sie einnehmen, wirkt – verzeihen Sie den Ausdruck – gewissermaßen verrohend, und das äußert sich zunächst in der Sprechweise, in einer Geringschätzung der ästhetischen Form, weiterhin in einer Ueberschätzung der eigenen Bedeutung, schließlich in einer schon das ethisch Statthafte überschreitenden Selbstherrlichkeit. Ja, ich habe leider einzelne Fälle beobachtet, wo man direkt von einer Psychose sprechen kann, ich möchte sie geradezu den "Erdkoller" nennen.] (Laßwitz 1979, 671)

The parallelism of physiological and psychical degeneration marks how the bacillus motif lies at the very centre of the novel's aesthetic and narrative unity.

Some points in conclusion on this admittedly narrow basis about the relation of literature and medicine in the threshold epoch around 1900, drawing on thoughts of Walter Erhard, Martina King and others (Erhard 1997; King 2008, 141–154; Schonlau 2005; Strowick 2009). Laßwitz, although no biologist, is clearly well informed about the latest developments in bacteriology. His gragra bacillus thus is foregrounded to possess a particular life-cycle, moving like the anthrax bacillus (discovered by Koch) strategically from the vegetable to the animal environment, becoming resurgent when unfavourable old conditions are replaced by new, and seemingly able to adopt a more virulent form, which undoes evolutionary-adaptive gains in immunity. This proto-narrative of the bacterial life-cycle from the world of medical-pathological discourse is evidently coupled by Laßwitz with his wider knowledge of Darwinian evolutionism to inform the aesthetic teleology of the novel. The rhythmic pulse of the bacterial life cycle psychophysically threatens cultural progress with regression. Cultural and biological sequences are suggested to function in parallel. *On Two Planets*, then, is not one of those novels which merely exploit some externalised feature or element of medical discourse and link medical or literary cognition in mechanical terms. Here, rather, one can speak of genuine interdisciplinarity: the transfer of generic and semantic energies from one discourse to another; at least in one direction, from the science to the art. But surely also from the arts to the sciences too, in that the scientific elements are shown to be factually embedded in cultural processes of communication which are in their turn susceptible best to narrative analysis of the kind the novel *eo ipso* enacts. It is no coincidence that the novel – in hitherto unacknowledged measure a self-reflective, proto-modernist novel about communication – so closely thematises the link between contagion of disease and degeneration of communication into little more than mass suggestion. A deep-structural parallelism between psychical and physiological malaise as the outcome of evolutionary maladaptation is thus surely intended.

References

Anz, Thomas. "'Gesund' und 'krank'. Kriterien der Kritik im Kampf gegen die literarische Moderne um 1900." *Ethische contra ästhetische Legitimation von Literatur.* Eds. Walter Haug and Wilfried Barner. Tübingen: Niemeyer, 1986. 240–250.

Bergson, Henri. *Schöpferische Entwicklung.* Tr. Gertrud Kantorowicz. Jena: Diederichs, 1912 [original French 1907].

Bölsche, Wilhelm. "Bazillusgedanken." Wilhelm Bölsche. *Vom Bazillus zum Affenmenschen. Naturwissenschaftliche Plaudereien.* 4th ed. Jena: Diederichs, 1906 [1900]. 3–39.

Bölsche, Wilhelm. "Das Märchen des Mars." Wilhelm Bölsche. *Vom Bazillus zum Affenmenschen. Naturwissenschaftliche Plaudereien.* 4th ed. Jena: Diederichs, 1906 [1900]. 301–321.

Brecht, Christine, and Sybilla Nikolow. "Displaying the Invisible: 'Volkskrankheiten' on Exhibition in Imperial Germany." *Studies in History and Philosophy of. Biological and Biomedical Sciences* 31 (2000): 511–530.

Conway Morris, Simon. *Life's Solution. Inevitable Humans in a Lonely Universe.* Cambridge: Cambridge University Press, 2003.

Cornils, Ingo. "The Martians Are Coming! War, Peace, Love, and Scientific Progress in H.G. Wells's *War of the Worlds* and Kurd Laßwitz's *Auf zwei Planeten.*" *Comparative Literature* 55 (2003): 24–41.

Erhard, Walter. “Medizingeschichte und Literatur am Ende des 19. Jahrhunderts.” *Scientia Poetica* 1 (1997): 224–267.

Esselborn, Hans. “Science Fiction als Lehr- und Forschungsgegenstand interkultureller Deutschstudien.” *Jahrbuch Deutsch als Fremdsprache* 18 (1992): 87–107.

Fischer, William B. *The Empire Strikes Out: Kurd Lasswitz, Hans Dominik, and the Development of German Science Fiction.* Bowling Green, Ohio: Bowling Green University Popular Press, 1971.

Gould, Stephen Jay. *Wonderful Life: The Burgess Shale and the Nature of History.* Harmondsworth: Penguin, 1991 [1989].

Gradmann, Christoph. *Krankheit im Labor. Robert Koch und die medizinische Bakteriologie.* Göttingen: Wallstein, 2005.

Gradmann, Christoph. “Unsichtbare Feinde. Bakteriologie und politische Sprache im deutschen Kaiserreich.” *Bakteriologie und Moderne. Studien zur Propädeutik des Unsichtbaren 1870–1920.* Eds. Philipp Sarasin, Silvia Berger, Marianne Hänseler, and Myriam Spörri. Frankfurt a. M.: Suhrkamp, 2007. 327–353.

Guthke, Karl S. *Der Mythos der Neuzeit. Das Thema der Mehrheit der Welten in der Literatur- und Geistesgeschichte von der kopernikanischen Wende bis zur Science Fiction.* Berne, Munich: Francke, 1983.

Kerslake, Patricia. *Science Fiction and Empire.* Liverpool: Liverpool University Press, 2007.

King, Martina. “Von Mikroben und Menschen. Bakteriologisches Wissen und Erzählprosa um 1900.” *Scientia Poetica* 12 (2008): 141–180.

King, Martina. “Inspiration und Infektion. Zur literarischen und medizinischen Wissensgeschichte von ‘auszeichnender Krankeit’ um 1900.” *Internationales Archiv für die Sozialgeschichte der Literatur* 35 (2010): 61–97.

Kittler, Friedrich W. “Dracula’s Legacy.” *Literature, Media Information Systems.* Ed. John Johnston. Amsterdam: G+B Arts, 1997. 130–146.

Laßwitz, Kurd. *Auf zwei Planeten.* Roman in zwei Bänden. Ed. Rudi Schweikert. Frankfurt a. M.: Zweitausendeins, 1979 [1897].

Lowell, Percival. *Mars.* Boston, New York, NY: Houghton Mifflin, 1896.

Lowell, Percival. *Mars and its Canals.* New York, NY: Macmillan, 1906.

Mann, Thomas. *The Magic Mountain.* Translated from the German by H.T. Lowe-Porter. London: Vintage, 1999

Müller, Götz. *Gegenwelten. Die Utopie in der deutschen Literatur.* Stuttgart: Metzler, 1989.

Penny, H. Glenn. *Objects of Culture. Ethnology and Ethnographic Museums in Imperial Germany.* Chapel Hill: University of North Carolina Press, 2002.

Rottensteiner, Franz. “Kurd Lasswitz: A German Pioneer of Science Fiction.” *SF. The Other Side of Realism. Essays on Modern Fantasy and Science Fiction.* Ed. Thomas D. Clareson. Bowling Green, OH: Bowling Green University Popular Press, 1971. 289–306.

Sarasin, Philipp. *Reizbare Maschinen. Eine Geschichte des Körpers 1765–1914.* Frankfurt a. M.: Suhrkamp, 2001.

Sarasin, Philipp. “Die Visualisierung des Feindes. Über metaphorische Technologie der frühen Bakteriologie.” *Bakteriologie und Moderne. Studien zur Propädeutik des Unsichtbaren 1870–1920.* Eds. Philipp Sarasin, Silvia Berger, Marianne Hänseler, and Myriam Spörri. Frankfurt a. M.: Suhrkamp, 2007. 427–461.

Schiaparelli, Giovanni Virginio. *Über die beobachteten Erscheinungen auf der Oberfläche des Planeten Mars.* Berlin: Gesellschaft Urania, 1888.

Schonlau, Anja. *Syphilis in der Literatur. Über Ästhetik, Moral, Genie und Medizin (1880–2000)*. Würzburg: Königshausen & Neumann, 2005.
Schweikert, Rudi. "Von Martiern und Menschen oder: Die Welt, durch Vernunft dividiert, geht nicht auf. Hinweise zum Verständnis von *Auf zwei Planeten*." Kurd Laßwitz. *Auf zwei Planeten*. Roman in zwei Bänden. Ed. Rudi Schweikert. Frankfurt a. M.: Zweitausendeins, 1979. 903–976.
Stoker, Bram. *Dracula*. Ed. Maud Ellmann. Oxford, New York, NY: Oxford University Press. 1998 [1897].
Strowick, Elisabeth. *Sprechende Körper – Poetik der Ansteckung. Performativa in Literatur und Rhetorik*. Munich: Fink, 2009.
Virchow, Rudolf. "Der Krieg und die Wissenschaft." *Archiv für pathologische Anatomie und Physiognomie und für die klinische Medizin* 51 (1870): 1–6.
Virchow, Rudolf. "Der Kampf der Zellen und der Bakterien." *Archiv für pathologische Anatomie und Physiognomie und für die klinische Medizin* 101 (1885): 1–13.
Weindling, Paul. *Health, Race and German Politics between National Unification and Nazism, 1870–1945*. Cambridge: Cambridge University Press, 1989.
Weindling, Paul. *Epidemics and Genocide in Eastern Europe 1890–1945*. Oxford: Oxford University Press, 2000.
Weindling, Paul. "Ansteckungsherde. Die deutsche Bakteriologie als wissenschaftlicher Rassismus." *Bakteriologie und Moderne. Studien zur Propädeutik des Unsichtbaren 1870–1920*. Eds. Philipp Sarasin, Silvia Berger, Marianne Hänseler, and Myriam Spörri. Frankfurt a. M.: Suhrkamp, 2007. 354–374.
Weinstein, Arnold. "Afterword: Infection as Metaphor." *Literature and Medicine* 22 (2003): 102–115.
Wells, H[erbert]. G[eorge]. *The War of the Worlds*. Ed. Patrick Parrinder. Harmondsworth: Penguin, 2005 [1898].
Wells, H[erbert]. G[eorge]. "The Stolen Bacillus." H[erbert]. G[eorge] Wells. *The Stolen Bacillus and Other Incidents*. London: Macmillan, 1904. 1–16.

Thomas Rütten

Genius and Degenerate? Thomas Mann's *Doktor Faustus* and a Medical Discourse on Syphilis

In 1902 Paul Julius Möbius (1853–1907), a neurologist working in Leipzig, published a study on "the pathological in Nietzsche" [das Pathologische bei Nietzsche]. The book's third edition (Möbius 1909) – identical with the second, slightly revised 1904 edition – was read by Thomas Mann on the evening of 27 October 1942, at his residence in Pacific Palisades – with, as his diary informs us, "the most intense interest" [mit stärkster Beteiligung] (Mann 1982, 490). He would forgive Möbius the "mental deficiencies" [geistige Manko] exhibited in his book. "[a]s though he were not right, from his point of view" [Alsob er nicht von seiner Seite recht hätte] (*ibid.*).[1] "His point of view" – that of Möbius – is that of degenerationism and hereditarianism; a medical point of view shaped by theories and nosology – the kind of view that had been enjoying great prominence since the *fin de siècle.* But at the same time it is the point of view of one who equates the 'average' with the 'normal,' and who suspects any departure from it as degeneracy. A summary of Möbius's thesis with regard to the 'pathography' of the recently deceased philosopher would go something like this: Friedrich Nietzsche was a *dégénéré supérieur,* that is to say one who was born with the hereditary illness of degeneracy. However, despite of the resulting character flaws and intelligence deficiencies, he was capable of high achievements in a specific area, whilst essentially remaining a dilettante in all other respects. The signs of his degeneracy were both bodily and, in Nietzsche's case at least, to a much greater extent mental in their nature. In the former category we find discrete signs, such as "small, but not significantly small" ears (Möbius 1902, 13, n. 1) and facial asymmetries (*ibid.*, 13).[2] In the latter, "irreligious individualism" [irreligiöser Individualismus] (*ibid.*, 35) or "lack of herd

1 Cf. also Thomas Mann's 1947 essay *Nietzsches Philosophie im Lichte unserer Erfahrung,* where he says: "The doctor Möbius has been heavily criticized for writing a book in which he presents Nietzsche's development, from a professional point of view, as a case history of progressive paralysis. I have never been able to share this indignation. What Möbius describes – in his own way – is nothing but the uncontestable truth." [Man hat es dem Arzt Möbius sehr verübelt, daß er ein Buch geschrieben hat, worin er die Entwicklungsgeschichte Nietzsches als die Geschichte einer progressiven Paralyse fachmännisch darstellt. Ich habe an der Entrüstung darüber nie teilnehmen können Der Mann sagt, auf seine Weise, die unbestreitbare Wahrheit] (Mann 2009, 189).

2 In Nietzsche's patient file from Jena [Jenaer Krankenjournal] bodily signs of degeneracy are explicitly mentioned (Volz 1990, 237).

instinct" [es fehlt ihm am "Herdensinne"] (*ibid.*, 30); one-sidedness of gifts [im höchsten Grade begabter, aber einseitiger Mensch] (*ibid.*, 29] (strong in music, poetry and language, weak in art, mechanics and mathematics) (*ibid.*, 14–18, 30); impulsive conditions of the soul (*ibid.*, 3); an unsettled way of life [Wanderleben] (*ibid.*, 62); lack of harmony (*ibid.*, 1, 29) and sôphrosunê (*ibid.*, 24, 30); instability (*ibid.*, 104) accompanied by a preference for composers and writers with nervous illnesses, such as Schumann and Wagner, Hölderlin, Stendhal, Flaubert, Dostoïevsky and Baudelaire (*ibid.*, 34). Fundamentally, Nietzsche was a "writer, through and through" [durch und durch Schriftsteller] (*ibid.*, 23), a "belletrist" [Belletrist(en)] (*ibid.*, 30 f.), one of the "writerly dégénérés" [schriftstellernde(n) Dégénérés] (*ibid.*, 34), in other words a type of character that "is usually designated 'modernity'" [(...) man bezeichnet diesen Charakter gewöhnlich als Modernität] (*ibid.*, 34 f.).[3] It was, then, on the basis of such hereditary degeneracy, and not independent of it, that Nietzsche had found himself in a brothel in Cologne in February 1865 – a visit which he recounted to his friend Paul Deussen (1845–1919) in the following way:

> I found myself suddenly surrounded by half a dozen apparitions in tinsel and glitter, who eyed me expectantly. I stood for a while, speechless. Then I moved away, instinctively, towards a piano, as towards the only entity in that company endowed with a soul; and played a few chords. These released me from my numbness, and I managed to regain the open air. [Ich sah mich plötzlich umgeben von einem halben Dutzend Erscheinungen in Flitter und Gaze, welche mich erwartungsvoll ansahen. Sprachlos stand ich eine Weile. Dann ging ich instinctmäßig auf ein Klavier als auf das einzige seelenhafte Wesen in der Gesellschaft los und schlug einige Akkorde an. Sie lösten meine Erstarrung und ich gewann das Freie.] (*ibid.*, 28)

Nietzsche, "a born moralist" [ein geborener Moralist] (*ibid.*, 28), had been "constrained by pure curiosity to eat of the apple" [...schon aus Wissbegierde vom Apfel zu essen gezwungen war] (*ibid.*, 28); and it was therefore no wonder that

> sources, which cannot of course be identified by name, relate that Nietzsche had had sexual intercourse even in Leipzig, when a student there, and that he later from time to time had relations with people who – it can't be helped – make themselves available for the fulfilment of men's needs. [Gewährsmänner, deren Name (sic) freilich nicht genannt werden soll, erklären, dass Nietzsche schon in Leipzig geschlechtlichen Verkehr gehabt habe und dass er später von Zeit zu Zeit mit den Personen, die nun einmal sich den männlichen Bedürfnissen zur Verfügung stellen, Beziehungen gehabt habe.] (*ibid.*, 28 f.)

---

3 The last quotation with its grammatically incorrect attribution of "modernity" to Nietzsche illustrates to what extent, throughout his works, Möbius views the philosopher as the representative or icon of the very movement he is criticising. For him, Nietzsche is the "modern artist (philosopher) par excellence" [moderne Künstler (Philosoph) par excellence], the "Cagliostro of modernity" [Cagliostro der Modernität] (Möbius 1902, 82).

In this context one cannot, of course, talk of love; it is simply a question of a "means of evacuation" [ein Mittel zur Entleerung] (*ibid.*, 30). In the process, as we learn from other passages scattered throughout the book, a 'poison' had entered his body – a poison which was to lead, fifteen years later, to the outbreak of disease, and in the end to mental breakdown, progressive paralysis and madness (*ibid.*, 2). But the 'poison' had had the effect, even before that, of aggravating Nietzsche's "inherited" [ein Erbteil (aus der väterlichen Familie)] (*ibid.*, 39) migraine; of opening the way to erroneous doctrines; and of enabling the philosopher to choose as his own divinity Dionysos, the "patron saint of hysteria" [(d)en Patron der Hysterie] (*ibid.*, 50). What Nietzsche's friends saw as the *furor poeticus* of *Zarathustra* Möbius interprets rather as a *furor poetico-paralyticus* (*ibid.*, 70). Although Möbius does not himself believe that a "brain illness" [Gehirnkrankheit] may increase the "intellectual capacities" [Geisteskräfte] (*ibid.*, 60), he does admit that colleagues have described such cases. It is not, in his view, unimaginable, considering that paralysis always seeks out "its places" [ihre Stellen] (*ibid.*, 61) in the brain in a very specific way. If inhibiting fibres in the brain were destroyed, this could result – Möbius concedes reluctantly, and in a purely hypothetical way – in a "failure of the sense of fatigue, and a euphoria" [Fehlen des Ermüdungsgefühls und Euphorie]. Hence an "increased capacity of the working parts" [eine gesteigerte Leistung der arbeitenden Theile] (*ibid.*, 61) might be expected.[4] It could also happen – again hypothetically, and without Möbius actually believing in such a possibility – that the stimulation might lead to a *hyperemia* which would "facilitate an increase in work" [dass die Hyperämie die Mehrarbeit begünstige] (*ibid.*). Such effects, Möbius relates, had been explained on the basis of an analogy with alcohol. "What alcohol brings about may also be brought about by paralysis [...]." [Was der Alkohol fertig bringt, dazu ist die Paralyse auch im Stande (...)] (*ibid.*). Nietzsche expresses himself, sometimes as "a youth excited by wine" [ein(en) durch Wein erregten Jüngling], sometimes as "a riotous drinker of Schnapps" [ein(en) zeternde(r) Schnapstrinker] (*ibid.*, 85). Fundamentally, and therefore in his overall analysis, Möbius, in a sort of thought experiment, puts Nietzsche on trial[5], warning the reader at the end of his book,

4 Despite his reluctance here to concede such a scenario in Nietzsche's case, Möbius later in his book explicitly mentions "failure of the sense of fatigue, and a euphoria alternating with sad or irascible dysphoria" [Fehlen des Ermüdungsgefühls, Euphorie im Wechsel mit trauriger oder zorniger Verstimmung] (Möbius 1902, 97) as manifestations of Nietzsche's paralysis prior to 1888.

5 "Supposing we lived in a country whose legislation would prohibit such [i.e. Nietzsche's] works, and a trial had raised the question of mental capacity, the expert witness for the prosecution would have to reply the following." [Gesetzt wir lebten in einem Lande, in dem die Gesetze solche Schriften verböten, und im Strafprozesse wäre die Frage nach der Zurech-

which finishes, as it were, with the final speech for the prosecution: "Be suspicious: because this man has a sickness of the brain." [Seid misstrauisch, denn dieser Mann ist ein Gehirnkranker] (*ibid.*, 106).

Whether Thomas Mann also read Möbius's book shortly after its publication has so far been impossible to establish. There are, however, some indirect indications that he may have done so. First, there is the outline of *Doktor Faustus*, the so-called *Sieben-Zeilen-Plan*, which appears in Thomas Mann's *Notebooks* (Mann 1992, 121 f.) and dates from 1904:

> Figure of the syphilitic artist: as Doctor Faustus and as one assigned to the devil. The poison has the same effects [on him] as intoxication, stimulant, inspiration; he may create wonderful works of genius in a state of enraptured enthusiasm; the devil himself guides his hand. In the end, however, *the devil comes for him:* paralysis [Figur des syphilitischen Künstlers: als Dr. Faust und dem Teufel Verschriebener. Das Gift wirkt als Rausch, Stimulans, Inspiration; er darf in entzückter Begeisterung geniale, wunderbare Werke schaffen, der Teufel führt ihm die Hand. Schließlich aber *holt ihn der Teufel:* Paralyse.] (Mann 2007, 10.2, 13; Mann 1992, 121)

This note reads like a reaction on the part of the author to Möbius's book and to the picture of Nietzsche that it contains. Indeed, even the reference to the devil appears in Möbius:

> In questions of truth, the effect of alcohol can only be detrimental; where, however, what is in question is the poetic feeling, or aesthetic aspect, of speech, where a certain degree of unclarity is acceptable, here even the devil may be of assistance. [Handelt es sich um Wahrheit, so kann der Alkohol nur schaden, handelt es sich um poetische Gefühle und um den Schmuck der Rede, wo es auf ein Bischen Unklarheit nicht ankommt, so kann auch der Teufel helfen.] (Möbius 1902, 61)

In this context it is worth mentioning that Thomas Mann's outline sketch to which we have alluded, the *Sieben-Zeilen-Plan*, is the revision of a still earlier one (Mann 2007, 10.2, 13), in which there is no mention of the devil.

When considering the evidence for Thomas Mann's knowledge of Möbius's pathological picture of Nietzsche during the early phase of the conception of *Doktor Faustus*, we should also mention that he consulted certain of Möbius's works even when writing *Buddenbrooks*. In particular, Mann shows a familiarity with the 1882 publication *Die Nervosität* – and through it with the French doctrine of degeneracy of Bénédict August Morel (1809 – 1873) and especially of Valentin Magnan (1835 – 1916) (Max 2008, 101 – 135). Thirdly, 1904 is the year of Tho-

nungsfähigkeit erhoben worden, so würde der Sachverständige etwa Folgendes zu antworten haben] (Möbius 1902, 104).

mas Mann's engagement to Katia Pringsheim, and of his first meetings with her grandmother, Hedwig Dohm (1831–1919) (Mendelssohn 1996, 950), who had recently – in 1902 – reacted to Möbius's *On the Physiological Feeblemindedness of the Woman* [Über den physiologischen Schwachsinn des Weibes] (Möbius 1900), with a rebuttal entitled *The Anti-Feminists* [Die Antifeministen] (Dohm 1902).

Finally, in his comments on Thomas Mann's essay entitled *Nietzsche's Philosophy in Light of our Experience* [Nietzsches Philosophie im Lichte unserer Erfahrung], Herbert Lehnert has pointed to the fact that the copy of the third edition of Möbius's book from 1909, in the Thomas Mann Archive, appears to have been bought secondhand, since "the signs of use that the book contains do not correspond to its significance for Thomas Mann" [dessen Benutzungsspuren nicht mit der Bedeutung des Buches für Thomas Mann korrespondieren] (Mann 2009, 227). The fleeting appearance of Möbius's book in Mann's diary points to a previous acquaintance with the work. For all of these reasons I agree with Lehnert's view that Möbius's book "will have spurred Thomas Mann on to the early plans (1904) for a work about a syphilitic artist" [(...) wird Thomas Mann zu den frühen Plänen (1904) eines Werkes über einen syphilitischen Künstler angeregt haben] (*ibid.*).

Before we jump to the conclusion that *Doktor Faustus* has been written in stark opposition to Möbius's provoking book, let us consider where Thomas Mann seems to be walking in the neurologist's footsteps. He certainly never agreed with those who fiercely disputed the diagnosis of syphilis given by Nietzsche's Basle and Jena doctors and confirmed vigorously by Möbius – first and foremost the philosopher's sister, Elisabeth Förster, who spoke of a "disgusting accusation" [ekelhafte Verleumdung] (as in Volz 1990, 4). She had in fact hired Möbius specifically to write a pathography of her brother, but was shocked by the result and the "vile insinuations" it contained (quoted in Peters 1977, 184). Right up to her death in 1935 she missed no opportunity of vehement denial. Thomas Mann also uses the brothel experience as Deussen and Möbius described it, in the sixteenth chapter of his novel. In a letter from Adrian Leverkühn, the main protagonist, written to the narrator, Serenus Zeitblom, and dated 2 February 1905 – or 1906, depending on how the inconsistencies that Thomas Mann left in the chronology of the narrated time of the novel are resolved (Mann 2007, 10.2, 400)[6] – Leverkühn tells of his early days as a student in Leipzig in the previous winter semester, when a tourist guide took him into a "bawdyhouse" where a "nut-brown lass, in Spanish jacket, with large mouth, stubbed nose, and al-

6 When reading Gennerich's book on syphilis (Gennerich 1921), Thomas Mann might have had the year 1905 in mind, as he highlights a case history from this year in the margins of Gennerich's text. See Gennerich 1921, 36. On p. 28, however, he also marked a case history of a man who, in 1914, infected himself in a brothel in Wilhelmshaven.

mond eyes" stroked his "cheek with her arm," before Leverkühn was able to flee the "hell-hole of lusts" (Mann 1999, 152; see also Mann 2007, 10.1, 209).

The story of the Leipzig doctors who said they knew of Nietzsche's syphilis was also used by Thomas Mann, but with significant modifications. There were certainly more gaps to be filled in the perceived narrative, as Möbius had neither named his source nor specified the spatio-temporal coordinates of Nietzsche's infection. Since Kurt Hildebrandt and Erich Podach had justifiably doubted the syphilis diagnosis in books only published in 1926 and 1930, respectively, and the rumour was only brought up again in Wilhelm Lange-Eichbaum's Nietzsche book, which appeared in the same year as *Doktor Faustus*, Thomas Mann was left with almost nothing to build on. That Möbius was the only rather meagre source, is confirmed by Lange Eichbaum. "In 1930," so he wrote in 1947,

> a Berlin neurologist told me that Nietzsche had infected himself with syphilis in a Leipzig brothel during his time as a student there, and that he had been treated for syphilis by two Leipzig physicians. (quoted in Sax 2003, 53)

Lange-Eichbaum went on to say that the Berlin doctor had received this information from Möbius and that he, Lange-Eichbaum, had talked to the brother of Dr. Möbius as well as the son of one of the two Leipzig physicians, both of whom confirmed the story. By that time letters proving the story had been destroyed (*ibid.*).

Thomas Mann accepts the rumour, but turns it into a very different story. Instead of credible expert witnesses whose identity is concealed by colleagues sworn to secrecy and confidentiality, we encounter rather dubious characters who are not only named and whose names are all over town – Leverkühn claims to have found them in a street directory –, but who even die almost in the open and are led away in handcuffs by the vice squad in broad day light (Mann 1999, 168). What is more, because of their ending, they hardly apply their trades (they used mercury, as the devil knows, probably in combination with iodine and bismuth[7]). They are thus not only poor healers, as a number of similar pairs of doctors in Thomas Mann's work, but here do not even have an opportunity to show their ultimate incompetence. They are also marked by signs of degeneracy; one of them, "a heavyset man with a red face and black goatee," "had a way of puffing air between his pouted lips" (Mann 1999, 166; see also Mann 2007, 10.1, 228), while the other suffered from "a kind of tic that lifted one cheek and a corner of

---

7 Salvarsan was only discovered in 1910 by Paul Ehrlich (1854–1915) and Sahachiro Hata (1873 –1938). For a period of ten to twelve weeks mercury had to be injected once a week. This procedure was then repeated twice with a month's interval in between each treatment. The devil confirms the mercury therapy in Mann 2007, 10.1, 341–2.

the mouth, while the eye joined in with a squint" (Mann 1999, 168; see also Mann 2007, 10.1, 230). They represent the more conservative and the more progressive specialist doctor, a variant of Mann's typical pairing of physicians (Elsaghe 2010, 57 f.). With regards to syphilis and its origin, fiercely debated between teutonic-nationalist Protestant and liberal-progressive Jewish physicians, particularly in Leipzig at the time, it is safe to assume that Zimbalist belonged to the camp of the Americanists, who believed in an import of syphilis from the New World into Europe at the end of the 15th century, whereas Erasmi who lived in "a rather gloomy building in the old city" and employed a "maid" (Mann 1999, 167; see also Mann 2007, 10.1, 228) belongs to the opposite camp of the Anti-Americanists who tried to prove the continuous endemic presence of syphilis in Europe from ancient to modern times and blamed periods of moral laxity for its epidemic flair-ups. More importantly, neither of the two physicians appears to be a disciple of Asclepios, but rather delegates of the devil, which is indicated by the colour red of Erasmi's face and Zimbalist's hair. Their quite literal disappearance may be an ironic allusion to all the secrecy mentioned above. That Leverkühn "had found the address listed in a street directory" (Mann 1999, 166; see also Mann 2007, 10.1, 228), is mentioned twice more in the novel (Mann 1999, 167 and 249; see also Mann 2007, 10.1, 229 and 341), and as the first mention was added to the manuscript by hand (Mann 2007, 10.2, 431) this information can be seen as a clear signal – a further ironic jab – that shows how simple it would be for anyone to discover the hidden identity of these doctors, and also just how irrelevant that is.[8] Dermatologists are, after all, quite superfluous when it comes to Thomas Mann's real interest in syphilis, as it shall be shown.

The disappearance of the doctors also enables Thomas Mann to question the dividing line that proponents of the theory of degeneration, such as Möbius, drew between the healthy on the one hand and the insane, the criminal, the prostitute and the artist on the other. Echoing Max Nordau and his triad of mysticism, ego-addiction, and realism as the main causes of degeneracy, Möbius, in his Nietzsche book, further defines the latter category of artists as "Parnassisists and diabolists,

---

8 Incidentally, in his book on Nietzsche, Möbius also mentions the "Leipzig street directory" [Leipziger Adressbuche] (Möbius 1902, 11, n. 1). He consulted the 1902 edition to search for residents whose surname was identical with, or similar to, Nietzsche's in order to substantiate his claim that the "Saxon population generally contains many Slavic elements" [dass die sächsische Bevölkerung überhaupt sehr viel slavische Bestandtheile enthält] (*ibid.*). The randomness of such statistically insignificant evidence is perhaps parodied in Thomas Mann's usage of the Leipzig street directory in his *Doktor Faustus*. While Möbius is gathering Slavs from the Leipzig street directory, Adrian Leverkühn is gathering physicians from it.

[...] decadents and aesthetes" [Parnassier und Diaboliker, (...) Decadente(n) und Aestheten] (Möbius 1902, 35),[9] thereby including the entire literary avantgarde. Mann turns the table by presenting both doctors not only as marred by degeneracy, but introduces one of them as a criminal, which may indeed evoke historically justifiable facts on the readers' part, should they recall the cases of Franz v. Rinecker (1852) or Albert Neisser (1900) who had both been convicted of unethical conduct in connection with human experiments to do with syphilis (Elkeles 1985). Mann's fictional version of a dubious episode in Nietzsche's life also makes it possible to omit the realm of sexuality, which would have been impossible to neglect when it came to discussing the primary stages of syphilis. "A localized infection" (Mann 1999, 166; see also Mann 2007, 10.1, 228) is all that the author has to say on the topic. Contrary to Möbius and his lubricious inuendos, Thomas Mann is less interested in syphilis as a sexually transmitted disease that at least temporarily manifests itself on the sexual organs, than in the infectious disease that ultimately attacks the brain and thus relates to the fields of neurology and psychiatry, for which Mann himself had a far greater affinity. That syphilis is also an affliction of the soul and the intellect can also be seen in Adrian's actual infection experience. In direct contrast to Möbius, the narrator Serenus Zeitblom insists that it might have been possible that love was involved,[10] when Leverkühn first visited

9 To Nordau, "degeneracy" [Entartung] was a hereditary disease increasingly exacerbated through stress generated by modern urban life. Humans had to adapt to their environment in order to survive. Due to a "biochemical and biomechanical fault" [biochemischen und biomechanischen Störung] of the neurones and brain cells, the "degenerate" [Entarteten] lacked the pre-conditions of all adaptation and refinement: "attention" [Aufmerksamkeit], "will power" [Willensstärke] and "reason" [Urteil]. The "degenerate" were "not always criminals, prostitutes, anarchists and confirmed lunatics, but sometimes writers and artists" [nicht immer Verbrecher, Prostituierte, Anarchisten und erklärte Wahnsinnige. Sie sind manchmal Schriftsteller und Künstler]. 'Degeneracy' manifested itself, so the start of Nordau's string of verdicts, in "mysticism" [Mystizismus], "ego-addiction" [Ich-Sucht] and "realism" [Realismus]. The most objectionable mystics were the English pre-Raffaelites, the French symbolists, Tolstoi, Wagner and Maeterlinck; they were united in their "blurred and incoherent reasoning, the tyranny of their association of ideas, the occurrance of obsessive ideas, their erotic excitability, their excessive religious enthusiasm" [das verschwommene oder unzusammenhängende Denken, die Tyrannei der Ideen-Assoziation, das Auftreten von Zwangsvorstellungen, die erotische Erregbarkeit, die Glaubens-Schwärmerei]. The worst ego-addicts were the parnassicists (especially Baudelaire), the aesthetes (Huysmans, Wilde), Ibsen and Nietzsche – each of whom "a morally insane, a pessimist, an anarchist, a hater of humankind" [ein sittlich Irrsinniger, ein Pessimist, ein Anarchist, ein Hasser der Menschheit]. The worst realists were Zola and his followers who excelled in their "deliberate cultivation of pessimism and bawdiness" [absichtliche Pflege der Schwarzseherei und Unflätigkeit] (Nordau 1895; see also Schulte 1997, 233–252; Hartung 1997; Krummel 1998, 270–271).

10 "And, good heavens, was it not love as well [...]" (Mann 1999, 165; see also Mann 2007, 10.1, 226).

his "hetaera Esmeralda," and even followed her to "Pressburg, or Poszony as the Hungarians call it," after she "had to leave her former place of employment to undergo hospital treatment" (Mann 1999, 164; see also Mann 2007, 10.1, 225). Entirely in contrast to contemporary stereotypes of syphilitic prostitutes as the donors or perpetrators of the disease, and the man as the recipient or victim (Spongberg 1997), in the novel the initiative is taken by the man. And instead of a degenerate, amoral, depraved representative of a homogenous profession that must be policed and subjected to health controls, readers encounter a prostitute who has "heart" [Gemüt] (Mann 1999, 165; see also Mann 2007, 10.1, 225), tender emotions and a certain sense of responsibility. Esmeralda expressly warns Leverkühn to be wary of her body, and this information is italicised in the novel. It also strikes the narrator Zeitblom, as he goes on to say:

> [...] and does not that imply a gratifying disparity between the creature's higher humanity and that physical part of her, the vile commodity of trade cast to the gutter? The hapless woman warned the man who desired her against "herself" – and that means an act of the soul freely elevating itself above her pitiful physical existence, a humane act of distancing herself from it, an act of compassion, an act, if I may be permitted the word, of love. (Mann 1999, 165; see also Mann 2007, 10.1, 225 f.)

Here the humanist Zeitblom is speaking, someone who learned to talk of the individual and not the collective, who associates love and empathy with the object of his thoughts and writing, and who meets that object with respect and tact and with an open mind. How different is Möbius's self-empowerment, when, as a doctor, he declares a whole epoch – modernism – to be a patient, and as a medical expert takes this whole epoch and its representatives to task. How different his talk of "evacuation" in connection with Nietzsche's apocryphal brothel experience.

Now, Leverkühn contracts syphilis, but with the pathogenic agent [Erreger] he receives what Thomas Mann described as "intoxication, stimulant, inspiration"; the capacity to create "wonderful works of genius in a state of enraptured enthusiasm" (Mann 1992, 121), something that Möbius, according to his own testimony, had never seen in patients and of which experts he had asked would have none (Möbius 1902, 60). What in Mann's initial formulation of the novel's plot in his *Sieben-Zeilen-Plan* and, incidentally in Möbius's book (Möbius 1902, 1, 2, 49, 50), had been called "poison" will be called *Spirochaeta pallida*, or *Treponema pallidum*, as of 1905 when the bacterium was identified and named by the zoologist Fritz Schaudinn (1871–1906) and the dermatologist Erich Hoffmann (1868–1959). In *Doktor Faustus*, central motifs are interlinked through both terms – poison and spirochaete. Thomas Mann is, after all, a master in the simultaneous evocation of different historical periods.

Why are spirochaetes capable of stimulating Leverkühn's brain? A partial answer is because they are neurotropic. Let us listen to the devil, to whom Leverkühn has sold his soul for the acquisition of genius in his musical output even before having slept with Esmeralda:

> In short and plain, metaspirochaetosis, that is the meningeal process. And I do assure you that it is indeed as if some certain of these small folk may have a passion for the uppermost, a special estimation for the region of the head, the meninges, the dura mater, the tentorium, and the pia, which defend the tender parenchyma within, and would swarm ardently thither from the moment of that first general infection. (Mann 1999, 249; see also Mann 2007, 10.1, 340)

"Liebhaber der zerebralen Sphäre" (Mann 2007, 10.1, 341) – "brain specialists, whose pastime is the cerebral sphere" (Mann 1999, 249) in John E. Woods' excellent translation[11] – in these words, the devil resorts to a medico-scientific discourse of the early 20th century about the existence of a *virus nerveux*, that is, about the question, whether a special 'neurotropic' variety of the spirochaete exists which affects predominantly the nervous system in contrast to the ordinary 'dermotropic' variety which involves the skin and other tissues. The neurologist Max Nonne (1861–1959) reformulated this question by asking whether "the syphilitic toxin has, in general, in certain predisposed individuals, or in certain conditions as yet unexplained, a specially poisonous influence upon the nervous tissues" (Paul 1909, 353) and devotes an entire chapter of his 1909 monograph *Syphilis and Nervous System* to its discussion (Nonne 1909, ch. 3). Is there a *lues nervosa*, a *syphilis à virus nerveux?* The author is inclined to answer the question in the affirmative, but suspends final judgement. The notion of a *virus nerveux* or of a syphilitic toxin is not to be found in Möbius, but Thomas Mann was familiar with this debate, as its key term – *virus nerveux* – is explicitly mentioned in the novel (Mann 2007, 341). He read about it in considerable detail in Wilhelm Gennerich's[12] (1877–1951) book *Die Syphilis des Zentralnervensystems*

---

11 For a harsher view on Woods' translation skills, see Buck 2002, 245–247.

12 Wilhelm Ferdinand Claus Gennerich received his physician's licence on 1 February 1901, became a consultant [Facharzt] for skin and venereal diseases in 1907/08, worked from February 1917 until March 1918 in the rank of a Major in the medical corps of the navy as the chief physician at the Fort Military Hospital in Kiel Ravensberg, before becoming the head of the dermatological department of the navy hospital Kiel Wik. Gennerich joined the National Socialist Party (NSDAP) on 1.5.1933 (membership no.: 2730621), became a member of the National Socialist German Association of Physicians [NSD-Ärztebund], an assessor at the Hereditary Health Court [Erbgesundheitsgericht], opened a medical practice in Kiel and was promoted to Lieutenant Colonel [Generaloberarzt]. I am grateful to Ms S. Langner from the Bundesarchiv in Berlin for providing photocopies of documents preserved in the former Berlin Document Center and in the Reich's inventory of doctors [Reichsärzteregister]. Why Thomas Mann chose Gen-

[The Syphilis of the Central Nervous System] published in 1921. Gennerich considered meningeal syphilis an important link between primary syphilis and metalues of the central nervous system. In Thomas Mann's copy of Gennerich's book, which survives in the Thomas Mann Archive in Zurich (TMA, Thomas Mann 4982), we find those passages underlined[13] that support the thesis of a neurotropic and neurophilic property of *spirochaeta pallida:* Gennerich's initial question whether a *virus nerveux* exists, that is to say "a virus with a particular penchant for the meninges" [mit einer besonderen Vorliebe für die Meningen] (Gennerich 1921, 3) is not only marked in the margin, but also underlined, suggesting a high degree of relevance, according to Thomas Mann's personal technique of marking passages for verbatim incorporation into his own writings. The same is true of Gennerich's phrase "increased sowing of spirochaetes towards the head region" [einer vermehrten Spirochätenaussaat nach der Kopfregion] (*ibid.*, 5) and his conclusion "that all diseases of the central nervous system

---

nerich's rather widely distributed and much discussed book as a source book for his novel, illustrate the first lines of a review (Anon. 1921, 462): "Gennerich has produced a monograph on syphilis of the central nervous system considered from the point of view of the syphilologist who looks on central nervous system involvement as merely one incident in the course of syphilis. His is not the point of view of the neurologist; he is not interested especially in symptomatology or nosology or even to any large extent in pathology. What he has done is to attempt to study the life history (Ursachen) of syphilis as it affects the central nervous system from the primary stage until the end of life of the individual."

13 This is at least the *opinio communis.* See Mann 1982, 1944–46, 352. On p. 20 of Thomas Mann's copy of Gennerich's book, however, in the left margin, there is a handwritten comment in pencil ("Unterschied // kann an // Kranken liegen?" [difference may be attributable to patients?]), which definitely does not show Mann's characteristic hand. This observation raises the question, whether all underlinings and annotations to be found in Gennerich's book can be attributed to Thomas Mann. It seems to me that all underlinings made with the help of a ruler as well as the combination of underlining a passage and highlighting it in the margin reveal Thomas Mann's reader response, whereas highlighting via arrows or unevenly drawn lines should be attributed to a prior owner of this copy. Martin Gumpert could be a candidate. In Thomas Mann's extant notes to his novel, we find excerpts, paraphrases or summaries of paragraphs to be found in Gennerich's book. In the cases of such parallels, it is safe to attribute the respective underlinings and highlighting in the margins to Thomas Mann. See Zurich, Thomas Mann Archiv, "Notizen zum Doktor Faustus", Ms 33, ff. 167v-168. I am grateful to Dr Katrin Bedenig and Ms. Gabi Hollender from the archive for making copies of this handwritten material available to me. The quote from Gennerich 1921, 38 given above appears in Thomas Mann's notes (Ms 33, f. 168) as: "Durch Syphilis verursachte Erkrankungen des Z.N.S. reichen auf die Infektion der zerebralen Pia u. zwar zumeist ihrer basalen Teile zurück." The quote from Gennerich 1921, 46 appears in these notes (Ms 33, sheet with letter head of The Library of Congress inserted between f. 167 and f. 168) as: "Die über 1–2 Jahrzehnte sich erstreckende schleichende syphilitische Meningitis (histologische Hirnlues) ist Grundlage und Vorstadium der Paralyse."

caused by syphilis can be traced back to the inflammation of the cerebral pia [mater], mostly its basal parts" [daß alle durch Syphilis verursachten Erkrankungen des ZNS zunächst auf die Infektion der zerebralen Pia und zwar zumeist ihrer basalen Teile zurückreichen] (*ibid.*, 38). Thomas Mann even uses an exclamation mark plus underlining after having read Gennerich's further conclusion "that syphilitic meningitis lasting and lingering for up to two decades [...] is the basis and prodromal stage of general paralysis" [daß in erster Linie die über viele Jahre (1–2 Jahrzehnte) sich erstreckende schleichende syphilitische Meningitis (...) Grundlage und Vorstadium der Paralyse bildet] (*ibid.*, 46). Gennerich interprets the metalues or metasyphilis, both of which he uses as umbrella terms for tabes dorsalis and general paralysis, as a meningitis of the convexity of the cerebrum, the symptoms of which include (according to Otto Heubner):

> a modest disgruntlement or irritability swiftly exacerbating into, respectively, melancholy or mania, occasionally also followed by considerable impairment of intelligence and weakness of memory, as we see them in paralytic dementia. The pronounced mood swings, the almost simultaneous weeping and laughing, the pliability of the intellect, the fleetingness of intellectual ideas, and the slowness of thought processes are all characteristic of these mental disorders caused by syphilis. [in einer mäßigen Verstimmung oder Gereiztheit, die aber auf der einen Seite in Melancholie, auf der anderen in Manie schnell übergeht, zuweilen auch bald von einer erheblichen Intelligenz- und Gedächtnisschwäche gefolgt ist. Diese letztere hat Ähnlichkeit mit derjenigen, wie sie bei der Dementia paralytica beobachtet wird. Die große Veränderlichkeit der Stimmung, das Weinen und Lachen oft in derselben Minute, die Biegsamkeit und geringe Fixierung aller geistigen Vorstellungen, die Langsamkeit des Denkens zeichnen diese syphilitischen Geistesstörungen besonders aus]. (*ibid.*, 70)

Given Thomas Mann's highly artistic blending in *Doktor Faustus* of the motifs of syphilis and paralysis on the one hand and melancholy on the other, it is not surprising that the writer also marked this passage in the margins of Gennerich's book. Such signs of use illustrate that the writer felt medically authorized to ascribe the sort of 'cerebrosity' to the spirochaetes that the devil is talking about.

Another passage from the devil's speech in chapter 25 of the novel highlights a medico-scientific debate that to some extent replaced the discourse on a particular neurotropic strand of spirochaetes after the 1910s and is hence also absent from Möbius's book. Let us listen to the devil again whose pronouncements are the fruits of Thomas Mann's further medical studies and enquiries:

> It is rather contrariwise. It is the brain that lusts after a visit and waits expectant for theirs. [...] There you have it, the disposition, the readiness, the invitation is all. (Mann 1999, 249; see also Mann 2007, 10.1, 341)

In the 1920s opposition against orthodox bacteriology had grown. This opposition shifted the emphasis from the agent causing syphilis and the laboratory where it was studied, to the people that were seen to host the agent and to the hospitals where carriers and patients were diagnosed and treated. Disposition and constitution became the catch phrases of a faction who considered neither bacterial agents nor humans statically caught in a stimulus response model. The new trend was highly critical of the monocausal, unilateral and reductionist thinking in the realm of their discipline. In the wake of such altered modes of thinking, the clinical case took centre-stage again and the hospital started reclaiming its previous role as a hub for generating new medical knowledge and increasing the efficacy of medicine.[14] Instead of mapping pathogenic agents or systematizing diseases into nosologies – both predominant activities of orthodox bacteriologists – the new trend favoured the systematisation of constitutional types. Such endeavours facilitated a new holism in medicine that led to a new vitalism and humoralism (Berger 2009, 291–390). Syphilis, according to this seemingly simple message, doesn't exactly equate to syphilis. Thomas Mann could not have agreed more. He was clearly concerned with a specific, individual course of disease, not with a paradigm. He was concerned with a 'patient,' not a disease. The painter Baptist Spengler and the composer Adrian Leverkühn are not comparable, despite sharing the syphilitic disease and heading towards general paralysis. The devil knows and informs Leverkühn that in Spengler's case,

---

14 Vgl. Wawrzik, 1938, 661: "Ohne mich in Einzelheiten dieses an Spekulationen immer sehr reichen Gebietes zu verlieren, möchte ich nur andeuten, dass wir heute wieder prinzipiell nicht wesentlich fortgeschritten sind gegenüber den Beobachtungen und Konsequenzen Charcots, Erbs und anderer Forscher der Vorspirochätenzeit, die sämtlich im konstitutionellen Moment die wesentliche Ursache [der Metalues] zu erblicken glaubten – eine Ansicht, die unter dem Eindruck der Lues-Tabes-Lehre und insbesondere des Nachweises der Spirochäten im Gehirn und Rückenmark mehr und mehr an Bedeutung verlor, um schliesslich eine Zeitlang der Lehre vom Virus nerveux ganz den Platz einzuräumen. Heute hingegen hat man bei Durchsicht der Literatur der letzten 20 Jahre den Eindruck, dass in der Aetiologie der Metalues, der angeborenen sowie der erworbenen, der Schwerpunkt wieder auf das endogene Moment gelegt wird." [Without getting bogged down in details on this field highly charged with speculations, I would like to merely indicate that today we are essentially not fundamentally advanced, compared with the observations and conclusions of Charcot, Erb and other researchers of the pre-spirochaete era who all considered the constitutional factor to be the main cause (of metalues) – a point of view, which became less and less important in the face of the lues-tabes doctrine and especially the detection of spirochaetes in brain tissue and in the medulla, until eventually, if only temporarily, it gave completely way to the doctrine of the virus nerveux. When going through the literature of the past twenty years, one gets the impression that, as far as the aetiology of metalues is concerned, both in its congenital and acquired form, the emphasis is placed again on the endogenous factor.]

"no metastasis [dissemination] to the metaphysical, metavenerial, metainfectious" (Mann 1999, 248; see also Mann 2007, 10.1, 340) will occur. As a result of his disease, the devil continues, even Spengler had "grown a bit cannier, more given to the intellect" (Mann 1999, 248; see also Mann 2007, 10.1, 339) but apart from such seeking refuge in "free thought, in books, in study" (*ibid.*) he was a "dull and humdrum case, without least consequence" (*ibid*). In short a

> man of the world, lightly singed and stale, of demi-interest, nothing more. He will cripple along with liver, kidneys, stomach, heart, and gut, and one day be all hoarse of voice or deaf and after a few years will perish inglorious, a sceptical jest upon his lips – but what else? There was nothing to it, there was never an illumination, enhancement, and excitation, for it was not of the brain, was not cerebrose, you see – our small folk had no concern for his noble, uppermost part, which parently had no allurement for them [...] (Mann 1999, 248; see also Mann 2007, 10.1, 339 f.)

Leverkühn's disposition is in stark contrast with Spengler's: according to the devil, Leverkühn is "a case of favourable disposition, out of which, presupposing but a little enkindling, incitement, and inebriation, something lustrous might be made" (Mann 1999, 244; see also Mann 2007, 10.1, 334). "A little tickle of hyperemia" (Mann 1999, 252; see also Mann 2007, 10.1, 345) not only sweeps away weariness, it even leads to authentic inspiration, to "genuine, ancient, primal enthusiasm," to "holy rapture" (Mann 1999, 252; see also Mann 2007, 10.1, 346). Leverkühn represents a *typus cerebralis,* whose disposition yearns for the visitation of the cerebrose spirochaetes and whose headache [Hauptweh] predisposes him for such visitation, whilst also revealing, why "Erreger" are called "Erreger" (the German word 'erregen' means 'arouse', 'excite', 'energize', 'stimulate'). The devil speaks the truth when claiming to keep continuously informed about the latest medico-scientific developments. This is as much true of the debate around the *virus nerveux*, the obsoleteness of which the Devil acknowledges with his reservation, "Item, several *doctores* would claim and swear by all swearing's worth..." (Mann 1999, 249; see also Mann 2007, 10.1, 341), as it is of the more recent developments in constitutional medicine.

Our considerations have now sufficiently facilitated a better understanding of a related medical debate to the extent that I would now like to sketch briefly in the remainder of this essay: the genius-releasing properties of syphilis *strictu sensu*. Quite surprisingly, this debate brings us back to Möbius's book. Even this motif, the popularity of which in non-medical literature has been noted by a number of scholars, has a medical *fundamentum in re*. Long before the identification of the spirochaete and its isolation from brain tissue, physicians seriously discussed whether syphilis was capable of increasing the cognitive, intellectual and affective faculties of those afflicted, at least temporarily.[15] The French physician Victor Parant (1848–1924) devoted an entire article to this question which was published in 1887 in the *Annales médico-psychologiques,* incidentally one of the few publications referenced in Möbius's book on Nietzsche (Möbius 1902, 60, n. 2). In this article, Parant assembled a number of case histories of patients from the Maison de Santé in Toulouse, of which he was medical director (Parant 1887, 36–49). These case histories seemed to confirm the thesis of a "suractivité intellectuelle" during the prodromal phase of general paralysis, as it circulated in the research literature of the time. In a second part of his article (*ibid.*, 212–232; see also Terrisse 1984, 277), Parant provides an overview of the state of research at the time and mentions in chronological order Jacques Joseph Moreau (1804–1884) (Moreau 1859), Jules Falret (1824–1902) (Falret 1866), Emmanuel Régis (1855–1918) (Régis 1879), Benjamin Ball (1833–1893) (Ball 1880) and Auguste Félix Voisin (1829–1898) (Voisin 1880) as proponents of the theory that the prodromal phase of general paralysis "is characterised, in some cases, by an intellectual overactivity, without delir or dementia" [est charactérisé, dans quelque cas, par la suractivité intellectuelle, sans délire et sans démence] (Parant 1887, 231 f.).[16] Based on the experiential evidence of his case histories, Parant advances the opinion that such enhancement of cognitive, intellectual and affective properties could continue over a longer period of time than generally assumed, did not necessarily build on pre-existing abilities, and was frequently associated with alcoholism. In some people, alcohol apparently worked hand in hand with the syphilitic poison in stimulating people rather than numbing them. Pathophysiologically, he contemplates functional changes in the brain and speaks, just like the devil in *Doktor Faustus* (Mann 1999, 252: "We stimulate and, with but a little tickle of hyperaemia, we sweep away weariness – be it small or large, private or that of the age."), much more confidently than Möbius of hyperemia (Parant 1887, 224). The debate about the genius-releasing properties of syphilis needs

15 An example of such an offshoot provides Jules Audrain (b. 1867) in *La syphilis obscure.* Paris: O. Doin, 1911, as quoted in Quétel 1990, 173: "The increased appetite becomes bulimic [...] The psycho-intellectual functions are generally or partially enhanced. It produces the archetypal cripple endowed with superior intelligence – Velasquez' [sic] dwarf with the most penetrating gaze that painting has ever reproduced."

16 To cite just one quotation from the works evoked by Parant, Ball writes in his *Leçons* (Ball 1880, 706): "During this period of exaltation or functional dynamism, one sees in sufferers [of early stages of paralysis] a stimulation of their intellectual capacities, which seems to make them more intelligent and more brilliant than they have ever been." [Pendant cette période d'exaltation ou de dynamie fonctionelle, on constate chez les malades [...] une stimulation des facultés intellectuelles, que semble les rendre plus intelligentes et plus brillants qu'ils ne l'avaient jamais été.].

to be seen in the context of the Société Médico-Psychologique founded in 1852 and the concept of *folie raisonnante*, a delusional form of any psychosis marked by a thought process that seems logical but lacks common sense, which featured highly on the Society's research agenda (Haustgen, Bourgeois 2002, 733). The debate about a *virus nerveux* or a syphilitic toxin can be considered later offshoots of discussions within the Société Médico-Psychologique on the superactivité intellectuelle. Möbius distanced himself from it in unambiguous terms, Thomas Mann seems to have embraced it.

To conclude, let us consider what the "grand mythe syphilitique" (Goens 1995, 152) and its medical authentication, as shown, does in the context of the poetological conception of Thomas Mann's novel. First of all, it is a clear counter-myth of Möbius's – and later the National Socialists' – negative myth of syphilis. Thomas Mann mobilises those trends within medico-scientific research and discourse that enable him to support his ambition to write a story of rise and decline instead of the linear story of biologically destined decline provided by Möbius. Quite ironically, Möbius's book starts with the line "Friedrich Nietzsche, a man of genius [...]" [Friedrich Nietzsche, ein genialer Mensch (...)] (Möbius 1902, 1).[17] From such a beginning, there is only one direction: downwards.[18] Let us remember that chapter one of Thomas Mann's *Magic Mountain* starts with the line "An ordinary young man" (Mann 2005, 3). As such, the protagonist can develop, can go on a quest for his innermost being, find out who he is, grow with the tasks he is given and the encounters he makes, become a true individual in whose name the reader gets interested. Secondly, the positive syphilis myth, in all its fictitiousness, represents one side of a coin, the verso of which was the negative myth of syphilis à la Möbius, Nordau and others, whose degenerational and hereditarian underpinnings of syphilis had been unmasked as equally fictitious, at least by the time Thomas Mann was writing his novel. Behind this verso's medico-scientific façade there was nothing left but story-telling, emplotment, and evoking emotions on the reader's part. Even when it came to medical matters, the medical prose writer appeared by no means more credible or more objective than the narrator of fiction. Both had landed in the same boat, which we would now call the boat of narration or, more

---

17 On p. 13, Nietzsche has already been 'downgraded' to an "unhappy human being of genius" [unglücklich genialen Menschen].

18 Unless "genius" is meant here by Möbius in the same derogatory sense delineated on p. 29 of his book: "The lack of harmony, the uneven development of individual faculties generally defines great talents and men of genius: in this sense, they all are pathological and results of degeneracy." [Der Mangel an Harmonie, die ungleichmässige Entwicklung der einzelnen Fähigkeiten ist das Merkmal der grossen Talente und der Genies überhaupt: sie sind in diesem Sinne sammt und sonders pathologisch und Ergebnisse der Entartung] (Möbius 1902, 29).

specifically and technically, of imaginative writing. Only Thomas Mann, as millions of readers of his *Doktor Faustus* would agree, rows it so much better than Möbius. The positive myth also allows Thomas Mann enormous historical depth, as he continuously links it with the tradition of melancholy, from which the debate about genius and madness [Genie und Wahnsinn] originates. I have only to mention the famous ps-Aristotelian Problema 30,1 translated into the early modern world by Marsilio Ficino whom Thomas Mann quotes (Rütten, 2002). Again Möbius, by contrast, had explicitly stated that Nietzsche had not been melancholic (Möbius 1902, 31). Furthermore, the positive myth of syphilis outweighs the burden of degenerationism and hereditarianism, which Thomas Mann accepted throughout his life as determining factors of human life. But this did not render him a determinist. Even under the aggravating conditions of a Devil's pact, he was interested in room for manoeuvre left to an individual who kept striving for humanity, integrity, dignity. He was interested in the "all the same" [Dennoch] that unites most of his protagonists, in their perseverance [Durchhalten], in their attempts to achieve something in life against all odds. In this context, story-telling is not, as Möbius would have argued, the auto-erotic satisfaction of a "compelling writer's drive" [Schriftsteller-Triebe] (Möbius 1902, 16), or a "yearning for applause" [Beifallsliebe] (*ibid.*, 23), a sign of graphomania or moral insanity. Rather, it is an essential way of breaking free from the factors that seem to determine our lives, limit our freedom and chances to develop into more humane human beings. Möbius's Nietzsche fills the reader with disgust. Leverkühn arouses compassion, and respect for the dignity of a human caught in a tragedy and for his work. The medical set-pieces Thomas Mann chose to incorporate, primarily in opposition to, and at times playful, humorous dissociation from, Möbius clearly helped to give that impression.

References

Archival sources

Berlin, Bundesarchiv, membership cards of Wilhelm Gennerich in the membership files of the NSDAP [NSDAP Gaukartei] and the Reich's Chamber of Physicians [Reichsärztekammer] and entry from the Reich's register of physicians [Reichsärzteregister].

Zurich, Thomas Mann Archiv. "Notizen zum Doktor Faustus". Ms 33, ff. 167v-168.

Printed material

Anon. "Die Syphilis des Zentralnervensystems. Ihre Ursachen und Behandlung (Syphilis of the central nervous system. Its pathogenesis and treatment)." *Archives of Neurology and Psychiatry* 6.4 (1921): 462–466.

Audrain, Jules. *La syphilis obscure.* Paris: O. Doin, 1911.

Ball, Benjamin. *Leçons sur les maladies mentales.* 2nd ed. Paris: Asselin, 1880.

Berger, Silvia. *Bakterien in Krieg und Frieden. Eine Geschichte der medizinischen Bakteriologie in Deutschland 1890–1933.* Göttingen: Wallstein, 2009.

Buck, Timothy. "Mann in English." *The Cambridge Companion to Thomas Mann.* Ed. Ritchie Robertson. Cambridge: Cambridge University Press, 2002. 235–248.

Dohm, Hedwig. *Die Antifeministen: Ein Buch der Verteidigung.* Berlin: Dümmler, 1902.

Elkeles, Barbara. "Medizinische Menschenversuche gegen Ende des 19. Jahrhunderts und der Fall Neisser. Rechtfertigung und Kritik einer wissenschaftlichen Methode." *Medizinhistorisches Journal* 20 (1985): 135–148.

Elsaghe, Yahya. *Krankheit und Matriarchat. Thomas Manns* Betrogene *im Kontext.* Berlin, New York, NY: de Gruyter, 2010 (= Quellen und Forschungen zur Literatur- und Kulturgeschichte. V. 53).

Falret, Jules. *De la folie raisonnante au folie morale, programme de questions à étudier. Discours prononcé à la Société médico-psychologique dans la séance du 8 janvier 1866.* Paris: E. Martinez, 1866.

Gennerich, Wilhelm. *Die Syphilis des Zentralnervensystems. Ihre Ursachen und Behandlung.* Berlin: Springer, 1921.

Goens, Jean. *De la syphilis au sida: Cinq siècles des mémoires littéraires de Vénus.* Brussels: Presses Interuniversitaires Européennes, 1995.

Hartung, Stefan. *Parnasse und Moderne: Théodore de Banvilles "Odes funambulesques" (1857). Parisdichtung als Ästhetik des Heterogenen.* Stuttgart: Steiner, 1997.

Haustgen, Thierry, and Marc-Louis Bourgeois. "Cinquante ans d'histoire des psychoses à la Société médico-psychologique (1852–1902)." *Annales médico-psychologiques, revue psychiatrique* 160 (2002): 730–738.

Hildebrandt, Kurt. *Gesundheit und Krankheit in Nietzsches Leben und Werk.* Berlin: Karger, 1926.

Krummel, Frank. *Ausbreitung und Wirkung des Nietzscheschen Werkes im deutschen Sprachraum vom Todesjahr bis zum Ende des Ersten Weltkrieges: Ein Schrifttumsverzeichnis der Jahre 1901–1918.* 2nd rev. and augm. ed. Berlin, New York, NY: de Gruyter, 1998.

Lange-Eichbaum, Wilhelm. *Nietzsche: Krankheit und Wirkung.* Hamburg: Lettenbauer, 1947.

Mann, Thomas. *Tagebücher 1940–1943.* Ed. Peter de Mendelssohn. Frankfurt a. M.: Fischer, 1982.

Mann, Thomas. *Notizbücher 1–14.* Ed. Hans Wysling. 2 vols. Frankfurt a. M.: Fischer, 1991–92. Vol. 2. 1992.

Mann, Thomas. *Doktor Faustus. Das Leben des deutschen Tonsetzers Adrian Leverkühn, erzählt von einemm Freunde.* Eds Ruprecht Wimmer and Stephan Stachorski. Text and Commentary in 2 vols. Frankfurt a. M.: Fischer, 2007 (= Thomas Mann. Große kommentierte Frankfurter Ausgabe. V. 10.1 and 10.2).

Mann, Thomas. *Essays VI. 1945–1950.* Ed. Herbert Lehnert. Text and Commentary in 2 vols. Frankfurt a. M.: Fischer, 2009 (= Thomas Mann. Große kommentierte Frankfurter Ausgabe. V. 19.1 and 19.2)

Mann, Thomas. *Doctor Faustus: The Life of the German Composer Adrian Leverkühn As Told by a Friend. Translated from the German by John E. Woods.* (New York, NY: Alfred A. Knopf, 1997) New York, NY: Random House, 1999.

Mann, Thomas. *The Magic Mountain: A novel. Translated from the German by John E. Woods.* (New York, London, Toronto: Alfred A. Knopf, 1995) Everyman's Library, No. 289, 2005.

Max, Katrin. *Niedergangsdiagnostik: Zur Funktion von Krankheitsmotiven in "Buddenbrooks".* Frankfurt a. M.: Klostermann, 2008 (= Thomas Mann Studien. V. 40).

Mendelssohn, Peter de. *Der Zauberer. Das Leben des deutschen Schriftstellers Thomas Mann.* Frankfurt a. M.: Fischer, 1996.

Möbius, Paul J. *Über den physiologischen Schwachsinn des Weibes.* Halle a. S.: Marhold, 1900.

Möbius, Paul J. *Ueber das Pathologische bei Nietzsche.* Wiesbaden: J. F. Bergmann, 1902 (= Grenzfragen des Nerven- und Seelenlebens, 17).

Möbius, Paul J. *Nietzsche.* 3rd ed. Leipzig: J. A. Barth, 1909 (= Ausgewählte Werke. V. 5).

Nonne, Max. *Syphilis und Nervensystem: 19 Vorlesungen für praktische Ärzte, Neurologen und Syphilidologen.* 2nd rev. and enl. ed. Berlin: Karger, 1909.

Nordau, Max. *Degeneration. Transl. from the 2nd ed. of the German Work.* 5th ed. New York, NY: D. Appleton, 1895.

Moreau, Jacques Joseph. *La psychologie morbide dans ses rapports avec la philosophie de l'histoire, ou De l'influence des névropathies sur le dynamisme intellectuel.* Paris: V. Masson, 1859.

Parant, Victor. "De la suractivité intellectuelle sans délire ni démence." *Annales médico-psychologiques* (1887): 34–49, 212–232.

Paul, Eden P. "Syphilis and the Nervous System [Syphilis und Nervensystem]. By Dr. Max Nonne. Berlin: S. Karger, 1909." *The British Journal of Psychiatry* 55 (1909): 350–360.

Peters, Heinz F. *Zarathustra's Sister: The Case of Elisabeth and Friedrich Nietzsche.* New York, NY: Crown, 1977.

Podach, Erich. *Nietzsches Zusammenbruch: Beiträge zu einer Biographie auf Grund unveröffentlichter Dokumente.* Heidelberg: Kampmann, 1930.

Quétel, Claude. *The History of Syphilis.* Tr. Judith Braddock and Brian Pike. Baltimore, MA: Johns Hopkins University Press, 1990.

Régis, Emmanuel. *De la dynamie ou exaltation fonctionnelle au début de la paralysie générale.* Paris: Donnaud, 1879.

Rütten, Thomas. "Krankheit und Genie: Annäherungen an Frühformen einer Mannschen Denkfigur." *Literatur und Krankheit im fin-de-siècle (1890–1914).* Ed. Thomas Sprecher. Frankfurt a. M.: Klostermann, 2002. 131–170.

Sax, Leonard. "What was the cause of Nietzsche's dementia?" *Journal of Medical Biography* 11 (2003): 47–54.

Schulte, Christoph, *Psychopathologie des Fin de siècle. Der Kulturkritiker, Arzt und Zionist Max Nordau.* Frankfurt a. M.: Fischer Taschenbuch Verlag, 1997.

Spongberg, Mary. *Feminizing Venereal Disease: The Body of the Prostitute in Nineteenth-Century Medical Discourse.* New York, NY: New York University Press, 1997.

Terrisse, Arnaud. "La psychiatrie en France dans le miroir de la thèse: l'évolution des thèses de médecine psychiatrique françaises du début du XVIIème siècle à 1934 d'après le

fichier des thèses de médecine de la Bibliothèque Nationale." *Histoire, économie et société* 3 (1984): 247–292.
Voisin, Auguste Félix. *De la mélancolie dans ses rapports avec la paralysie générale.* Paris: G. Masson, 1880.
Volz, Pia Daniela. *Nietzsche im Labyrinth seiner Krankheit. Eine medizinisch-biographische Untersuchung.* Würzburg: Königshausen & Neumann, 1990.
Wawrzik, Fritz. "Ueber konsanguine juvenile Tabo-Paralyse." *European Archives of Psychiatry and Clinical Neurosciences* 108.5 (1938): 661–667.

Luis Montiel*

Aweysha: Spiritual Epidemics and Psychic Contagion in the Works of Gustav Meyrink

1 Introduction

Almost twenty years ago I began studying the work of Gustav Meyrink (1868–1932), intrigued by the striking correspondence I noticed between his esoteric thinking and the analytical psychology of Carl Gustav Jung, developed at best in parallel with the Austrian writer's novelistic output, and often later (Montiel 1998). Since then, I have become more and more convinced that Meyrink is a much more interesting writer than is commonly recognized. I recently tried to show, I think successfully, that his way of imagining – and living – the occult, and his dissemination of it through his novels, authentic best-sellers in the early decades of the twentieth century, sensitized European society towards the new field of psychoanalysis.

In any case, Meyrink's world-view must be considered as occupying a position far on the fringe of the dominant ideas of his time and also of today. However much we may be able to rescue a large part of his message for intellectual orthodoxy, there still remain sections in it which are totally inconsistent with this orthodoxy. However, the surprising fact noted at the beginning – that the pseudoscience of the occult could unexpectedly lead to valuable, socially recognized although controversial knowledge – prevents me from ignoring those other areas of his thinking that are more difficult to incorporate into our way of seeing the world. If I have argued in the book mentioned at the outset that Gustav Meyrink discovered for himself the psychic event that Jung called the "individuation process" and reflected it in his novels, I inevitably have to ask myself whether his idea of psychic contagion could actually have some significance for us, the non-occultists. This is the objective of this paper.

* History of Medicine. Faculty of Medicine. Complutense University of Madrid (Spain). This study was sponsored by the research project HAR2008–04899-C02–02.

2 On Magic as a "Force of the Soul," and the Energetic and Material Condition of the Psychic

In the pages of the most detailed and committed of his texts dedicated to the description and evaluation of his occult experiences, *Die Verwandlung des Blutes* [The Transformation of the Blood][1], there is a phrase which for me is of great value from the point of view of this paper. The phrase in question represents a criticism of the unilateral nature of the intellectual progress of Western thought. Our culture, says Meyrink, has made great advances in terms of the explanation of natural laws; but not only has it not made similar progress, but it has actually regressed in so far as "instinct" is concerned. He goes on to declare that in contemporary thinking "whatever has to do with magic and the other occult forces of the soul, he believes wrongly either does not exist or has no importance" [(...) was mit Magie und den andern verborgenen Kräften der Seele zusammenhängt, wähnt er, dergleichen existiere überhaupt nicht oder sei gering zu schätzen] (Meyrink 1981 [ca. 1928], 205).

Note that the writer has not associated magic with supernatural powers, or at least not with powers outside man himself, as happens in the traditional interpretation, but considers it to be one among several "occult forces of the soul": a psychic ability. Indeed, only from this point of view does his criticism of science have any meaning, since science appears to take for granted the fact that magic is none of its business but is, at best, the business of religion: a diabolical or divine subject. Clearly, Meyrink is not alone in his way of interpreting phenomena which are considered as magic; occultism as a whole is a more or less specific attempt to erase the frontiers between the actual human being and what may be generically referred to as "the beyond" (Treitel 2004, 8, 14–16). But this declaration should be taken as a starting point to interpret Meyrink's work correctly, and we should also note that, in this phrase, not all the alleged occult forces of the soul fall under the name of "magic": divination, premonition, visionary ability, all of which are documented by Meyrink in various of his writings, are not, as I understand it, "magic" for him. Otherwise, why make such a distinction in the phrase quoted? Magic must be, although he does not say so explicitly, the ability to modify reality without the mediation of any material agency; in other words, by means of what has been classically known – and considered to be the essence of magical activity – as "actio in distans" (Rothschuh 1978, 107). But in Meyrink's opinion this involves no pact with

1 This is a text of uncertain date, very probably written in 1927 or 1928. It was only published after the death of its author.

the underworld, but simply spiritual activity; so inevitably we have to ask ourselves what exactly the writer means by "spirit".

Indeed – this is a word too laden with meaning, even with meanings that change over history and depend on the beliefs of each individual. So it is easy to understand different things when it is said or written; and what is worse, each of us adapts it to our own way of thinking. A clue to help us understand what Meyrink meant whenever he referred to this aspect of humanity is to be found in his article entitled *Fakirpfade* [The Paths of the Fakirs]. Here, he describes the result of his own ecstatic experiences resulting from the practice of yoga. These ecstasies, which he refers to in the text more crudely and less grandly as "catalepsy," are experienced as a radical separation, in which the human is divided into a bodily part and a shapeless force. He tells us that this is, ultimately, the real situation of any person, who is continuously surrounded by invisible figures that, when they become visible – for example, by the use of hallucinogenic substances or through yoga – are wrongly thought to be spirits of the dead. When this division takes place, and one becomes aware of it, it is because an unknown spiritual force has been released, bringing these images to life in the same way – he says – as electricity affects frogs in Galvani's experiment. But with yoga exercises, he adds, these figures are eliminated, as Hercules eliminated the heads of the Hydra (Meyrink 1993 [1907b], 236).

From the outset we can see in this declaration how the author disassociates himself explicitly – and radically – from what we might call the hard core of the occult: spiritism. The disembodied presences that some observe are not the spirits of the dead, but spiritual – I think we might say "psychic" – emanations from the person himself or herself; emanations which, in the logic of the concept of psychic energy that Meyrink believes in, are always present even though they are only seen in very special circumstances. And in this way we begin to understand what "spirit" means for him: something which accompanies the material body in an extremely subtle way – so much so that it is generally not perceivable – and secretly fluid, moving not only within him but also in his surroundings, as if it were an emanation of the body itself. Or is the body rather an emanation of the spirit in a coarse but also ephemeral form?

I think this is the opinion, the belief, of Gustav Meyrink, as shown by a reference he makes to one of the great figures of the Western Hermetic Tradition:

> The medieval magician Agrippa von Nettesheim coined this phrase: '*nos habitat non tartara sed nec sidera coeli: spiritus in nobis qui viget, illa facit*' [...] It dwells within us, not in the nether world, nor in the stars of the heavens: the Spirit which lives within us does it all. [Der mittelalterliche Magier Agrippa von Nettesheim hat den Satz geprägt: '*nos habitat non tartara sed nec sidera coeli: spiritus in nobis qui viget, illa facit*' (...) Nicht Gestirn noch Unterwelt: in uns allein der Geist ist's, der alles bewirkt.] (Meyrink, 1993 [ca. 1928], 281)

But this principle is far from clear: "the spirit *which lives within us*" [emphasis mine]. Once again we have to turn to his criticisms of spiritism to see just how demanding is his concept of the human condition, following neither purely materialist theories nor those which are purely spiritualist. In the text entitled *An der Grenze des Jenseits* [On the Borders of the Beyond] he once again writes about these figures which are only perceptible in special situations, which spiritists identify as ghosts, maintaining that they are just as material as the bodies of human beings, and belong to the realm of the material just as Röntgen's X-rays do (Meyrink 1993 [1923], 372–373). So, where does this leave us? Are they spiritual or are they material?

The answer must be: both. What happens is that both thought and word are insufficient to represent these phenomena which, by definition, are marginal. They are spiritual, but emanating from the "spirit which lives within us," an embodied spirit which is, and at the same time is not, what is called "the spiritually pure" [Reingeistig(en)], "the eternal cause" [Ewige(n) Ursache] (Meyrink 1993 [1923], 372–373). These "spiritual" phenomena are so inseparably linked to the material, that they can be said to be "as material as X-rays"[2]: "hidden forces of the soul"; and, as the Western tradition well knows, the soul is the wonderfully subtle amphibious entity that lives at the same time in the spirit and in the body and which, by living, gives life to both in temporal terms, on this side of a supposed eternity.

We have been able summarily – although helped by the certainty of being able to refer to the writer's own words – to explain just how Meyrink sees magical ability; a concept that, although not exclusively, is firmly based on the psychic seen as something purely natural. This is what distinguishes his world view from what we may call "popular" occultism, but which also gives him a very special singularity when compared to the "scientist," who is reluctantly limited by the rules of the game of materialistic experimental science (Treitel 2004, 8–12). Meyrink will need no laboratory equipment to argue his belief in this controversial spiritual domain, referring in the last instance to his own experiences, of which the only guarantee is his own objectivity and, in some cases, the observations of others.[3]

Only from this point of view can we consider worthy of our interest his conviction that certain convulsions in the history of humanity should be interpreted, in the most literal sense of the word, as psychic epidemics; let me stress "literal",

2 This mention of Röntgen's X-rays is probable connected with a public experiment carried out in the Urania Theatre in Berlin within the context of what we might call scientific spiritism (Boyd 2005, 71–72).

3 As an example we may take Meyrink 1993 [1927].

and not metaphorical, for the theory underlying this belief is that there really exists what might be called a psychic infection: a contagion caused by an agent on a passive organism by means of something so subtly material as that embodied spirit that lets him understand magic as "an occult force of the soul". This idea does not seem altogether strange, after we have seen the force, commonly called 'magnetic', exercised by the totalitarian regimes of the last century, in particular that of Hitler.[4] Our understanding of this psychic contagion, however, does not go beyond mere suggestion, a concept underlying the nineteenth-century rationalisation of the controversial animal magnetism by converting it into therapeutic hypnotism. Meyrink is more ambitious, for suggestion is not, nor can it be magic, understood as *actio in distans* in a more or less broad sense: in order to induce suggestion one must be, in one way or another, nearby; there has to be contact, even if it is only verbal, optical or gestural, between the agent and the patient, whereas Meyrink's idea is that this contagion is much more diffuse – environmental, if you will – and his idea of contagion would thus be closer to the miasmic theory that predominated prior to bacteriology than to the microbial theory prevalent today. He could hardly be more old-fashioned.

Or at least so it seems.

3 War as a Psychic Epidemic (or as a Symptom of such an Epidemic)

Gustav Meyrink barely had time to see Adolf Hitler in action, since he died in 1932. Nor did he need to in order to formulate his epidemic theory of war; for him, it was enough to be a spectator of the so-called "Great War," the First World War. Many years later the acknowledgement – always metaphorical, of course – of the feverish nature, the arousal, the mercurial excitement of the masses of young people took place who all over Europe enlisted and set off in trains towards a battle-front that was seen as a jamboree. But few contemporaries considered this attitude to be particularly unhealthy, in the strictest sense of the word. Meyrink did, and this, together with his radical antimilitarism, high-

4 Hitler actually on occasion described himself as a "somnambulist," in the sense popularised by animal magnetism (Kershaw 1999, 517). As early as the Romantic period, when animal magnetism was at its height in medicine, the writer E.T.A. Hoffmann gave a largely political interpretation of the figure of the magnetiser in his short story *Der Magnetiseur* (Barkhoff 1995, 197–210). One of the Romantic doctors most committed to the study of animal magnetism also suggested the risk of its use for political ends (Kieser 1826, 442–443; Montiel 2003, 143–170).

lighted in many of his satirical short stories published in the widely-read magazines *Der liebe Augustin* and *Simplicissimus*, brought him serious persecution and a boycott which threatened his and his family's survival in the middle and final years of the war (Binder 2009, 162–181). But, I repeat, over and above his sociological criticism, shared by other writers, we must stress his conviction that the origins of war lay in something more than what the most convinced critics could contemplate; and that "something more" belonged to the world of the spirit, in the sense we have described.

In one of the essays already cited Meyrink notes that many have felt occultism to have been a moral consequence of the war. They are wrong, he maintains, and not only for obvious chronological reasons, but also because both phenomena, occultism and war, are the product of the same "hour" (Meyrink 1993 [1923], 374). This is the term he uses, and I believe it must be understood in a historical sense. There must have been something, then, in the environment responsible for the appearance of both illnesses, or both symptoms of the same illness.

Occultism, understood as a mass phenomenon – this from someone who had been, at least for a time, an occultist – is for him "a psychic epidemic which is at our doors," comparable to the mediaeval and Renaissance outbreaks of collective madness (Meyrink 1907a, 230). He uses the same term for another type of movement whose relationship with violence and war is much more explicit – "what we call spiritual epidemics, such as Bolshevism" – (Meyrink 1981 [ca. 1928], 218). For him, occultism and revolution share an origin: the blind search in the world of the spiritual; for, based on his own experience, he is convinced that certain esoteric practises may destroy the mental health of those who carry them out; and not only this, but they may also act unconsciously on the "invisible world of causes," introducing into the world a sort of poison for the mind responsible for these "epidemics" (Meyrink 1981 [ca. 1928], 218).

Psychic epidemics. Metaphysical-religious in one case, ideological-political in the other, they are at base two manifestations of the same imbalance in the collective physiology; for we have seen that in this case the psyche cannot be divorced from physiology. With Bolshevism we move more clearly towards war than with occultism, although for Meyrink, as we have just seen, it is a fallacy to separate the two phenomena. In fact, Bolshevism represents the visible motive for war, or more specifically for bloody insurrection, in his 1917 novel *Walpurgisnacht* [Walpurgis Night], although this novel in particular insists on the more remote, even unconscious, origins of that ideology and of the slaughter, the stage of which, in the story, is a Prague more dreamlike than real.[5] Before beginning to analyse the novel, I think it would be good to outline Meyrink's position not only relative to "Bolshevism," but also in general to the political ideologies prevalent in the same context.

As I have already said, the writer not only distanced himself from the reactionary style of militaristic nationalism that formed the cultural atmosphere of "Germanness" in the early decades of the last century, but literally confronted it; but, as has also been clear from the foregoing, he felt that its extreme alternative, Communism, was an epidemic, too. Apparently he once declared that he longed for an *Unabhängige Egoistenpartei* [Independent Egoist Party] (Harmsen 2009, 145), which should not be taken to mean a comfortable distancing from politics; the above mentioned satirical short stories, some fragments of his novel *Das grüne Gesicht* [The Green Face] (1916) and the one we are dealing with now, *Walpurgisnacht*, are each evidence of his personal commitment to a subject as serious, particularly at that moment, as the ideological struggle. An American author has gone so far as to maintain that Gustav Meyrink's two stories most closely related to the First World War, *Das Grillenspiel* [The Game of the Crickets] (1915) and *Die vier Mondbrüder* [The four Moon Brothers] (1915) represent a criticism, veiled under an esoteric disguise, of the powers who benefit from war (Boyd 2005, 186). But I beg to differ from this opinion: I think that this way of getting involved in the conflict could not be unaffected by his most deeply-held beliefs; and proof of this lies not only in his literature, which may in any case owe much to perfectly legitimate artistic license, but also in some of the anecdotes about his life, such as his prophecy about the fate of his friend and fellow-writer Erich Mühsam. When the latter was called to arms and sent to the front, Meyrink told him not to fear for his life, since he had always been opposed to war; but this phrase, which sounds like a strange form of consolation, carried with it a warning: be more afraid of the revolution you carry in your blood, for this can indeed kill you. Well, Mühsam did survive the Great War, and he took an active part in the abortive project of the *Räterepublik* of Bavaria, which ended in a bloodbath; and with this record, when the Nazis came to power he was interned in the Oranienburg concentration camp, where he died in 1934 (Harmsen 2009, 144–145).

I think, then, that it is incorrect to limit the scope of Meyrink's analysis to the purely metaphorical domain. Another thing altogether is the fact that, in his writing devoted to the subject, it is necessary to wade through some metaphors and try to discover their meaning in order to understand his point of view and the message he

5 "It is not a historic novel in the usual sense, but a work that throws light on the history of Prague" (Harmsen 2009, 143).

is trying to put across; this is what I set out to do in an article devoted to *Das Grillenspiel* (Montiel 2004). But I am convinced that, although we may find it disturbing, either because it might reinforce the image of an "irrationalist" Meyrink, or because he confronts us with hypotheses that are difficult to digest, we can only be faithful to the text if we give it an almost literal interpretation – with the stress on almost. Let us say, once and for all, that Gustav Meyrink firmly believed that the First World War and Communism had their origin, or at least one of their origins, in an ill-fated conjunction of spiritual forces, magical in the sense we have explained above; that is, when all is said and done, psychic. We shall see how he presents these forces in *Walpurgisnacht* and whether they can be interpreted in a way that makes Meyrink's 'magic' seem less remote from a contemporary rationalistic-materialist mode of thinking than might be expected.

4 The Vampire Past (History as a "Haunted House")

From the very first lines of the story its author confronts us with a concept of history which will be confirmed as the story unfolds. This concept, present in the majority of novels written at the same historical period, is that of the end of a stage, even of an age, which shows the clearly-identifiable features of decadence; which, moreover, seems to have been a generalised feeling among Europeans (Blom 2010, 13–16, 28, 29–38, 552–553). Almost all the characters belong to the nobility of Bohemia, or to the government employees in their service, as in the case of the main character, the physician Taddhäus Flugbeil; or they have a close, often unrecognised, relationship with it, like young Ottokar Vondrejk, the unacknowledged son of Countess Zahradka. They all live in the ancient district of Hradčany, in voluntary seclusion. At the beginning of the novel one of the characters comments with admiration, tinged with horror, that the Court Counsellor has been "in the world" [In der Welt!] (Meyrink 1985 [1917], 7), by which he means in Prague, but outside the castle district; to this the Countess replies that she has never been in that place where her ancestors were beheaded, a reference to the Thirty Years' War, and maybe even to the fourteenth-century religious wars which, through the evocation of the figure of Jan Žižka, play such a part in the story. In Zahradka's statement there is a meeting of the two elements making up the warp and weft of life: space, as we have just seen, and time: "never," she says. And this is because, for her, it is as if the violent death of her ancestors "had happened today" [ich denk es noch wie heite (sic)] (Meyrink 1985 [1917], 9). In a certain sense, the noble protagonists are dead: in a place which no-one leaves and, at least as far as they are concerned, outside time. Or perhaps it would be more accurate to say that they have decided to live like the dead, for time – history – is going to burst violently into their lives.

The physician, Flugbeil, only partially shares this situation, for in his youth he had a dalliance with a prostitute, nicknamed Liesel the Bohemian [die böhmische Liesel], who now, ravaged by old age, lives in the neighbourhood significantly known as "the New World" (Boyd 2005, 220). The reencounter of the two characters in the Countess's palace at the beginning of the story will lead Flugbeil to leave his seclusion in order to find out how the woman he once fell in love with is living, although he immediately protects himself from this wish by running away and forgetting. This amphibious condition – if we can call it that – of Flugbeil is what gives him his position as the central figure of the story, for he is the only one who is not on only one side of the frontier; a frontier which, as we shall soon see, may perfectly well be compared to a mirror.

In fact it is precisely Liesel who holds the key of the sense of history on which the story is based; or at least of the diagnosis of the historical disease to which Meyrink seeks to alert his contemporaries. When she is visited by young Ottokar, due to her fame as a witch and fortune-teller, Liesel emphatically pronounces her diagnosis of the end of the age: "there is no future" [Es gibt doch gar keine Zukunft!] (Meyrink 1985 [1917], 46). And this lack of a future has to do with a pathological past whose roots lie in darkness: "Bohemia is the cradle of all wars" [Böhmen ist der Herd aller Kriege] (Meyrink 1985 [1917], 47), and this is because

> [...] everyone in Prague is mad [...] I think it is due to the mysterious vapours that emanate from the ground [...] [In the Hradčany] there is another kind of madness [...], a sort of petrified madness. [(...) in Prag alles wahnsinnig is (sic) (...) Ich glaub, das kommt von der geheimnisvollen Luft, die aus dem Boden steigt (...) (auf dem Hradschin) da is (sic) eine andere Art Wahnsinn (...) So – so mehr ein versteinerter Wahnsinn.] (Meyrink 1985 [1917], 50 – 51)

These "mysterious vapours that emanate from the ground" cannot fail to evoke the miasma theory of contagion, defended until the end of the nineteenth century by such an authority in the field of public health as Max von Pettenkofer (1818 – 1901); a theory overthrown in the scientific debate over cholera by the bacteria theory defended mainly by Robert Koch (1843 – 1910) on the basis of his discovery of the *vibrio cholerae* in 1883. So why does Meyrink choose it at such a late date as 1917?

No doubt because in this case we are dealing with a non-material contagion, the contagion of "madness"; and in the writer's opinion it would be a mistake in this instance to rule out the "miasmic" or "environmental" hypothesis, since in history it is the mephitic atmosphere which is responsible for the epidemic; or at least, as we shall see, one of its causes. The place – Prague as a whole, and the Hradčany in particular – is contaminated, and contaminated by the seeds of the past: as far as Bohemia is concerned, war; as to the castle, murder, as the novel will show as it unfolds. The place in which the protagonists of the tragedy live – the city, the castle – is thus a "haunted house"; and the ghosts which haunt it and plague its inhabitants are the spectres of the past, of history, who live on, like vampires, at the expense of the blood of their descendants. This situation is represented in the novel in a particularly explicit way by the figure of the young Polyxena, who sees herself as being inhabited by her terrible forebear, the murdering Countess Polyxena Lambua (Meyrink 1985 [1917], 111–112). She and Ottokar will fall in love, despite the incestuous implications of the relationship – remember that the young man is the son of Countess Zahradka, and Polyxena is her niece; but even before he met the real Polyxena the young man had fallen in love with the figure of her ancestor, preserved in a portrait kept in a closed room, as if it was intended to imply that the ancestor is in some way reincarnated in the body of the contemporary young woman.[6] This belief, moreover, discredits the notion, so highly valued by Western thought, of free will; it represents a novel version of the classical concept of *fatum* or *ananke*, where the force that we know as destiny appears to have less to do with the superhuman than with the human unconscious, both on an individual level but also, and perhaps above all, collectively: a 'miasmic' theory of the activity of the spirit.

But there is more: according to medical theory one of the possible origins of miasmas is the putrefaction of corpses underground, which gave rise to the practice of moving cemeteries outside the towns. I have already mentioned that Countess Zahradka killed her husband, who lies buried beneath the floor of his mansion, explaining the "plague of flies" – the sudden appearance of dense swarms of flies in the palace – which takes place just before the outbreak of the revolution and, with it, the bloody dénouement of the story (Meyrink 1985 [1917], 165). Other corpses, on the other hand, are not so easily buried, as I explained in the case of Polyxena's ancestor. The writer tells us that when her young descendant saw her portrait shut away in the family gallery, she felt

> [...] the eerie feeling that this was not a painting of a dead person, but the reflection of a being that must really exist somewhere, of a being *much more alive than anything she had ever seen* [...]. In some way, the portrait that hung on the wall was herself [...] to someone, the only thing that can appear more alive than anything in the world is oneself. [(...) das unheimliche Gefühl, als sei es gar kein Gemälde einer Verstorbenen, sondern der Widerschein eines Wesens, das irgendwo in Wirkichkeit existieren müsse, viel lebendiger als irgend etwas, was sie je gesehen (...) das Bild, das dort an der Wand hing, war gewissermas-

6 The conviction that successive generations are in some way present in each individual forms one of the key points of another of Meyrink's novels, *Der weisse Dominikaner* [The White Dominican] (1921) (Montiel 1998, 137–178).

> sen sie selber (...) lebendiger als irgend etwas anderes in der Welt kann aber nur der Mensch sich selbst vorkommen.] (Meyrink 1985 [1917], 109 – 110)

But in this case the miasmas behave like the *seminaria* imagined by the Italian humanist physician Girolamo Fracastoro (1483 – 1553): as their name indicates, these were seeds which were only waiting to fall on an appropriate ground in order to germinate: and this is also the metaphor used by Meyrink:

> In some way, the portrait that hung on the wall was herself. Just as the seed carries within it the image of the plant which it will one day become, clearly shaped in all its organic peculiarities, though hidden to the five senses; so that portrait had hung in her since her childhood as the predetermined mould into which her soul was meant to grow with every fibre and every cell, until the smallest crevice of the form was filled by it. [Das Bild, das dort an der Wand hing, war gewissermassen sie selber – so, wie ein Samenkorn das Konterfei der Pflanze, die es dereinst werden soll, in sich trägt, verborgen den äusseren Sinnen, und dennoch in allen organischen Einzelheiten klar umrissen, so hatte jenes Bild in ihr seit Kindheit an gehangen, war die vorbestimmte Matrize, in die ihre Seele hineinwachsen musste mit jeder Faser und Zelle, bis auf die kleinste Vertiefung der Form von ihr ausgefüllt sein würde.] (Meyrink 1985 [1917], 109 – 110)

Common history as a miasma; then individual history as a *seminarium* – a seedbed. And the history of medicine tells us that, in time, Fracastoro's purely speculative theory would be shown to be in a sense prophetic, for science would discover that indeed there are germs – and what is a germ without a seed? – that infect bodies, causing individual and collective disease. But in the case in point, these germs, although they have to do with history – for they have history – are not, strictly speaking, history itself. History provides the noxious environment. Humans transmit pathogens by contact, *contagium*, although, in the present case, the contagion does not occur between bodies, but between souls: psychic contagion.

5 *Aweysha:* Psychic Parasitisation

In *Der Golem* Meyrink, the insatiable student of the mystical tradition, had already paved the way for the idea that an alien psychic principle could take over the mind of a human being, based on the Cabbalistic doctrine of the *Ibbur*, "the impregnation of the soul," in this case to trigger a spiritual evolution within him.[7] This same idea becomes the key to the explanation of the "Bolshevik" revolution depicted in *Walpurgisnacht* in the form, this time, of another kind of infiltration; in this case parasitic, unlike what occurs with *Ibbur*; and this he calls *Aweysha*, referring obscurely to the esoteric world of Asia.[8]

Once we understand how to interpret what *Aweysha* means, we realise that it has been present in the whole story, acting, directing the actions of all the characters, right from the start; for its instrument is the actor/sleepwalker Zrcadlo – the word means "mirror" in Czech – with whose sudden arrival in Countess Zahradka's salon the story begins. The circumstances in which Doctor Flugbeil receives the revelation of the existence of *Aweysha* from the lips of Zrcadlo himself could hardly be more significant. At night, in the private room of a restaurant, the reclusive doctor looks at his image in a mirror and ponders, remembering what he has learnt about the laws of reflection: "It is so strange that in just one tiny point so very much more can happen than in the largest of spaces!" [Merkwürdig genug, dass in einem so winzigen Punkt so ungeheuer viel mehr geschehen kann als in ausgedehnten Räumen selbst!] This thought proves so upsetting that he stops thinking about it, for fear of

> [...] coming to the painful conclusion that man is absolutely incapable of undertaking anything from a conscious will – rather, he is merely the helpless machine of an enigmatic point in his inner being. [(...) zu der peinlichen Schlussfolgerung kommen, der Mensch sei überhaupt unfähig, irgend etwas aus bewusstem Willen heraus zu unternehmen – sei vielmehr nur die hilflose Maschine eines rätselhaften Punktes in seinem Innern.] (Meyrink 1985 [1917], 82–83)

In these circumstances Zrcadlo, the mirror, appears to him, adopting the features of Flugbeil as a child, and identifies himself, in a long poetical tirade, as his "innermost self", even when later he says he is a "Manchu," using Zrcadlo's body as a mere instrument. Flugbeil is not disposed to believe it, so the other has to remind him that a moment ago his, Flugbeil's, "innermost self" had spoken to him from the body of the actor, because for many years it had been denied, confused with the old body – and orderly mind – of a court physician:

> A little while ago you wondered... or rather, *thought:* "Has my own I left me, then, and moved over to the actor?" My answer is this: the true "I" is only visible by its *effects*. It

7 I have dealt with this subject in Montiel 1994; 1998, 36–37. The information I have used in both texts on the concept of *Ibbur* comes from Scholem 1962, 203–237.

8 I have been unable to find any information on the origin of the term, nor its meaning other than in the novel; I therefore do not know if it is an invention of the author or if it comes from one of the esoteric sources he consulted.

has no extension, and precisely because it does not, it is – everywhere. [...] It should not surprise you that your so-called own I speaks more clearly from another than from yourself – you are, unfortunately, like most people, steeped in the delusion since childhood of considering your "I" to be your body, your senses, your rationalness [...] The "I" flows *through* man, so a re-education in thinking is required to be able to find oneself in one's own I. [Sie haben vorhin gefragt, oder, besser gesagt, Sie haben sich *gedacht:* "Hat mich mein Ich denn verlassen und sich auf den Schauspieler übertragen?" – Ich antworte Ihnen darauf; das wahre "Ich" ist nur an der *Wirkung* zu erkennen. Es hat keine Ausdehnung; und eben, weil es keine hat, ist es – überall (...) Es darf Sie nicht wundern, dass Ihr sogenanntes eigenes Ich aus einem anderen deutlicher spricht als aus Ihnen selbst – Sie sind leider, wie fast alle Menschen, von Kindesbeinen an in dem Irrtum befangen gewesen, unter "Ich" ihren Körper, Ihre Sinne, Ihr Denkvermögen (...) zu verstehen (...) Das "Ich" fliesst durch den Menschen *hindurch*, deshalb ist ein Umlernen im Denken nötig, um sich selbst im eigenen Ich wiederfinden zu können.] (Meyrink 1985 [1917], 98–99)

The "I" flows – notice that Meyrink always writes "I" in inverted commas, as if to show that it is only a manner of speaking; an incorrect way of speaking – and because it flows it can take control of the body of someone who, so to speak, does not have much "I": the body of a sleepwalker, or someone brain-dead, a "zombie" [ein Scheintoter]; a little later this is stated by another character who has the task of giving a more specific definition of *Aweysha*, the Turk Molla Osman, who works as a stable boy in the palace (Meyrink 1985 [1917], 116). It would be very tempting to give Molla Osman's beliefs an allegorical interpretation, to allow us to fit them within our logic; as, in fact, does Polyxena, one of those to whom the explanation is addressed, when Molla Osman attributes war to *Aweysha:*

Polyxena: So would it be possible for war...? [Da wäre es ja möglich, dass der Krieg...]

Molla Osman: Certainly! [...] Everything men do against their will comes from the Aweysha [...] If men one day fall upon each other like tigers, do you really think they would do so if someone had not done Aweysha with them? [Gewiss (...) Alles, was die Menschen gegen ihren Wunsch tun, kommt aus dem Aweysha her (...) Wenn die Menschen eines Tages übereinander herfallen wie die Tiger, meinst du, sie täten es, wenn nicht irgendwer Aweysha mit ihnen gemacht hätte?]

P: They do it, I think, because... well, because they are just excited about... about something; about an... idea perhaps. [Sie tun es, denke ich, weil sie – nun, weil sie eben begeistert sind für – für irgend etwas; für eine – Idee vielleicht.]

MO: There you are, that is precisely Aweysha. [Nun, das ist doch Aweysha.]

P: So are excitement and Aweysha the same thing? [Also ist Begeisterung und Aweysha dasselbe?]

MO: No, first comes Aweysha; then excitement follows [...] Some people can produce Aweysha in others, merely by giving a speech [...] [but] nobody in the world can make Aweysha with someone who relies only on himself. [Nein, zuerst kommt Aweysha. Daraus entsteht dann Begeisterung [...]

> Manche Menschen können Aweysha bei anderen machen, bloss indem sie eine Rede halten [...] Mit jemand, der sich nur auf sich selbst verlässt, kann kein Mensch auf der Welt Aweysha machen.] (Meyrink 1985 [1917], 117–118)

Read a century later, these statements seem less incredible, when we consider the extent to which they are prophetic: remember, they were written in 1917, or ten to fifteen years before the most powerful shaman of the century performed his *Aweysha* with unprecedented success on hundreds of thousands of *Scheintoter.* Science is no fonder of prophecies than it is of this theory of psychic contagion that Meyrink proposes in his novel, but we shall have to acknowledge the lucidity – might I even say "clairvoyance"? – he shows in the last sentence of the quote. But there is no cause for alarm. In the same way that we can rationalise Gustav Meyrink's prophetic powers, at least partially – and at least in this case, for there are others, considerably more difficult, we can certainly make an interpretation which is more acceptable to our sensibility of the concept of "psychic epidemic," based on the notion of possession/parasitisation known in the novel as *Aweysha.* And it is notable that the way it is obtained may be classified, at least in part, as Freudian.

Watching over the massacre with which the book ends is the Devil; a devil who plays a historic – maybe legendary – drum; which of these is unimportant for my argument. It is the drum that, it is said, the dying Jan Žižka ordered to be made with his own skin after his death. It is no coincidence that this image was chosen for the cover of the first edition of the novel.

Not long before, this same Devil presented himself before Thaddäus Flugbeil, promising him rebirth, his dearest wish; a wish that the Devil is more aware of than him because, he declares,

> I am the only one of the gods to gird my loins; the others are sexless.
> Only I can understand wishes; one who is truly sexless has forgotten for ever what wishes are. The unrecognisable, deepest root of every wish rests always in our sex. [Ich bin der einzig Gegürtete unter den Göttern; die andern sind geschlechtslos. Nur ich kann Wünsche verstehen; wer in Wahrheit geschlechtslos ist, der hat für immer vergessen, was Wünsche sind. Die unerkennbare, tiefste Wurzel jedes Wunsches ruht stets im Geschlecht.] (Meyrink 1985 [1917], 155)

On the one hand, this devil rather resembles the devil in Baudelaire's *Litanies of Satan:*

> I am the only merciful one among the gods. There is no wish I cannot hear and fulfil instantly. [Der einzige Erbarmer unter den Göttern bin ich. – Es gibt keinen Wunsch, den ich nicht auf der Stelle hörte und erfüllte.] (Meyrink 1985 [1917], 155)

On the other hand he differs from the former in one essential aspect:

> But it is only the wishes of the soul that I hear and bring to the light: hence my name is *lucifero.* [Aber nur die Wünsche der Seelen höre ich und bringe sie dem Lichte. Darum heisse ich: luci- fero.] (Meyrink 1985 [1917], 155)

In the case of the physician the desire which is deep-rooted in his soul – so deep-rooted that even he is not aware of it, as happens with his "innermost self"– is what the text refers to as "eternal youth," about which this devil of the unconscious allows us to make no simple interpretations:

> Eternal youth is eternal future; and in the realm of eternity the past also wakes again as an eternal present. [Ewige Jugend ist ewige Zukunft, und in dem Reich der Ewigkeit wacht auch die Vergangenheit wieder auf als ewige Gegenwart.] (Meyrink 1985 [1917], 156)

Elsewhere I have tried to explain, in the light of C. G. Jung's analytical psychology, what this means in the psychological field: renewal, the discovery of the innermost depths of the personality, which Jung called *Selbst* and which is no doubt equivalent to the "innermost self" announced by Zrcadlo in *Walpurgisnacht.* As we near the end of the story, when the physician is making his final preparations to leave Prague, he receives the successive visits of his old friends – Baron Elsenwanger and Countess Zahradka – who come to bid him farewell. And this is what he feels as he finds himself alone again:

> The ghosts of my life say farewell to me! It's dreadful. Dreadful! A city of madness and crime has surrounded me and eaten my youth! – And I have neither heard nor seen! I was deaf and blind. [Die Gespenster meines Lebens nehmen Abschied von mir! – Entsetzlich. Entsetzlich. – Eine Stadt des Irrsinns und des Verbrechens hat mich umgeben und meine Jugend gefressen! – Und ich habe nicht gehört und nicht gesehen! War taub und blind.] (Meyrink 1985 [1917], 169)

Now he has opened his eyes to another reality. Alas, things are different in the case of the rest of the characters, named and nameless, of the novel. They do not seek to cultivate their "innermost self," of whose very existence they are unaware, or which they deny (Polyxena); but they allow and even encourage the insinuation of the miasmas and the shoots of the *seminaria* of the past; to the obsessive rhythm of the devil's baneful drum, they allow the contagion of madness and death to spread.

Incidentally – where did this drum come from? From history, we are bound to reply. From that poisonous, ill-digested history that I introduced above as a *haunted house.* From the history of nations and religions; from the history of wars and slaughter. Is it not, then, the famous drum of Žižka?

But the unconscious has also emerged. From a wild unconscious, evoked in error, which is manifested not as the "innermost self" but as a ghost. Liesel the Bohemian explains it clearly to her beloved Flugbeil on her last visit:

> Can you hear it? Can you hear it? They're coming!... Quickly! Hide!... Do you hear them drumming?... There! Again!... It's Žižka! Jan Žižka of Trocnov!... Zrcadlo! The devil!... He stabbed himself to death... They pulled off his skin. In my house! In my room!... It's what he wanted... And they stretched it over a drum... The tanner Havlik made it. [Hörst du's, hörst du's? Sie kommen! – Rasch! Versteck dich! – Hörst du sie trommeln? – Da! Wieder! – Der Zizka! Jan Zizka von Trocnov! – Der Zrcadlo! Der Teufel! – Erstochen hat er sich. – Die Haut haben sie ihm abgezogen. Bei mir! In meinem Zimmer! – Er hat's so gewollt. – Und auf eine Trommel gespannt. – Der Gerber Havlik hat's getan] (Meyrink 1985 [1917], 177–178)

So the drum is made of the skin of someone who was no-one and could be anyone, everyone. And the unfortunate tanner Havlik played it only for a short time. Shot dead, he would be replaced by its true owner, who is only seen by Polyxena:

> [...] the shadowy figure of a man who scurries along [...], sometimes emerging, soon disappearing again, now here, now there. He is naked, it seems, and wears a mitre on his head, although she cannot see him clearly. He moves his hands over his chest as if beating an invisible drum. [(...) einen schattenhaften Menschen dahinhuschen (...) bald auftauchend, bald wieder verschwindend – bald da, bald dort. Er ist nackt, wie mir scheint, und trägt eine Mitra auf dem Kopf, doch kann sie ihn nie genau unterscheiden. – Er bewegt die Hände vor der Brust, als rühre er eine unsichtbare Trommel.] (Meyrink 1985 [1917], 207)

The devil? Of course. But also, as Polyxena understands,

> He is the serpent who lives in men and sheds his skin when they die. [Er ist die Schlange, die in den Menschen wohnt und sich häutet, wenn sie sterben.] (Meyrink 1985 [1917], 208)

The devil. Zrcadlo. The unconscious. The Lord of *Aweysha.*

References

Barkhoff, Jürgen. *Magnetische Fiktionen. Literarisierung des Magnetismus in der Romantik.* Stuttgart: Metzler, 1995.

Binder, Hartmut. *Gustav Meyrink. Ein Leben im Bann der Magie.* Prag: Vitalis, 2009.

Blom, Philipp. *Años de vértigo.* Barcelona: Anagrama, 2010.

Boyd, Amanda Ch. *Demonizing Esotericism: The Treatment of Spirituality and Popular Culture in the Works of Gustav Meyrink.* Doctoral thesis. University of Amherst, MA, 2005.

Harmsen, Theodor. *Der magische Schritsteller Gustav Meyrink, Seine Freunde und sein Werk.* Amsterdam: In der Pelikaan, 2009.

Kershaw, Ian. *Hitler, 1889–1936.* Barcelona: Península, 1999.

Kieser, Dietrich Georg. *System des Tellurismus oder thierischen Magnetismus*. Leipzig: Herbig, 1826.
Meyrink, Gustav. "Die Verwandlung des Blutes." *Fledermäuse*. Ed. Eduard Frank. Munich: Langen Müller, 1981 [ca. 1928].
Meyrink, Gustav. *Walpurgisnacht*. Berlin: Verlag der Nation, 1985 [1917].
Meyrink, Gustav. "Fakire." *Das Haus zur letzten Latern*. Ed. Eduard Frank, Frankfurt a. M., Berlin: Ullstein, 1993 [1907a].
Meyrink, Gustav. "Fakirpfade." *Das Haus zur letzten Latern*. Ed. Eduard Frank, Frankfurt a. M., Berlin: Ullstein, 1993 [1907b].
Meyrink, Gustav. "An der Grenze des Jenseits." *Das Haus zur letzten Latern*. Ed. Eduard Frank, Frankfurt a. M., Berlin: Ullstein, 1993 [1923].
Meyrink, Gustav. "Haschisch und Hellsehen." *Das Haus zur letzten Latern*. Ed. Eduard Frank, Frankfurt a. M., Berlin: Ullstein, 1993 [1927].
Meyrink, Gustav. "Magie im Tiefschlaf." *Das Haus zur letzten Latern*. Ed. Eduard Frank, Frankfurt a. M., Berlin: Ullstein, 1993 [1928].
Montiel, Luis. "De la Cábala al psicoanálisis a través de la literatura. La vivencia de *Ibbur* y su significado en *El Golem*, de Gustav Meyrink." *Actas del XXXIII Congreso Internacional de Historia de la Medicina. 1–6 septiembre 1992*. Eds Juan L. Carrillo and Guillermo Olagüe de Ros, Seville: Sociedad Española de Historia de la Medicina, 1994. 417–424.
Montiel, Luis. *La novela del inconsciente. El proceso de individuación en la narrativa de Gustav Meyrink*. Barcelona: MRA, 1998.
Montiel, Luis. "Primera Mirada sobre el lado oscuro del magnetismo: *El magnetizador* (1813) de E.T.A. Hoffmann." *En ningún lugar. En parte alguna. Estudios sobre la historia del magnetismo animal y del hipnotismo*. Eds Luis Montiel and Ángel González de Pablo. Madrid: Frenia, 2003. 143–170.
Montiel, Luis. "Una consideración intempestiva sobre los orígenes de la guerra: *das Grillenspiel*, de Gustav Meyrink". *Frenia, III*-2 (2004): 33–53.
Rothschuh, Karl Eduard. *Konzepte der Medizin in Vergangenheit und Gegenwart*. Stuttgart: Hippokrates, 1978.
Scholem, Gershom. *Von der mystischen Gestalt der Gottheit. Studien zu Grundbegriffen der Kabbala*. Zurich: Rhein, 1962.
Treitel, Corina C. *A Science for The Soul: Occultism and the Genesis of the German Modern*. Baltimore, MA: Johns Hopkins University Press, 2004.

Rudolf Käser

Living with Rats and Mosquitoes: Different Paradigms of Cohabitation with Parasites in a German Narrative of Contagion around 1930

This paper focuses on Ernst Weiss' novel *Georg Letham, Arzt und Mörder* [Georg Letham: Physician and murderer] published in 1931. The first part of the novel narrates the story of a medical doctor who, trained as a bacteriologist, becomes the murderer of his wife. The second part presents a process of recovery: how the protagonist, deported to a penal colony in a tropical area, finds a new meaning for his existence in the fight against yellow fever and in the realisation of large scale hygienic measures to control its live vector, the mosquito Stegomyia fasciata. This project of sanitation is depicted in contrast to the exterminatory war of men against rats. Rats play a major role in the first part of the novel. Georg Letham senior's expedition to the North Pole is a failure because of the exponential multiplication of rats on his ship and because of his crew not being able to adapt to this situation adequately. The main purpose of Weiss' novel, as I suggest reading it, is to show the possibility of changing the values from a social Darwinist notion of confronting parasites destructively to notions of symbioses and controlled cohabitation. Weiss chooses examples of different human forms of conduct towards parasites as literary metaphors to criticize National Socialism and – more precisely – to imagine an alternative to Hitler's concept of the radical extermination of the other.

The author Ernst Weiss was born in 1882 as the second son of a Jewish cloth merchant in the Moravian city of Brünn. He studied medicine in Prague, Vienna, Berne and Berlin and, in 1911, worked at the surgical division of a Viennese hospital. Suffering from a lung disease, he had to quit and accepted the position of a ship-doctor with Austrian Lloyd. In this position, he travelled to India and Japan. In 1913 he moved to Berlin and tried to live as a writer. In the same year he met Franz Kafka, who later helped him publish his first novel. In 1914 he was summoned by the Austro-Hungarian army, where he worked as a military physician of an infantry unit at the military base and at the East front. After World War I, from 1919 to 1920, Weiss worked again as a surgeon in Prague. He then went back to Berlin, where he lived as a productive novelist for more than ten years. In 1933, he left Berlin for Prague in order to take care of his severely ill mother. After her death in 1934, Weiss emigrated to Paris. On June 15 1940, one day after the invasion of German troops in France, Weiss committed suicide.

1 Plot and Plot Structure

The novel is written in a first person perspective. The protagonist, Georg Letham junior, presents his own life in retrospective view. He is a medical doctor, son of a leading public official. He lives as a bacteriologist and gynaecologist in a big European metropolis. He is a man deeply traumatized by both the social-darwinist framework of education his father imposed on him and by his later experiences of World War I at the East front. After the war, he marries a wealthy widow; their relationship, however, develops into a desperate sado-masochistic drama. As a bacteriologist, Letham works on the aetiology of Scarlet Fever. He succeeds in isolating the 'Scarlet toxin' in crystalline shape. But instead of publishing his success, he kills his wife with a dose of this poisonous substance.[1] This could have been the perfect crime, but his subconscious desire to be punished causes a Freudian slip: he forgets to dispose of the small bottle that contained the poison. Immediately after his deed, Letham rushes to his father to tell him what he has done. But his father denies his son and flees in panic. Letham junior is arrested by the police. The punishment for the murderer is a lifelong deportation to the penal colonies.

The second part of the novel narrates the deportation on a vessel and the poor life of the detainees. During the deportation Letham recapitulates his life from childhood to his deed. He explains his unhappy life as being the result of the methods of education his father applied on him. The reader learns that this father, a trained scientist, guided an expedition to the North Pole in his younger days. He would have reached the pole before Nansen did, very much with the same method Nansen used, but the success of his expedition was destroyed by the exceeding multiplication of rats on his boat. Traditional rat-hunting methods do not work. Letham senior, the trained scientist and observer, becomes aware of growing signs of scurvy among the members of his crew. He observes their growing apathy, many signs of psychological regression, e.g. their dwindling zeal for fighting the ever growing number of rats. But he also observes his dog Ruru. The dog is still entirely healthy, fair looking and alert, he hunts every rat that dares show up on deck. Feeding on their blood and flesh

1 The psychodynamic evolution of characters in Weiß' fiction is oftentimes designed along the concepts of inferiority complex vs. hypercompensation as developed by Alfred Adler. See Käser 1998, 267–321.

is obviously good for the dog's health. Letham senior makes the experiment himself: he hunts rats, he drinks their blood and eats their meat as a medication against scurvy, and his health stays perfect. He therefore suggests to his crew that they overcome the traditional cultural prejudice against rats, imitate the behaviour of the dog, conceive the unwanted passengers of their boat to be a kind of living stock and feed on their fresh meat and blood. But he fails. The cultural prejudices against the allegedly "pestiferous" rats prevail: "Kill – yes. Eat – no. They shun the repulsive animals like the plague, a plague of rats [...]" (Weiss 2010, 197). A finally self-destructive war of extermination against the parasites begins. The crew decide to kill the rats by means of gas. The first attempt is made by an evaporation of arsenic and sulphur, both chemicals being on stock on the boat: "Poison gas warfare had been invented long before the Great War" (Weiss 2010, 185). But the attack fails, because the gas, lighter than air, does not get into the vessel, but almost suffocates the crew waiting on deck. The second attempt is made with carbon oxide. But the rats attack the smoking coal buckets placed inside the ship, tip them over and thus the ship is set on fire. Among the crew waiting outside on the ice, a merciless, utterly brutal battle for survival of everybody against everybody begins. Only Letham senior and one of his colleagues survive, all the others kill each other or die in the ice. The narrator comments on this episode of self-destructive warfare against the parasites with a rhetorical question: "How can they be eradicated without also eradicating the people to whom they have adapted themselves" (Weiss 2010, 192)?[2]

For the rest of his life, Letham senior lives as a disappointed misanthrope in the constant thought of taking revenge on the rats, and he converts his experiment with the rats into the educational programme for his son. He buys a house infected with rats, he forces his son to spend day and night together with rats in the same room, he catches rats in carefully constructed traps, he sets male and female rats in the same trap and urges his son to observe their behaviour, their excessive eating as long as there is food around, their excessive sexual copulations and their ruthless killing attacks on each other when starvation sets in. The father wants his son to look at all this in order to lose all emotional prejudices, to lose all illusion about love and life of both animals and men. He wants to show him that the struggle for survival and the survival of the physically most powerful who control and kill the less powerful is the essential truth one has to know about life in order to maintain oneself. The sadomaso-

2 The German text emphasizes the symbiotic aspect: "Eingliedern" – "incorporate" – draws the reader's attention to the formation of a single socio-biological system involving at least two species.

chistic perversion of the young man's sexual drive is made understandable by the detailed narration of the scenes of these educational "experiments on living souls" (Weiss 2010, 9). This lesson on inhumanity is reinforced by the experience of World War I, during which Letham junior serves as a military physician for several months. The war experience sets the seal on the desperate nihilism in which Letham junior has been brought up by his father.

Weiss treats the fight against rats as a metaphor of social and political relations among human beings and among states. The desperate nihilism of social Darwinist ideology is seen as the result of the education by father and fatherland alike.[3] It is important to observe therefore that the reconstruction of the experience of Letham senior in the retrospective of his son contains not only the social Darwinist solution that leads to nihilism and to the affirmation of brutal power, but is also reminiscent of traces of an alternative solution, which unfortunately could not been put into practice so far. Letham senior, by close observation of the behaviour of his dog, begins to experiment with a pattern of conduct I would like to call the paradigm of nutritional symbiosis: rats feed on food stock, humans feed on rats.

This ambivalence in the value system of his father, however, allows the son a differentiated evaluation of his relationship towards his father. On the one hand, he has to free himself of the social Darwinist interpretation his father has given to his experience, and, on the other hand, he has to understand that the alternative solution, which his father had in mind but was not able to put into practice, would indicate the path to a more viable solution not based on power, domination and extinction. Letham junior's finding of a third and viable pattern of conduct towards parasites, the paradigm of controlled cohabitation, is told in the second part of Weiss' novel.

Letham knows that the penal colony to which he is deported is a place of repeated outbreaks of yellow fever. The fact that "this sun of Yellow Fever" does not make any moral difference and "shines on just and unjust alike" (Weiss 2010, 98) is of some consolation to him. The government constitutes a small team of medical scientists to explore the unknown causes of this infectious disease. The team consists of two persons: Dr. Carolus, a military physician in the rank of a general who is quite knowledgeable in statistics, and Walter, a bacteriologist, who is very skilled in laboratory experimentation. After his arrival in the penal colony, Letham is assigned to this group as an assistant for experimental work in the laboratory and as a medical assistant to yellow fever patients who

3 See Weiss 2010, 15: "He – my father – and my country, too."

are under quarantine. In both fields of action, Letham junior makes experiences that change his notions of identity, of meaning and of human values.

For the trained medical professional and bacteriologist Georg Letham, the confrontation with death caused by yellow fever is first a challenge to his self-control, to his emotional reaction of disgust:

> The smell, an outrageous, abominable stench utterly beyond description, something purely sensory yet beyond what the nervous system could make sense of, made me, believe it or not, cry. Shed tears, to be more precise. I wanted to vomit but did not allow myself to. I had to manage that much self-control. I needed to live up to the upbringing my father had given me, and I did. (Weiss 2010, 274)

These few lines are, in several respects, characteristic of the novel, of its plot structure, of its system of values and of the basic concepts of Weiss' poetology in general. With his criminal act and the ensuing deportation, Letham junior breaks with his father and with his fatherland. But nevertheless, the transformation of his identity into a different paradigm draws on some of the values his father stands for and implements them even more consequently than his father did. Self-control and scientific observation are persistent values. But self-control does not mean inurement and cynical nihilism any longer for Letham junior, as it did for Letham senior. The objective reality is experienced as utterly and aggressively meaningless. The acute experience of this lack of meaning is the opposite of cynical distance. Weiss' depictions of the corpses of yellow fever victims are masterpieces of "Neue Sachlichkeit," but they are masterpieces of expressionist prose at the same time. The drastic aspects of the depicted facts express the powerlessness and the despair of the beholder. The most impressive passages in Weiss' writing are those in which objective existence and emotional meaning of things and situations are completely but provocatively negative. The contagious disease yellow fever is constructed by Ernst Weiss as a power that demonstrates to the human beings their utter powerlessness, their insignificance. There is no way to make any sense of the disease at all. Death by yellow fever shows the 'stupidity' and terrifying gruesomeness and inhuman indolence of nature. There is no way of aestheticizing the aspect of the dead body as an allegory of meaning.[4]

---

4 The aesthetically overpowering presence of the meaningless is represented in the original text in a very dense stylistic climax: "Der Geruch, der rein sinnliche, nein widersinnige, empörende, ganz unbeschreiblich abscheuliche Gestank" (Weiß 1982, 245). The objective fact ("rein sinnlich"), the emotional meaning ("widersinnig "), the subjective resistance against the negativity of the coincidence of fact and meaninglessness ("empörend") and the breakdown of (poetic) language in this constellation ("ganz unbeschreiblich") are expressed in utter literary intensification. It is one of Weiss' poetological ideals to create situations in which "Sinn" and "Be-

But the experience of yellow fever in the colonies offers, in addition to the lesson of the mortuary, yet another lesson to Letham junior: the lesson of loss and mourning at the bedside of a beloved person. One of the patients put under quarantine in the hospital is a young Portuguese girl. Letham is touched by the beauty and the suffering of this young patient. He is deeply moved by the signs of trust communicated by her. The convicted murderer, who has considered himself to be emotionally dead, falls in love with her and is tempted to use euthanasia in this situation of helpless despair.[5] But Letham withstands this temptation; the death of the beloved young patient is turned into a profound lesson in active passivity for the physician and for the reader. In this situation, the most difficult task to learn is not to be doing anything and accept passivity and helplessness as facts of life. In Weiss' narrative, this experience is presented as a crucial step in the process of psychic healing. Letham becomes capable of emotionally participating in the experience of a dying person. He loves and he goes

deutung," objective facts and subjective meaning, are aesthetically identical: "The elementary force, the psychological insight, the all-encompassing love of the creative person advances further to the basic grounds of existence, where this existence cannot be restricted any longer within words or conditions but where it is something and means something at the same time. This coincidence of being and meaning is called mythic." ["Die elementare Kraft, die psychologische Einsicht, die umfassende Liebe des Schaffenden dringt weiter zu den Urgründen des Daseins, wo dieses Dasein sich nicht mehr in Worten und Zuständen begrenzen läßt, sondern wo es zu gleicher Zeit etwas ist und etwas bedeutet. Man nennt diese Zusammentreffen von Sein und Bedeutung mythisch."] (Ernst Weiß: Die Kunst des Erzählens, 292). The aesthetically most powerful realizations of this poetological principle in Weiss' work are, however, to be found in the depiction of situations lacking meaning completely, a literary procedure which implements, so to speak, the paradoxical rhetoric figure of 'myths of negativity.' Weiss' representations of victims of yellow fever are most elaborately inscribed in a discourse on realism and religious faith that begins with Dostoïevsky's comment on the representation of the dead body of Christ by Holbein. In Dostoïevsky's novel *The Idiot*, Prince Myschkin expresses his feeling that the observer of such a corpse and the beholder of such a realistic painting will necessarily lose faith in resurrection. In other words: if the dead body of a human being is to be understood in the context of religious faith as an allegory of resurrection, the realistic detail ought not be too gruesome. As Käser (2004, 213) and Orell (2005, 180) argue, Weiss' hyper-realism in depicting the victims of yellow fever blocks any kind of allegorical transcendent meaning of death. Yellow fever, the contagious disease that destroys and disfigures the human body completely, cannot be a message of God, not even a message in the sense of punishment for sinful conduct or call for repentance, as contagious diseases so often have been interpreted in the context of religious literature from Abraham a Santa Clara to Jeremias Gotthelf and beyond.

5 The loving physician at the bedside of a dying patient is a topical scene in literature. The physician in Storm's *Ein Bekenntnis* [A Confession] is overwhelmed by compassion and uses euthanasia to help his beloved wife escape from suffering. For a contextualized interpretation cf. Käser 1998, 150–178.

through a deep mourning process – and at the end of this process, he is capable of accepting yellow fever as a challenge to his professional skills. On the other hand, his professional skills are not any longer the results of a completely distanced, emotionless, and misanthropic notion, but they are underpinned by the experience of love and mourning, which both imply the attribution of a human value to the existence of another person and therefore, an affirmation of the meaningfulness of life as such.

This is the result of Letham's experience as a physician in confrontation with the death of an infected patient. What are then his experiences in the field of scientific bacteriological research? The team of medical scientists first concentrates on the infectious agent of the disease and tries to isolate and visualize the pathogenic germ in the blood or in the tissue of the victims by microscopic methods and then transfers the infection to laboratory animals. The affiliation to this team of researchers gives some meaning to his shattered existence:

> For the first time in years, I was absorbed, knew no fatigue, I had a truly pervasive feeling that there was a constructive reason for me to exist, and the others. (Weiss 2010, 276)

But their research is not successful. No germ can be discovered and visualized in the myriads of scrutinized specimens. The transfer of infected blood to laboratory animal shows no effect. Desperation and lethargy begin to grow among the team. Carolus, however, the statistician, does not stop calculating the statistics of the cases of infection. He can demonstrate that the infection develops in waves, a high density of cases is followed by intervals with low case numbers. He also looks at the spatio-temporal distribution of the cases: the disease does not spread in close neighbourhood, it seems to hop from one place to the other. This does not make any sense to anybody at all at that time. In this situation, Letham remembers an episodic encounter he had on the first day of his presence at the hospital. The old town physician of the colony came to visit the researchers, and he told them his old theory about mosquitoes being the 'causes' of yellow fever ever. He even brought with him some eggs of Stegomyia fasciata. Nobody took him seriously, yellow fever was not malaria, and the old man had already been ventilating his ideas for years without being able to deliver any scientifically acceptable proof. But suddenly, Letham sees a possible connection between the hitherto meaningless statistics of Carolus and the equally meaningless twaddle of the old town physician. What if a mosquito transfers the infection from victim one to victim two? This could explain the spatial distribution of the cases. And what if the infectious agent had to 'ripe' for some days inside the mosquito? This would explain the distribution of the cases in time. Two meaningless observations seen together seem to form a meaningful hypothesis, which can be empirically tested without exactly identifying the agent of the disease. Letham now wants to perform these experiments. As it has been impossible to transfer the infectious agent to laboratory animals, this experiment would include human beings: the researchers will have to accept to be bitten by mosquitoes which have fed on the blood of infected patients before. Letham junior, trained by his father to live with rats, is prepared to accept this situation of nutritional symbioses and he is able to persuade his fellows of the necessity of this passive activity, i.e. of being the live hosts of the parasites. Letham is infected with the disease. The construction of yellow fever in the mind of the scientific team has dramatically changed. In this part, the narrative is structured by the logic and the precisely defined questions and uncertainties of bacteriological knowledge and experimental practice. Much of the aesthetic tension the reader may experience is due to the literary dramatisation of experimental bacteriological knowledge and the logical structure of its methods:

> My Y.F. had meaning. For the first time since this terrible illness had begun afflicting and killing people, it had meaning. The experiment was a necessary one, whose result would be that things would change. It had great significance. Though I lay powerless in the grip of this awful disease, my mind and my will made me superior to it. (Weiss 2010, 426)

The series of experiments is performed even during Letham junior's illness and recovery. All cases seem to corroborate the hypothesis of the mosquito being the life vector of yellow fever. A subsequent series of experiments excludes further ways of transmission (by excrements, clothing, direct contact etc.).

These experiments are successfully performed when Carolus and Letham learn that another research team of different nationality pretends to have discovered the active agent of yellow fever in the form of a spirochaete. Carolus is disappointed. In Letham's understanding of the situation, the two results fit together like the two halves of a sheet of paper torn apart. The two teams meet and exchange their information. Carolus and Letham accept the spirochaete-theory, but the other crew denies the validity of Letham's experiments and does not accept the mosquito as a live vector. The identification and visualization of the infectious agent being the more prestigious scientific achievement, the career of the mosquito theory seems to be blocked. But the story takes a further surprising turn.

Carolus arranges a meeting with the recently installed governor of the penal colony. This young official is not interested in the scientific discussion of methods and prestige; his understanding of truth is not academic, but pragmatic. He understands that the identification of the infectious agent has relatively little consequences for the actions that the government may take; the identification of the life vector, on the other hand, opens a large field for hygienic sanitation. He defines a two-year-project for the area of the penal colony that aims at eliminating all pools with standing water where the mosquitoes lay their eggs. In this administrative measure the governor sees first of all the possibility to create employment for the prisoners. With his statistics Carolus can prove that cases of yellow fever have drastically diminished in the sanitized areas. The project is prolonged. After a certain time, Letham junior, being granted a reprieve, is appointed the successor of the old town physician who first had the idea of Stegomyia fasciata being the vector of yellow fever. In this function, he is involved in a large scale sanitation project of the colonial government, in the context of which an area "larger than Europe" (Weiss 2010, 559) is freed of the attacks of yellow fever.

There is one detail still to be mentioned, which is important for my interpretation of the novel: The young governor who gives a chance to the sanitation project is a former protégé of Georg Letham senior. Later, however, the brilliant young man becomes a threat to the power position of the senior official, who cynically manages to sidetrack his career in the metropolis. Two victims of Letham senior thus cooperate successfully in the colonies: On the axiological level of the narrative, this coincidence signals once more the difference between the destructive, social Darwinist power play of the rat-man Letham senior in contrast to another, pragmatic attitude of the younger generation of the mosquito-controllers, who are able to renounce a position of absolute dominance, who abandon projects of radical eradication of the other, who adapt, however, to situations of cohabitation and start projects of pragmatic cultural progress.

It is only after many years of practicing colonial medicine as a humble official that Georg Letham junior writes down the history of his life. The beginning of this narrative is a psychological novel. Inner monologue is often used to give insight into the inner experience of the protagonist. The style of writing changes but later. The text turns more and more into a factual report of external events. At the end, the narrator confesses to have used a pseudonym. Letham is not his real name, but an acronym of Hamlet. In this context, Hamlet is seen as the prototypical European, who becomes a murderer because he is hunted by his father's shadow. This period is over. Family names do not matter anymore. His real name does not even figure among the authors of the scientific report of the Stegomyia experiments, there is only a patient No. 5. The novel ends with the following lines:

> We stamped out Y. F. here. Others followed us. The battle to eradicate the mosquitoes and develop the fertile region was a fascinating one that lasted for years and turned out well. The territory flourished.

> This is where I leave the scene.
> I disappeared into the crowd, and that is for the best. (Weiss 2010, 559f.)[6]

2 Facts and Fictions: The Problem of the Frames of Reference

Letham's experiments to identify Stegomyia fasciata as the live vector of yellow fever are not pure literary fiction. Weiss' imagination draws on historical facts to some extent. But the factual extra-literary information is not represented with historical, referential accuracy. Weiss' appropriation of historical facts is highly selective and highly transformative. The comparison of the facts and their literary transformations may provide us with some more insight concerning the genuinely literary intentions of Weiss' novel, especially with respect to the axiological tendencies of its persuasive strategies and of their ideological background. Let us therefore have a short look at the historical facts of the human efforts to control yellow fever.[7] They are closely linked to the history of colonialism. It begins with the record of a failure. In 1888, the French project to connect the Atlantic and Pacific oceans by building the canal of Panama was brutally stopped by the deaths of more than 20.000 workers caused by the epidemics of yellow fever and malaria. After the war between the United States of America and Spain in 1898, the island of Cuba came under US-American control. In the same year, the American army physician William C. Gorgas was appointed Chief Sanitary Officer in Havana to control an epidemic outbreak of yellow fever. He took sanitary measures based on a theory of the Cuban physician Carlos Finlay, who first had the idea that Stegomyia fasciata transmitted yellow fever in 1881. These sanitary measures were quite successful. In 1900, the US-American surgeon Walter Reed and his team where mandated by the American government to examine all questions related to the causes and the transmission of yellow fever. The Reed com-

6 Rotenberg's English translation does not follow the German text very closely. It introduces the notion of "eradication" in close connection with the mosquitoes, which is, as this paper wants to demonstrate, inappropriate to the logics of the sanitation project conceived in the context of this novel. The mosquitoes are not "eradicated" as a species, but only controlled by the local sanitation of their breeding places.

7 On the history of Yellow Fever see Crosby 2006. We further consulted Wikipedia: History of Yellow Fever (2012), Wikipedia: William C. Gorgas (2012), Wikipedia: Noguchi Hideyo (2012), Wikipedia: Max Theiler. Compare also the website of the National Library of Medicine entitled "Profiles in Medicine. The Wilbur A. Sawyer Papers: The Yellow Fever Laboratory: Rockefeller Foundation 1928–1937". On Walter Reed, see Bean 1982.

mission proved Finlay's Stegomyia theory to be true, and it proved other theories of transmission by water, air, clothes, contact etc. to be wrong. The Reed commission was not successful, however, in identifying the causal agent of the disease. But the success of Gorgas' sanitary measures was convincing. Gorgas presented his method at the 11th International Sanitary Conference in Paris in 1903, where he urged the international community to abolish international quarantine regulations with regard to yellow fever and to adjust sanitary measures to the newly developed knowledge. In November 1903 US Military forces occupied the southern part of Columbia, declaring this area to be the independent State of Panama. The USA revived the former French project of the Panama Canal in 1904. In the same year, William Gorgas became the Chief Sanitary Officer of the Canal Zone. Due to the sanitary measures he installed, yellow fever was almost banned from that region by 1906. The construction of the Panama Canal was completed in 1914. But there was still no certain knowledge concerning the infectious agent of this disease. In 1918, the Japanese bacteriologist Noguchi, a specialist on spirochaete as the infectious agent of syphilis, was mandated by the Rockefeller foundation to develop a vaccine against yellow fever. Noguchi started his work in Ecuador, and after a few weeks of laboratory research, he pretended to have discovered the infectious agent of yellow fever in the form of a spirochaete. But in 1926, Andrew Sellard and Max Theiler, two researchers of the US-American Rockefeller Institute, proved Noguchi's hypothesis to be wrong. Noguchi had discovered the agent of another disease causing serious liver conditions, Weil's disease. In 1927, the same team of the Rockefeller Institute isolated the virus of the African yellow fever. They then proved the causal agents of African and of South American virus strands to be immunologically identical. This knowledge formed the basis of the development of a vaccine by Max Theiler ten year later in 1937.

This is a brief and quite superficial summary of the medical history of yellow fever. But it is sufficient to show some of the characteristic aspects of Weiss' methods of literary appropriation of historical facts. The Stegomyia experiments of Letham and his crew are depicted in close analogy to the experiments performed by the US-American army physician Walter Reed and his team in Cuba in 1900. The sources that Weiss used are not yet comprehensively identified, we only know that he used the presentation of Walter Reed and his Stegomyia experiments in Paul de Kruif's book *Mikrobenjäger* [Microbe Hunters], which was first published in English in 1925 and in German translation two years later. It had been a bestseller of popular literature for many years. But this historical information is not transposed into a literary, fictional narrative without substantial transformation. How did Weiss proceed as a writer of fiction and what is the significance of this poetic licence?

Letham junior mentions the sanitation project carried through by himself and the governor called "La Forest" in an area "larger than Europe" (Weiss 2010, 559). This is very clearly an analogy to Gorgas' activities. In Weiss' novel, the Canal of Panama is mentioned early as a place, where yellow fever takes its tribute among coloured workers and white engineers alike (Weiss 2010, 98), but the historical connection of Gorgas' fight against yellow fever with the building of the Panama Canal is never explicitly mentioned. The factual information is abstracted from the original frame of reference in time and space. The Stegomyia experiment is post-dated from 1900 to an indefinite, fictional point of time in the 1920s: "It was five thirty on ..., 192..., a weekday: Tuesday, I believe" (Weiss 2010, 377). The location is not Cuba any more, but the small city of "C.," the main site of a penal colony, which makes the reader rather think of Cayenne and the French penal colony in French Guayana. Weiss is deliberately ambiguous about the geographical location of the narrated plot. "C." is said to be an "island or peninsula" (Weiss 2010, 97). Weiss establishes some similarities between the names of some real persons involved in the Reed Commission and the names of his fictional physicians: the fictional "Walter" corresponds to the factual Walter Reed, the fictional Carolus might allude to the factual James Carrol; Felizian v. F., the town physician of C., is set in analogy to Finlay. There actually is an anonymous patient No. 5 in Reed's records etc. But all the bacteriologists involved in Weiss' fiction are not US-American citizens any longer, but they all studied at the "Pasteur Institute" (Weiss 2010, 142), which, in reality, is a French institution. Walter's wife and his children, however, return from the colony to London (Weiss 2010, 345, 440). The power structure of administration Letham senior lives in seems to be rather German or Austrian, neither specifically French nor British, but clear indications are not given in this respect either. What is the significance of this repeated blurring of national identities?

Some knowledge that the narrator-instance Letham junior uses seems to be scientifically outdated, not only in the perspective of today's knowledge, but even in the context of the late 1920s, when the novel was written. This is the case as far as the discovery of the infectious agent of yellow fever is at stake. At this point Ernst Weiss draws on the hypothesis of Noguchi from 1919, which was refuted by the research of Sellard and Theiler in 1926. Did the author Ernst Weiss know about this fact, was it his intention to make the reader realize that some of the knowledge used by Letham and his team is outdated and flawed?

What is the lesson we learn from cross-reading contemporary historical and medical knowledge about yellow fever with its literary appropriation in Weiss' fictional novel? We observe that Weiss' method of transformation is highly selective towards historical facts and that he uses an irritating technique of blurring referential identities of information in space and time and an irritating technique of syncretism, of melting together bits and pieces of locally and chronologically heterogeneous frames of reference. Weiss' literary technique of blurring the national identities of the persons involved can probably be read in this context as a literary statement. In reality, the progress of bacteriology was highly invested with feelings and the rhetoric of national competition and national pride. But the problem that Weiss wants to discuss in this novel should not be seen within the frame of a nationalist discourse. Weiss probably wanted to address a cultural frame he considered to be European, i.e. Occidental, not national, and he addresses a reader who is willing to adopt this contra-factual perspective. It is not a national project in which Letham junior reconstructs his new anonymous identity. His visions of science and civilization are kept universal and transnational.

The blinding out of the construction of the Panama Canal hints in the same direction: It allows to silently pass over the context of US-American Imperialism in Middle and South America and to avoid any confrontation with the realistic conditions of work during the construction of the Panama Canal. If we consider the selective appropriation of the historical context as a strategy of the model author, we may conclude that the plot of this novel is strategically set in the frame of a 'colonial idyll'. Obviously the text is not about historical truth. It is not a text with the polemic intention of an explicit, politically engaged criticism of nationalist and imperialistic rhetoric and practices. Weiss rather avoids discourses of nationalism and of colonialism; he tries to sidetrack them by blurring the historical references of his information. Within the frame of this 'colonial idyll' however, Weiss uses contemporary bacteriological and epidemiological knowledge to innovatively structure the plot of his narrative.

Weiss positively dramatizes the methods of empirical scientific research in bacteriology and of science-based hygienic practice as the frame of a new concept of a socially constructed identity of the modern individual. The contemporary methods of experimental research in its function of verifying and falsifying empirically testable hypotheses are widely and skilfully used. The scientifically creative synthesis of unrelated pieces of knowledge in the framework of a new theory of transmission and the design of a coherent series of experiments on people in order to empirically test this theory creates much of the aesthetic tension of this narrative. In this respect, Weiss is creative in transposing modern scientific methodology into a literary text. The reader may learn from this popularisation of science in literature that science is not the act of a single individual, but the result of a thoroughly enacted method of research. This methodological orientation remains true, even if a piece of positive knowledge used by one or the other researcher may actually be refuted. Weiss abstains from strategies of trivial glorification of the bacteriologist as an individual hero of splendid scientific geniality. His protagonists are all human beings with problematic traits of character.

They have their skills and their partial knowledge. But this knowledge is shown to be limited, they all make mistakes in their work, but together, they perform steps ahead in creating new knowledge. Weiss depicts scientific, medical and hygienic progress as the result of cooperation in a team. Even if not all of the presuppositions and results of the experiments narrated in this novel are and remain true in the horizon of an informed reader and in the horizon of later stages of scientific knowledge, the method of scientific research depicted in this novel remains valid because it implies a pragmatic criterion of validity and shows the path to empirically correct flawed pieces of knowledge. It is functionally adequate in this perspective, that Letham and his team partly use false and outdated medical knowledge in the construction of a functioning hygienic project and of a science-based concept of socially constructed subjectivity. Neither of these leading axiological concepts of the novel is dependent on factual truth of a single argument, but on the acceptance of scientific research as a method of acquiring and correcting knowledge in and for the community. In accordance with this pragmatic concept of subjective identity, Weiss chooses a narrator who is not beyond doubt, who is unreliable in many respects.

3 Contemporary Knowledge about Rats

After the comparison of Weiss' fictive construction of the fight against yellow fever with the medico-historical facts, we may ask analogous questions about the fight against rats. What was known and discussed concerning the control and eventual eradication of the rats in the late 1920s, when Weiss conceived and wrote his novel?

In Mai 1928, the "First International Conference on Rats" was held in Paris. This conference was organized by Gabriel Petit, member of both the French Academies of Medicine and Veterinary Medicine. It stood under the patronage of Raymond Poincaré, president of the French Republic, and Aristide Briand, Minister of Foreign Affairs. Official representatives of the public health systems of more than fifty nations gathered at the Sorbonne University. The echo in the international press was significant. The contributions to the conference, containing reports on the different practices of rat control all over the world, were published in print in 1931 (Petit 1931).

The rat is seen as a vector of numerous contagious diseases, especially of the pest, by all the participants of the conference. But it is also considered as a considerable threat to economic welfare because of the destruction of a substantial amount of food stock, mainly on ships and in the warehouses of the ports. The growth of the world market after World War I makes both aspects of rat populations an urgent topic of international coordination. More food stock is transported worldwide, and the danger of infectious diseases spreading around the globe is higher than ever before. Deratisation of ships therefore is the main focus of this international conference.

When it comes to discuss the measures to be taken, the conference is divided into two groups. There are some few advocates of the method of building rat-proof ships and warehouses. It is the delegate of the United States, Senior Surgeon Samuel B. Grubbs, who argues that all the measures of extinction never attain full success and are therefore doomed to failure because of the enormous proliferation rate of the rodents (Petit 1931, 78–81). He draws on biological observations of species having been extinguished, and he argues that this extinction has never been due to directly aggressive measures like hunting, but to the invasion of the habitat by other species or by mankind. He therefore pleads to adopt 'natural' measures, by which he means constructing ships and buildings that do not offer a favourable environment to rats for hiding, feeding and breeding. The strategy consists in changing the environment where human beings and parasites cohabitate in such a way that the conditions of reproduction of the parasite are changed. Thus, a direct aggressive killing attack on the parasite with its dangerous and incalculable side effects is avoided. The extinction of the biological species of the parasite is not the explicit target of these procedures. Grubbs explicitly mentions the possibility of survival of the targeted species as far as it is living apart from human settlements.[8] It is quite evident that this principle of rat control is similar to the methods and ideologies used by the US-American medical officers to control mosquitoes in the Panama Canal zone.

But the majority of the experts gathered in 1928 do not adopt and do not practice this US-American method. The rhetoric of warfare and extinction, of crusade against the enemy of mankind prevails. Some of the papers of the European experts draw a systematic overview of the techniques used for killing rats: dogs and other animals, mechanical traps of different types, solid poison, infection with bacteria, the "Système Ratin" which consists in a combination of poison and bacterial infection, or, most efficient especially for the deratisation of ships: fumigation with gas – with carbon oxide, oxide of sulphur, cyanide, hydronic acid and others. These methods of fumigation are widely discussed, practical experiences in avoiding accidents are shared; the delegates travel to the

8 It is quite obvious that Grubbs' argument is inscribed in an ideological context of "colonial idyll". In this perspective, the bison in North America, for example, disappeared because of the introduction of agriculture in the areas where the species lived and bread (cf. Petit 1931, 78). Grubbs does not mention the nutritional symbioses of bison and Native Americans. The genocide executed on American Natives is no topic in the framework of his argument.

port of Hague to look at demonstrations of some recently developed types of fumigation devices.

The reason of this preference has to be seen in the continuity of hygienic measures basing on the military experiences of World War I. It is the delegate of Great Britain, E.-C. Read, technical adviser for rat destruction in the Ministry of Agriculture and Fisheries, who most explicitly addresses this historical connection between rat destruction and Wold War I:

> Immediately after the war the question of asphyxiating gasses was examined with regard to their applicability in rat-destruction. Experiments were carried out with all sorts of gasses, especially those which had been used in the trenches, e.g. chlorine and chloropicrin. These gasses, undoubtedly very powerful in killing rats, were highly dangerous for the operators. Experiments made in order to find less dangerous gasses showed sulphur dioxide (SO2) to be most appropriate. Research recently done by private companies introduced various new forms of using asphyxiating gasses to the markets. The products are mainly of two types: 1. Sulphur compounds, 2. Calcium cyanide. [Aussitôt après la guerre la question des gaz asphyxiants fut mise à l'étude en ce qui concerne leur application à la destruction des rats. Des expériences furent faites avec toutes sortes de gaz, particulièrement avec ceux qui avaient été employés dans les tranchées, tels que le chlore et la chloropicrine. Ces gaz, sans contredit très efficaces pour la destruction des rats, présentaient de graves dangers pour les opérateurs, et les expériences faites dans le but de trouver un gaz moins dangereux démontrèrent que l'anhydride sulfureux (SO2) présentait les meilleures conditions. Les recherches faites récemment par des sociétés privées ont introduit sur le marché différentes manières d'utiliser les gaz asphyxiants. Les produits se divisent en deux catégories principales: 1. Les composés du soufre; 2. Le cyanure de calcium.] (Petit 1931, 226 f.)

The delegate of the Netherlands, Dr. Nicolaas Marinus Josephus Jitta, reports that the port authorities in Rotterdam recently made good experiences with Cyclone and Cyclone B – "qui nous vient de l'Allemage" (Petit 1931, 191), and Dr. Theodor Saling, delegate of the Prussian Institute of Hygiene, communicates the names and addresses of producer and distributor of this newly developed substance:

> Among the toxic gasses most frequently used for the fumigation of ships, the procedure 'Cyclone' of Degesch in Frankfurt-on-Main proved to be most efficient. [...] In Germany, the official decree on the usage of highly toxic substances against parasites applies to said procedure with prussic acid. Only two big enterprises, Degesch in Frankfurt-on-Main and Stabenow in Hamburg, are authorized to fumigate with prussic acid. [Parmi les gaz toxiques dont l'usage prévaut pour la désinfection des bateaux, le procédé 'Cyclone', de la Degesch, à Francfort-sur-le-Main, a fait ses preuves. (...) En Allemagne, l'ordonnance relative à l'emploi de substances très toxiques pour détruire les animaux nuisibles s'applique au procédé dit à l'acide prussique. La désinfection par l'acide prussique n'y est permis qu'à deux grandes maisons, la Degesch, à Francfort-sur-le Main, et Stabenow à Hamburg.] (Petit 1931, 144 f.)

In the context of holocaust research it is well known that Cyclone and Cyclone B were used in Auschwitz and other German concentration camps to kill hecatombs of Jews, Roma and other human beings seen as 'undesirable parasites' by the Nazi regime. After World War II, "Degesch," the "Deutsche Gesellschaft für Schädlingsbekämpfung" and "Testa," Tesch & Stabenow in Hamburg, were accused of producing and delivering Cyclone and Cyclone B to the concentration camps. Cyclone B thus became a symbol of the Holocaust.[9]

The simultaneous coexistence of at least two concepts of rat control in the international discourses of 1928 can be seen as characteristic for the broader context of epidemiological disease control and especially bacteriology by the end of World War I and during the interwar period. Bacteriology as developed by Robert Koch dominated the German military medicine and its approach to the control of contagious diseases during World War I. This paradigm of disease control is characterized by a strictly monocausal model of contagious diseases: it is the presence of a specific pathogenic agent which causes the disease. The presence of this pathogenic agent has to be demonstrated by strict laboratory methods. The measures of disease control are designed in order to stop the pathogenic agent from spreading. There is not much scientific interest in treating the ill and in respecting the socio-cultural contexts and traditions in which infected people live. There is some criticism of this strictly scientific approach and its impracticability in the field by officials of German military medicine during the war. But Koch's bacteriology is put into a severe crisis only by the end of World War I. The officials of military medicine feared and forecasted a severe epidemic outbreak of bacterial infection, especially typhus, caused by the uncontrolled remigration of soldiers form the Eastern Front and by the uncontrolled migration of populations of the East to the West. But these bacterial epidemics did not happen. Another, hitherto unknown and untreatable disease exploded almost simultaneously all over the World in 1918: the Spanish flue. It caused an estimate death-toll of about 30 million victims worldwide by the End of 1919, i.e. definitely more victims than the war did. Bacteriology was clueless in confrontation with this (viral) disease of which the agent could not be visualized and isolated by the methods then available and of which the ways of spreading were therefore unknown. The development of new virological concepts in bio-medical science was a long and tortuous process. The monocausal paradigm of Robert Koch was contested and partially replaced by other paradigms. The presence of the causal agent was not seen any longer as the necessary and sufficient cause for the

9 For the long medical history of gassing in the context of the attempts to control typhus in East Europe by delousing clothes of migrants cf. Weindling 2000. Weindling documents the growing function of Cyclone in this context and the genocidal turn given of this method of disease control under the Nazi regime.

outbreak of the disease. Notions of immunity entered the discussion. The presence of the pathogenic agent could be checked by other causal factors. The notion of balance was introduced into bacteriology: the outbreak of the disease was understood as the expression of a disturbed balance in the perennial symbioses of host and parasite. Environmental factors had to be taken into account in order to explain how balanced systems could be disturbed and how balance could be restored.[10]

But the reception and appropriation of this environmental and ecological arguments differed substantially along national and ideological borders. While the US-American discourse led by the Rockefeller Institute was rather open to 'liberal' interpretations of controlled cohabitation, the German military medical discourse remains rather oriented toward Koch's concepts and methods of strict, exterminatory control. This predilection for quarantine and aggressive cleansing has to be seen, as Weindling 2000 demonstrates, in the context of disease control in Eastern Europe and in the German attempt to control the immigration of Jewish and Roma populations from the East in the interwar period. Methods of shower-bathing of migrants, delousing their cloths by gassing and of cremation of dead bodies has been constantly used and developed as the technical standard between World War I and World War II. In the context of Nazi ideology, the environmental argument was again reinterpreted in terms of Nazi "Geo-Medicine," of "Lebensraum" and of racial supremacy of the Aryans. Paul Weindling shows in detail how the medical notion and the practices of disease control, especially of typhus control, became part of the genocidal practices in extermination camps.

We propose to read Ernst Weiss' novel in the context of contemporary bacteriology, which during this period went through a major shift from the Kochian paradigm to a not yet fully developed virology. Weiss began to work on this text in 1925. He then lived in Berlin. As a professional physician he had easy access to, and an informed understanding of, the ongoing discussion. Weiss obviously knew about the crisis of bacteriology and of the environmental arguments drawing on parasitological discourses which resurfaced in this context. Weiss certainly knew about the use of gas in World War I and the use of gas in the war against rats afterwards. And there are many signs in Weiss' novels and essays which hint at the fact that Weiss read Hitler's *Mein Kampf.* Weiss perfectly understood the death-threat that Hitler addresses to the Jewish minority in Germany, Austria and elsewhere. Hitler blames 'The Jew' to be the cause of every evil he thinks to identify as a sign of degeneration of the 'Aryan race'. Hitler metaphorically identifies 'The Jew' with any kind of parasite and of contagious agent imaginable

10 The complex and dynamic status of this discussion in the field of bacteriology after World War I has recently been reconstructed in Berger 2009.

and current in the discourses of his time. Jews are defamed in Hitler's rhetoric as contagious agents of syphilis, as mosquitoes and as rats. Weiss as a medical doctor and as a knowledgeable observer of bacteriology and hygiene of his time understood very precisely what these metaphors meant if understood in the context of a discourse of disease-eradication. In his essay *Bemerkungen zu den Tagebüchern und Briefen Franz Kafkas* [Notes on the Diaries and Letters of Franz Kafka], he wrote in 1938 on behalf of Kafka's notion of 'Gesetz':

> If we only knew what the commandment prohibits, something would then remain that is permitted (At least if it were not a commandment such as Hitler's towards the Jews. This one says: I want your best, gentlemen Jews, so much the best as you can only achieve in death; eradicate yourselves, please, be as polite; what does it matter to you; you are unable to change yourselves and it is impossible that you and we live together!) Yes indeed, it may be that Kafka's commandment is of this kind! [Wüßte man, was das Gebot verbietet, dann bliebe doch etwas, das es erlaubt. (Es sei denn, es wäre ein Gebot wie das Hitlers den Juden gegenüber, das sagt; ich will Euch wohl, meine Herren Juden, so sehr wohl, wie Ihr es nur im Tode haben könnet, löscht Euch aus, seid einmal so freundlich, was liegt Euch daran, ändern könnt Ihr Euch nicht, Ihr und wir können nicht zusammen leben!) Ja, vielleicht ist Kafkas Gebot doch etwas dieser Art.] (Weiss 1982, 419)

Weiss' reading of Kafka in the context of Hitler may be irritating, but it expresses Weiss' acute awareness of living under a cynical and inescapable death-threat.

4 Metaphors of Disease and Contagion

Hitler's application of metaphors of disease and contagion on human beings in the context of political demagogy is a life-threatening rhetorical strategy because the paradigm of extinction is dominant in the discourses of medical hygiene of the time. In Weiss' novel semantics of disease and of infection are mainly used in the literal, i. e. pragmatic sense of the word. Weiss' novel literally speaks of infectious diseases like scarlet and yellow fever within the framework of contemporary medical knowledge. The terms are used in their medical, bacteriological and epidemiological meaning. Thus, the metaphorical use of infection and infectious disease as a simile or as a metaphor in the sense of classical rhetoric is relatively rare in Weiss' text. There are some few instances of a metaphoric use of the term 'contagion,' when Letham depicts his tendency to involuntarily mimic the body language and conduct of another person with whom he communicates: yawning and laughter are "contagious," but also the habit of experimentally influencing the behaviour of other people (Weiss 2010, 47 and 76). There are some instances of a conventional use of illnesses as a metaphor, e. g. when Letham represents his own imbalanced character as "tugged this way and that by internal contradictions, like a malaria patient who sweats and shivers" (Weiss 2010, 8). Plague is used several times as a conventional metaphor, e.g. in the perspective of the members of Letham senior's expedition. They identify the rats with the plague: "They shun the repulsive animals like the plague, a plague of rats" (Weiss 2010, 197). On the deportation vessel, the officers "avoid the convicts like the plague" (Weiss 2010, 256). There is one quite unusual, innovative instance of metaphorical use of "plague" [Pest] in the text: "The mere appearance of order without order itself – this is the plague of mankind, enshrined in administration and government" (Weiss, 2010, 150).

If we want to look comprehensively at the narrative implementation of rats and mosquitoes and their possible metaphorical meaning in the fictional world of Weiss' novel, we have to shift from the interpretation of metaphors on a local level to the reading and interpretation of a semantic field that is richly differentiated and almost omnipresent in its ramifications throughout the text. We thus propose to consider an allegorical interpretation of Weiss' text, i.e. to read some selected constellations of its drastically factual surface as invitations to think about a second, more comprehensive meaning.[11] In an episode of the deportation camp, rats and convicts are put in close parallel in the context of a narrative episode: the tension among the convicts living under deck becomes more and more aggressive. The captain decides to evacuate the under deck and to blow hot steam into the caverns. After this demonstration, several cadavers of dead rats are detected and ostensibly thrown overboard, in order to demonstrate to the convicts that the same steam device could be used against them, if necessary (Weiss 2010, 266). The simile of rats = convicts is staged here not on the level of a conventional, local rhetoric trope, but as a textual plot that triggers the reader's emotions and his reflection on the axiological, ethical and political implications of the situation and the practices represented in the text.

In the fictional world of Weiss' novel, on the level of narrative and global signification, we identify the staging of three different paradigms of human conduct towards the live vectors of infectious diseases. We propose to read these three paradigms as allegories of different relations to otherness in human societies.[12]

The first paradigm can be labelled the paradigm of total warfare of extinction, the second the paradigm of controlled cohabitation, and the third the paradigm of nutritional symbiosis.

---

11 The pragmatics of allegorical reading are analysed by Zabka 2005. Weiss' poetics of the "mythic" identity of existence and meaning (see footnote 4) should be reconsidered in this context.

12 As an introduction to the ecocritical framework of this proposition cf. Hofer 2007.

The first paradigm, the total war of extinction, is dominant in the extratextual discourse. As instance of this paradigm we identify the aggressive life-threatening labelling of 'The Jew' as a parasite, as a rat and as a mosquito in the anti-Semitic discourse of the time and especially in Hitler's *Mein Kampf.* Hitler and the anti-Semitic National Socialist of his time are to be identified as advocates of a total war of extinction with the use of all technical means against the racial other seen as parasite. Weiss' novel gives an answer to this paradigm in narratively depicting the self-destructive consequences of a total warfare against a symbiotic parasite. This is the allegorical political meaning of the fictionally depicted experience of the gas war against rats invented by Georg Letham senior and his crew on their expedition to the North Pole. Letham junior comments on this self-destructive fight critically. On this level of interpretation, Letham senior's biography narrated by his son Letham junior can be read as a literary allegory of the political ideology which has lead to World War I and would lead to another aggressive and eventually self-destructive conflict in the near future.

The second paradigm, a social and ecological relation of human society towards the other, is presented in the novel: Letham junior's involvement in the control of the live vector of yellow fever. The pragmatic concept of truth, which is implied in the American way of looking at diseases and at the biology of their live vectors, is presented as an alternative to the Social-Darwinist concept of total eradication of the other. The paradigm of controlled cohabitation is free of any moral and cultural prejudices against parasites. Rats do not always mean pest. Mosquitoes do not always mean disease. They are both aspects of life and as such interesting and even beautiful phenomena.[13] Their behaviour is scientifically observed and to a large extent considered to be intelligent and functional. Human beings have to understand the life conditions of the parasite in order to intelligently alter the environmental condition: the area of human civilisation and colonisation has to turn into an unfavourable breeding place for parasites. This procedure is not aggressive toward the single individual, but prohibitive to the reproduction of the species. Total extinction is not the primordial aim of the intervention. In the protagonist's understanding of this paradigm, the self-destroying backslash of wars of extinction on human society is avoided. The extinction of the other is rather seen as an unwanted side effect of human civilisation, an unhappy coincidence. In principle, this paradigm tolerates the survival of the

---

13 Cf. the description of rats: "They gleam in the sun, well fed and plump, their fur is smooth, and they actually have a kind of beauty, such as is produced even in ugly individuals by proper nourishment and a feeling of being at one with the world" (Weiss 2010, 206) and of Stegomyia fasciata: "It is a graceful, lively insect of brown to blackish brown color punctuated by conspicuous white parts" (Weiss 2010, 366).

other in different places. In this paradigm of human conduct, the narrator of the novel, Georg Letham junior, finds a frame to physically and mentally survive as a useful and anonymous member of human society.

The third paradigm evoked in Weiss' novel is the paradigm of nutritional symbiosis. This paradigm is realized only by one person in the novel, and only experimentally, without finding the consent of the represented community: it emerges in the mind of Georg Letham senior who, as a scientist, observes the feeding behaviour of his dog Ruru on the rat ship, experiments privately with eating rat meat and drinking rat blood in order to prevent scurvy. For Letham senior, equilibrium of nutritional symbiosis between rats and human beings in the closed system of the expedition vessel is imaginable and practicable. But his crew categorically denies this opportunity and opts for the eventually self-destructive warfare of extinction. Letham junior remembers this unrealized possibility. To the reader of the novel, and probably to its model author as we propose to understand him, this would have been a way out of the crisis, a third possibility.

Readers living in the twenty first century might be prepared to reconsider these fictional constructions of the metabolic relation between human societies and their biological environment presented in Weiss' novel with more ecological understanding and more ecocritical sensibility. We propose to read Weiss' novel as a fictional text which respects the axiological demand that Paul Weindling formulates, it being the ethical result of his historical studies of epidemics and genocide: "All programs of disease eradication must be free from coercive experimentation and differential evaluations of human lives. Preventing disease should be accompanied by preventing the definition of any new species of infectious human parasite" (Weindling 2000, 427). We thus think of Ernst Weiss as of an author who writes the text of his fictional world in close connection with, and as a critical answer to, contemporary contexts of political discourse and its ethical implications.

References

Bean, William. *Walter Reed: A Biography.* Charlottesville: Univ. of Virginia Press, 1982.

Berger, Silvia. *Bakterien in Krieg und Frieden. Eine Geschichte der medizinischen Bakteriologie in Deutschland 1890–1933.* Göttingen: Wallstein, 2009.

Crosby, Molly Caldwell. *The American Plague: The Untold Story of Yellow Fever, the Epidemic that Shaped our History.* New York: Berkley Books, 2006.

De Kruif, Paul. *Mikrobenjäger.* Zurich, Leipzig: Orell Füssli, 1927.

Hofer, Stefan. *Die Ökologie der Literatur. Eine systemtheoretische Annäherung.* Bielefeld: Transcript, 2007.

Käser, Rudolf. *Arzt, Tod und Text. Grenzen der Medizin im Spiegel deutschsprachiger Literatur.* Munich: Fink, 1998.

Käser, Rudolf. "Wie und zu welchem Ende werden Epidemien erzählt? Zur kulturellen Funktion literarischer Seuchendarstellung." *Internationales Archiv für Sozialgeschichte der Literatur* 29.1 (2004): 200–227.
Orell, Esther Claudia. *Die Macht der Benennung. Literarische Seuchendarstellungen und ihre wertvermittelnde Funktion.* Zurich: Univ. Diss. 2005.
Petit, Gabriel (Ed.). *Première conférence internationale du rat. Paris-Le Havre 16–22 Mai 1928.* Paris: Vigot, 1931.
Weindling, Paul. *Epidemics and Genocide in Eastern Europe, 1890–1945.* New York, NY: Oxford University Press, 2000.
Weiss, Ernst. *Georg Letham. Physician and Murderer. Translated from the German by Joel Rotenberg.* Brooklyn, NY: Archipelago Books, 2010.
Weiß, Ernst. *Georg Letham. Arzt und Mörder. Roman.* Frankfurt a. M.: Suhrkamp, 1982 [1931] (Gesammelte Werke V. 10. Eds. Peter Engel, and Volker Michels).
Weiß, Ernst. *Die Kunst des Erzählens. Essays, Aufsätze, Schriften zur Literatur.* Frankfurt a. M.: Suhrkamp, 1982 (Gesammelte Werke V. 16. Eds. Peter Engel, and Volker Michels).
Zabka, Thomas. *Pragmatik der Literaturinterpretation. Theoretische Grundlagen – kritische Analysen.* Tübingen: Niemeyer, 2005.
Webpages:
Harvard University Library Open Collections Program. *Contagion: Historical Views of Diseases and Epidemics. Tropical Diseases and the Construction of the Panama Canal* [http://ocp.hul.harvard.edu/contagion/panamacanal.html (1.07.2012)].
National Library of Medicine. Profiles in Science. The Wilbur A. Sawyer Papers: The Yellow Fever Laboratory: Rockefeller Foundation, 1928–1937 [http://profiles.nlm.nih.gov/ps/retrieve/Narrative/LW/p-nid/138 (1.07.2012)].
Wikipedia. "History of Yellow Fever". [http://en.wikipedia.org/wiki/History_of_yellow_fever (1.07.2012)]
Wikipedia. "William C. Gorgas". [http://en.wikipedia.org/wiki/William_C._Gorgas (1.07.2012)]
Wikipedia. "Noguchi Hideyo". [http://de.wikipedia.org/wiki/Noguchi_Hideyo. (1.07.2012)]
Wikipedia. "Max Theiler". [http://en.wikipedia.org/wiki/Max_Theiler (1.07.2012)]

Yahya Elsaghe

Infectious Diseases in Max Frisch

1

Max Frisch was born in May 1911, at a time when tuberculosis was still the leading cause of death in Switzerland (Eidgenössisches Statistisches Amt 1947). May 1911 was also the month in which an author from Germany, about whom Frisch subsequently felt the usual anxiety of influence, began a holiday journey. The literary result of that journey is well known: *Death in Venice* became and remains one of the famous memorials which its author, like no other in the history of German literature, created to the profound fears of those infectious diseases which once flourished in the Western world – the fear not only of cholera, but also of typhoid, of tuberculosis and finally of syphilis. The cure for this last had already been found (Brandt 1993, 573–574) by the time Frisch himself began to make a name as an author – or the name under which he is still famous today.[1] But while Frisch was still working to consolidate and institutionalise that name, the fears of infection returned: In the year that his archive was established, acquired immune deficiency syndrome was documented for the first time. In the year that his collected 'Portraits, Sketches and Speeches' appeared under the title *Forderungen des Tages* [Demands of the Day], scientists succeeded in identifying the human immunodeficiency virus. And in the year that the final authorised edition of Frisch's works was published, the World Health Organisation established its wide-ranging Global Programme on AIDS (Mann 1987, 733).

In other words, Max Frisch – along with the generation of German-speaking authors of whom he is the best-known representative – has a remarkable significance in the *Mentalitätsgeschichte* of infection. In terms of the history of infectious diseases, the experience of Frisch and his generation extends from the 'Spanish' influenza (Schütt 2011, 63; Hieronimus 2006, 8; Thalmann 1968, 7) to the emergence of a completely new retrovirus, and thus encompasses not only the epoch of centuries-old – indeed, millennia-old – fears of infectious diseases, but also the era in which such diseases were alleviated, as well as the first years in which they reappeared in one form or another. There is no doubt that the traces of Frisch's generational position can be observed in his *Collected Works*; or that in a certain sense those traces *cannot* be observed in the *Collected Works*.

1 A key factor here is his *Diary 1946–1949*, which was published by Suhrkamp, and is significant because it was published by Suhrkamp.

For regardless of how powerful or how slight Frisch's fear of influence by Thomas Mann may have been, of how perhaps it is palpable as late as a Mannian title *Forderungen des Tages* or as the decision to establish an archive at none other than Zurich's Federal Institute of Technology: that fear does not seem to have touched – or at least to have touched substantially – infection as a fundamental and life-changing theme in Frisch's literary works. Frisch's œuvre testifies less, if at all, to the absence of fears of infection than – in accordance with his generational position – to the disappearance of those fears.

Frisch's heroes and anti-heroes grapple neither with cholera nor typhoid, nor with syphilis; and there is no question of them dying of those diseases. His heroes and anti-heroes do not even contract tuberculosis, notwithstanding that during the earlier years of his life this was "the most significant of all the chronic infectious diseases" [d(ie) wichtigste() aller chronischen Infektionskrankheiten] (Weygandt 1912, 91), to quote a medical journal of the time; though when Frisch himself finally died of illness, tuberculosis was no longer among the twenty most frequent causes of death (Bundesamt für Statistik 2010).

But on the other hand, it would be quite incorrect to assert that the major infectious diseases, and tuberculosis specifically, are nowhere to be found in Frisch's works. Rather, they are conspicuous in his œuvre by their retreat. Even in his famous novels – indeed, especially in those novels – one can observe *in actu* how tuberculosis in particular is first forced to the periphery of the fictional space, before withdrawing from it entirely.

Whenever and wherever tubercular infections occur in Frisch's fictional works, they appear in their most prevalent form, designated as consumption of the lungs (Frisch 1994a, 101), and only at the margins of – or outside – the text's true narrative or intellectual focus. Tuberculosis is never fatal, nor dominant, nor characteristic in any way of any protagonist. Instead, it always occurs as it were eccentrically. It is only ever one of the features associated with female characters, who at the very most are deuteragonists.

This continuing marginalisation of tuberculosis is readily demonstrated by reference to Frisch's three most famous novels: *I'm Not Stiller* (1954), *Homo faber* (1957) and *Gantenbein* (1964). All three clearly indicate the generation to which their author belonged, and how familiar he must have been, in particular, with the ideas about tuberculosis which had once held sway among the general public. And when the three novels are read in the order of their composition, they clearly show how during Frisch's lifetime *Schwindsucht* – to use the popular word – fulfilled the prophecy of its traditional name self-reflexively by disappearing gradually from the collective consciousness.

2

If any of Max Frisch's texts unambiguously reveals his fear of influence by Thomas Mann, it is the first of his texts to be translated into English, which thus brought him his international or intercontinental breakthrough, *I'm Not Stiller.* It is no coincidence that *Der Zauberberg* is "the only work by Thomas Mann" which Anatol Stiller possesses, however modestly his library may be stocked, and however careless the narrator may be about it (Frisch 1994b, 314; 58). In the "Second Notebook" of *"Part One"* the action of *I'm Not Stiller* moves explicitly to where *The Magic Mountain* was set, in a passage which occupies several pages, and which abounds in direct references to, and thematic echoes of, the earlier novel: "*art nouveau* veranda" (*ibid.*, 97, 103), "the unchanging veranda" [die immergleiche Veranda] (Frisch 1986, 3: 464), "wrapped up in a rug," "most of the new arrivals," and most importantly the "young sanatorium veteran," a "Jesuit" and "student from a Catholic seminary" who is a reincarnation of, or a younger counterpart to, Leo Naphta, but who dies of tuberculosis in his turn, avoiding a violent death like Naphta's (Frisch 1994b, 97–116).

The disease which determines everything in *The Magic Mountain* also plays a decisive, 'final,' yet not really central role in *I'm Not Stiller.* While the latter novel is not animated by tuberculosis, in a sense it is ended by tuberculosis. The illness afflicts neither the main character, nor only a minor character, but a – or the – deuteragonist, for it afflicts the protagonist's wife, Julika Stiller, *née* Tschudy.[2]

Julika Stiller-Tschudy's tuberculosis attacks the most susceptible organ, in its smaller half and on the 'feminine' side of the body: "It was her left lung" (*ibid.*, 83). "The whole [...] left lung" (*ibid.*, 354) must eventually be removed, and the patient dies as a result of the operation.

This much at least can be gleaned from *"Part Two"* of the novel, the "Postscript by the Public Prosecutor," although the postscript itself includes a lacuna which is repeatedly marked as such. Before the evidently very urgent operation, "the doctor" avoids giving his patient a "medical expression," although her "own common sense" supplies it for her; just as the narrator avoids giving the readers that "medical expression" (*ibid.*, 83, 354), although it seems that none of them have so far identified it with their own intellect. And the immediate cause of death is also a lacuna. It is more or less ostentatiously *not* mentioned, when

---

2 Her birth name admits an autobiographical interpretation, suggesting the forename of the woman to whom Frisch was still married at the time, Trudy *née* von Meyenburg.

the narrative says expressly that the protagonist is indifferent to it: "The medical report did not interest him" (*ibid.*, 384).

This death from tuberculosis, which in terms of calendar years is the last to occur in Frisch's works, seals the tragic ending of the story. But in the overall context of the novel, the disease's fatal consequence and narrative credibility seem somewhat ill-founded, or at least they are very surprising. For in "*Part One*" the – still autodiegetic – narrator did not initially treat his wife's illness with the seriousness which, if one reads retrospectively from the novel's end, it would have merited. He did not hesitate to challenge the diagnosis offered by the doctors. He then speculated that his wife was not ill, or not seriously ill, but only simulating serious illness to avoid his sexual demands upon her; and he even toyed with the idea that she had adopted her "hugely expensive" disease as a kind of status symbol: "One might be tempted to not entirely believe even the medically attested tuberculosis which cost her so much throughout her life" [man könnte versucht sein, nicht einmal ihre ärztlich beglaubigte und in ihrem Leben so ungeheuer kostspielige Tuberkulose ganz zu glauben] (Frisch 1986, 3: 450; Condrau 1993–1994, 222–223; Condrau 2001, 429–430).

But some pages later here in the "Second Notebook," when Julika Stiller-Tschudy "must go as quickly as possible to Davos" (Frisch 1994b, 82) – on the journey which initiates the allusions to *The Magic Mountain* – the narrator who such a short time ago was so sceptical and smug about his wife's illness suddenly adopts a completely different attitude. He now eschews all smugness and irony, but he does not remark on the inconsistency of his narrative position, let alone explain it, still less excuse it. Giving not the slightest indication of irony, doubt or his own unreliability, he records characteristic and clinically unambiguous consumptive sensations experienced by the patient, which he now attributes to her in the indicative mode, in the affirmative mode and without reservation, reporting that she "fe[els] her slender body burning up like tinder" [ihren grazilen Körper verbrennen fühlt wie Zunder] (Frisch 1986, 3: 482).

These bodily sensations are accompanied by a psycho-physical and no less typical sensitivity which amounts to a profound change in being. To understand the extent of this change, it is necessary only to recall the nature of the Stillers' marital difficulty, or at least of one of their marital difficulties. The fact that the husband could so recently suspect his wife of only assuming her illness in order to escape her spousal obligations casts a disturbing light on the couple's sex life; or at least it betrays how the husband regards his wife *in eroticis et sexualibus*.

According to Stiller, "[t]he beautiful Julika" had long been "a crystal water-fairy" (Frisch 1994b, 85; 93–94). In her bluntly described frigidity, she had "expressed disgust" [ekelte] at "male sensuality" [männliche Sinnlichkeit], openly or at least "always to some extent" [immer etwas] (Frisch 1986, 3: 449).

The narrator's remarkably frank and unrestrained words here also reveal the attitudes of his generation in sexual matters. For *Stiller* was published a year after the famous or infamous *Kinsey Report.* And the novel echoes questions and answers in this report, for example when Stiller "casually mention[s] the scientific theory that in the whole of nature no female, except the human woman, experiences the so-called orgasm" (Frisch 1994b, 85).[3]

During her summer in Davos, Stiller's hitherto frigid and thus – if one will – conspicuously natural wife undergoes a transformation which is as astonishing as it is confusing. More or less overnight, she becomes a nymphomaniac. She is suddenly plagued by a "hitherto unknown [...] hunger" – or "strictly speaking" a "hunger for men," (Frisch 1986, 3: 482) given that a long time ago she had also made a "few unsuccessful ventures into lesbianism" (Frisch 1994b, 86). She is now overcome by "a desire that [...] could not be banished," (Frisch 1986, 3: 482) and which apparently cannot even be spoken aloud, but is so unspeakable and compulsive that it can only be written down in letters which must never reach their addressees:

> A hitherto unknown and confusing hunger for men, the more she felt her slender body burning up like tinder, a desire which at least in dreams could not be banished, as well as the constant awareness that Stiller was being unfaithful to her in those same nights, all this drove poor Julika to write letters which were not to be posted, no, not under any circumstances. And she never dreamed about Stiller, strictly speaking, but about consultant physicians, bakers' boys and men whom Julika had never seen. [Ein bisher unbekanntes und verwirrendes Verlangen nach dem Mann, je mehr sie ihren grazilen Körper verbrennen fühlte wie Zunder, eine Begierde, die sich zumindest in Träumen nicht verscheuchen ließ, und dazu das stete Bewußtsein, daß Stiller in diesen gleichen Nächten sie betrog, all dies zwang die arme Julika zu Briefen, die nicht abzuschicken waren, nein, unter keinen Umständen. Sie träumte ja auch gar nicht von Stiller, genau genommen, sondern von Oberärzten, Bäckerburschen und Männern, die Julika nie gesehen hatte.] (Frisch 1986, 3: 482)[4]

These are purely sexual fantasies, in other words dreams that are entirely divorced from married life and spousal love (the kind of fantasies which a minority

3 Whether this – highly debatable – thesis derives from some kind of contemporary source – at second hand, third hand or even first hand – is of course of subsidiary interest and would be difficult to determine in any case. For Alfred C. Kinsey *et alii* remain vague here, indeed contradictory. They content themselves with a *non liquet,* although they admit various hypotheses (1953, 135, 627–631).

4 Bullock's translation (Frisch 1994b, 114–115) misses the point: Theoretically speaking, "Verlangen nach *dem* Mann" [emphasis mine] could be rendered by "for her husband"; but this translation contradicts what follows, i.e. dreams of "consultant physicians, bakers' boys and *men*" [emphasis mine]. For the best part of the English version many thanks to Geoff Wilkes, Brisbane.

of the women interviewed by Kinsey *et aliis* were willing to state for the record [1953, 667–668]). "Strictly speaking," the cachectic woman does not dream about her husband. She has either never seen the imagined agents of her sexual fantasies, or else – in dreams where the men have or could have some relation to the patient's lived reality – they seem to be reduced solely to their sexual function or position: They are "*Ober*ärzte" [doctors on top] and as it were vigorous attendants of the oven, bakers' boys (Frisch 1986, 3: 482 [emphasis mine]).

In purely psychological terms, this mutation in the sick woman seems likely to test the goodwill of even fairly naive readers; and it should definitely have raised questions for professional commentators. For the narrator spares not a single syllable for explaining the change to himself or others. He does nothing more than establish a simple parallel between the psychic transformation of the patient's personality and the course of her physical illness: "*the more* she felt her slender body burning up like tinder" [emphasis mine].

However, it is only outside the novel's historical context that the narrator's failure to trouble himself or the readers further about the causes of this female metamorphosis becomes an affront to the narrative's credibility. In its original context, the novel would probably still have been plausible on this point – though not in primary psychological terms, but rather in physiological or pathological terms.

Recontextualised within medical history, the apparent lack of an explanation simply indicates how matter-of-factly an author of Frisch's generation could assume that his readers were able to fill in the only notional blank themselves – because the author's generation evidently shared with the intended readers the same readily accessible general knowledge. Such knowledge and its currency are also palpable in the author to whom and the novel to which Frisch made his deepest obeisance in *I'm Not Stiller*'s Davos scenes. In an early chapter of Felix Krull's *Confessions,* which Frisch seems to have known (Frisch 2008, 47), the narrator can speak quite automatically about the "perverted longings" [krankhafte() Gier] and "sexual desires of weak-chested people" [Begehrlichkeit brustschwacher Leute] (Mann 1974, 7: 316). And in the novel with which the Davos scenes in *I'm Not Stiller* establish a direct and significant intertextual relationship, perhaps the most famous doctor in all German literature can blather just as automatically about how "*of course* phthisis is accompanied by increased concupiscence" [die Phthise *nun mal* mit besonderer Konkupiszenz verbunden ist] (Mann 2002– , 5.1: 628 [emphasis mine]).

This once common belief, which the literary topos of tubercular patients' increased sexual desire merely reflects, was supported at least partly by the medical knowledge of the time. That tuberculosis, of course, ignites the sexual feelings of those it afflicts seems to have been, if not *communis opinio*, then undoubtedly a widespread assumption in medical circles (Porter 1996, 106; Latimer 1999, 1016–1031; Gilman 1995, 187–188), as medical research of the earlier era indicates. In the year of Frisch's birth, for example, a Prof. Dr. W. Weygandt (Friedrichsberg Insane Asylum, Hamburg) seems to have conducted a survey among his colleagues, publishing the results under the title 'The Psychological Status of Tubercular Patients' in the *Medizinische Klinik*, a weekly journal for practising doctors. On the very first page of his article, Weygandt again adopts quite as a matter of course the ideas which are reflected in the novels of the pre-war, the inter-war and indeed the post-war eras, stating that among the "peculiarities" [Eigentümlichkeiten] for which "phthisis sufferers have been conspicuous since time immemorial" ["(s)eit alters (...) bei den Phthisikern aufgefallen"], "the great *libido sexualis* has earned a kind of popularity" [die große Libido sexualis() ha(t) geradezu eine gewisse Popularität gewonnen] (Weygandt 1912, 91 [emphasis mine]). In the remainder of the article, the durability of this popular belief is demonstrated by the way it asserts itself in the face of empirical evidence, given that such evidence as was gathered in the author's survey to confirm this specific peculiarity in the psychological status of tubercular patients did so, at the absolute most, only intermittently and anecdotally. Weygandt's conclusion thus seems to be less a clinically based insight than a cliché with wide-ranging implications for *Mentalitätsgeschichte*.

The fact that a narrator such as Stiller can invoke this supposed parallel between tuberculosis and man-madness so openly and matter-of-factly is presumably as significant as the toll which the supposition exacts from the narrator here. For – even leaving aside the patient's eventual death – the sensations of cachexia which are as characteristic as they are unmistakable here – like tinder – clearly contradict the only slightly earlier scene, in which that same narrator felt able to face his wife's ultimately fatal disease with equanimity. So if, in *I'm Not Stiller*, the tuberculosis which afflicts a single character can appear as two things simultaneously, as a deadly disease and as the affectation of a well-heeled female narcissist (Frisch 1994b, 86), then this inconsistency in the text can probably be interpreted as reflecting a turning point in the history of civilisation. It is no coincidence that the medical case narrated here is set years after tubercular diseases had ceased to be the leading cause of death in Switzerland. By the time that, according to the novel's chronology, Julika Stiller arrived in Davos, these diseases had declined to the fourth most prevalent cause of death (Eidgenössisches Statistisches Amt 1947), and by the time she died they were barely still included among the ten most prevalent causes (Eidgenössisches Statistisches Amt 1957).

3

The death of Julika Stiller, which “obviously c[a]me as a surprise to the doctor” (Frisch 1994b, 382), and with it the end of the novel, is dated in the year 1955, almost a full decade after her cure in Davos. To be absolutely precise, Julika’s death is supposed to occur in March (Frisch 1994b, 363), on Easter Monday, after she had still seemed to be recovering on the morning of Easter Sunday (Frisch 1994b, 362). So if Julika dies on a day which is fraught with symbolism in the Church calendar – and which demonstrably was chosen with such symbolism in mind, given that in 1955 Easter was to fall not in March, but rather in mid-April – then ten years earlier she travels to Davos during a summer which is noteworthy in secular history. The year of her arrival there is significant obviously, or even primarily, although not solely, in terms of war, peace or politics (Rohner 2013), because that year also marked an epoch in medical history and *Mentalitätsgeschichte*.

At the end of 1945, the Nobel Prize for Medicine was awarded to Alexander Fleming, Ernst Boris Chain and Howard Walter Florey. They received the Prize “for the discovery of penicillin and its curative effect in various infectious diseases” (The Nobel Foundation). The now world-famous “Penecillin” treatment, as Frisch regularly spelt it in the typescript of his next novel, provided a cure for the last of the major infectious diseases, syphilis, but above all the treatment also alleviated the visceral fear of these diseases.

The Nobel laureates had ‘discovered,’ or more accurately isolated, penicillin two years previously. At that stage, in 1943, the application of streptomycin had accomplished a final breakthrough in the battle against the infection which takes Julika to Davos, and which the town was once so famous for treating. The success of this battle against tuberculosis will be particularly noted by the narrator of Frisch’s next novel. Walter Faber defends the termination of pregnancy [Schwangerschaftsunterbrechung] as a necessity in an era which has overcome the “plagues” [Seuchen] (Frisch 1986, 4: 105–106). The sole example he offers is precisely the disease which the deuteragonist of the immediately preceding novel had been unable to escape:

> The reduction of tuberculosis, for example: through successful prophylaxis tuberculosis has been reduced from thirty per cent to eight per cent. God does the job with diseases, we have snatched the diseases out of his hand. The result: we must take procreation out of his hand as well. (Frisch 1994a, 108)

Although or because this narrator is presenting himself as one who has witnessed the victory over tuberculosis, his *Report* also clearly indicates that it was written by an author who must still have been very familiar with this disease and its associated topoi. And evidently he was also and particularly familiar with the topos of the erotic stimulation experienced by tuberculosis sufferers, or more precisely, *female* tuberculosis sufferers. Because although tuberculosis appears in *Homo faber* only marginally, and notwithstanding that it does not even appear under that name, it is still assigned to the other gender. And as a result of the particular disease, the femininity of that gender seems to assume palpably – indeed even more palpably – sexual characteristics here by comparison with *I'm Not Stiller*, where the patient only imagined her acts of adultery:

> I've really forgotten my first experience with a woman, the very first, that is to say I never remember it at all if I don't want to. She was the wife of a teacher of mine, who used to invite me to his house for weekends shortly before I took my final examination; I used to help him read the proofs of a new edition of his textbook, in order to earn some money. My dearest wish was a cheap secondhand motorcycle, it didn't matter how old the machine was as long as it went. I had to draw geometrical figures, Pythagoras's theorem and so on, in India ink, because I was the best pupil in mathematics and geometry. His wife, as she appeared to me at the age I was then, was a lady in the years of discretion, forty, I believe, consumptive, and when she kissed my boyish body she seemed to me like a madwoman or a bitch; and I continued to address her as "Frau Professor." (Frisch 1994a, 101–102)

Faber's "first experience" shortly before graduating from high school (called 'Maturität' in Swiss German) has extensive implications, which are unfolded rather more here than the development and plausibility of the plot might justify. For example, it seems superfluous for Faber to specify what he intended to buy with the money which he was earning in the adulterous woman's house. For the model pupil did not enter her territory in search of erotic adventures; the immediate object of his typically adolescent and pubescent desires was a purely material possession. But, well beyond the familiar sexual symbolism of motorcycles and riding motorcycles, this possession has an exact paradigmatic relationship to the female body which attracts Faber as an unexpected substitute.

In the same way as the motorcycle will be the protagonist's first motor vehicle, the teacher's wife is his first woman – and a symbol of how, for Faber and others like him, technical mobility and male sexuality are metaphorically interchangeable – "hips [...] like [...] the steering wheel of my Studebaker" (Frisch 1994a, 88). If the desired motorcycle may be 'second-hand' and however old, as long as it fulfils its sole and essential purpose of serving as a "vehicle," then Faber extends his expectations of this purely material object of desire *mutatis mutandis* to the woman of whose offer he takes advantage. *Mutatis mutandis*, but *paulo mutandis*, she also is "eine Occasion" [second-hand] (Frisch 1986, 4: 99), a typically Swiss German loan. As a married and "mature lady" [gesetzte

Dame] (Frisch 1986, 4: 99), she too is used goods, a second-hand functional object, reducible to the single role of being a woman. Nameless and faceless, she serves in effect as a mere vehicle for the sexuality of the man, who can then choose to expunge her from his memory entirely, even though in a sense it is she who first made him a man.

As the wife of a respected figure and father figure, the "Frau Professor" initially had the status of a mother, as it were of Jocasta. This suggests that the whole episode could be assigned to the readily recognisable and long recognised (Blair 1981) subtext of the Oedipus legend, and of its psychological ramifications and interpretations. And arguably this context could also provide a reading of the brutal end to the *affaire*, as poetic justice, or rather poetic injustice, given that the woman is destined to die "the same summer" (Frisch 1994a, 102). But – and this is where the psychoanalytical and especially the mythical approaches to the novel undeniably reach their limits – she succumbs to a chronic disease. Interestingly, Faber includes this in his list of her characteristics only incidentally, immediately after an estimate of her age which is conspicuously low in the light of the death which occurs soon after.

Despite everything, the narrator can remember quite clearly that she was said to have been ill, "with an illness of the lungs" [lungenkrank] (Frisch 1986, 4: 99). Regardless of whether this designation of her sickness was a common euphemism or simply a synecdoche which was automatically understood (Mann 1936, 133; 1988, 93; 1999a, 12; 1999b, 105) – it is no coincidence that Michael Bullock translated "lungenkrank" (Frisch 1986, 4: 99) in this passage unambiguously as "consumptive" – it is more than probable that Faber's first sexual partner suffered from tuberculosis of the lungs, which was still endemic in Switzerland at the time in question. In the mid-1920s, when Faber must have had his very first sexual experience, tuberculosis was just beginning its gradual descent in Switzerland's mortality statistics from the first most frequent to the second most frequent cause of death, being displaced in the first instance by cardiac diseases (Eidgenössisches Statistisches Amt 1947, 125).

In the figure of the teacher's wife, femininity and sexuality, sexuality and disease, disease and death thus unite in a textbook-like symbiosis. This symbiosis corresponds entirely with the theory which Mary Douglas proposed under the title *Purity and Danger*. Douglas's theory posits that anything which is in any way 'dangerous' can be separated, according to a hygienic code, from a 'pure' Self. In contradistinction to the Self, the dangerous Other reduces to a chaotic stew of concepts, whether of excrement and dirt, of death or disease, of the physical and animalistic in opposition to the intellectual, or of the other sex in opposition to masculinity, and to everything which can be connected unconsciously or associatively with masculinity (Douglas 1966).

In *Homo faber*, the already exemplary conflation of female sexuality and fatal disease is compounded by associations with the non-rational, irrational and animal-like, for the woman seemed to the high-school pupil "like a mad-woman or a bitch [...]." Later, Faber also repeatedly compares the final sexual partner of his life with a "dog" (Frisch 1994a, 123); a black cleaning woman in Houston has "animals' eyes" (*ibid.*, 185); and a Guatemalan landlady has "hair" which "resemble[s] plumage" (*ibid.*, 39).

Faber, however, becomes involved in the *affaire* as he is "the best pupil in mathematics and geometry." As the most abstract, most intellectual of all scholarly disciplines, "mathematics and [*sic*] geometry" are of course diametrically opposed to everything that the teacher's wife – in the truest sense of the verb – embodies. And in the older medical literature about *Consumption of the Lungs and the Nervous System*, mathematics appears as an antidote to the libido. Friedrich Jessen, who provided the real-life model for Thomas Mann's fictional doctor and blatherer, recommended mathematics "to men as a sovereign specific for suppressing desire" [Männern (...) als ein souveränes Dämpfungsmittel]. Significantly, the medical professional used a much more cautious and much less generalised formulation than his literary counterpart: "*should there be* excessive sexual desire" [(bei) *etwaiger* übermäßiger sexueller Reizbarkeit] (Jessen 1905, 40 [emphasis mine]). All this, for that matter, offers an intriguing backdrop to the play *Don Juan or The Love of Geometry*, which Frisch wrote immediately before *I'm Not Stiller.*

If one compares the representation of tuberculosis in that novel and in *Homo faber*, considerable and significant differences emerge. In *I'm Not Stiller*, as already noted, tuberculosis still affected the deuteragonist, even if initially only in the form of a dubious diagnosis, or at least a diagnosis which the narrator could doubt without subsequently having to withdraw his doubts explicitly, much less regret them. But then – curiously, yet it seemed unmistakably – the disease afflicted one whole side of the lungs. And finally tuberculosis caused the death of the patient – as it did of the Jesuit who was her companion in suffering. Thus tuberculosis ultimately occupied an important and ineradicable position in the script of the novel.

In *Homo faber*, by contrast, tuberculosis of the lungs is not even designated by its proper name, and the disease and its fatal consequences are removed in their entirety to the periphery of the novel's plot and *dramatis personæ*. It is shifted to the protagonist's "first experience [...], the very first," and more or less buried in the prehistory of the events narrated, where it is assigned to a character who is marginal and anonymous. And that character is by no means marginal only because she is a woman. The peripheral and unnamed woman comes from a completely different world, including in the etymological sense of the word. She belongs to a different generation from the main characters, to the next oldest generation, or even to the generation before that. When the story time proper begins, she has been dead for more than three decades.

And in Frisch's next novel, tuberculosis also belongs to that past, or in one respect to an even more distant past, and naturally it is attributed once more to a woman. Or rather, the disease as such no longer appears in the novel at all. For in a sense the narrator of *Gantenbein* achieves for good what Anatol Stiller had merely aspired to ten years previously. Pseudo-Gantenbein sustains the position which Stiller only adopted initially – if only in the form of a possibility and a convenient interpretation – before it was disproved catastrophically by the further and fatal sequence of events. Stiller's *ex post* and thus egregiously misguided suspicion that his wife was only simulating her tuberculosis in order to extort one or other advantage from it, probably a certain social cachet, and definitely respite from her marital responsibilities – the second part of that suspicion recurs *tale quale* in *Gantenbein*, but this time it is not even slightly inconsistent with any other aspect of the narrative:

> She [scil. Svoboda's wife and, by the same token, Enderlin's lover] is healthy, even robust, and at the same time delicate, so that one enjoys feeling a tender anxiety about her; an early tuberculosis has healed up, a memory that she only rarely uses to demand consideration, only in case of need. (Frisch 1967, 209)

Whereas Stiller had at least retained sufficient tact to reject his suspicions as a temptation, and then ascribe them to an anonymous and indefinite subject, moreover expressing them with the subjunctive of a modal verb which in itself was apt to deprecate them, and thus permitting them only partial validity – "*one might* be *tempted* to not *entirely* believe" (Frisch 1986, 3: 450 [emphasis mine]) –, pseudo-Gantenbein no longer feels constrained to take such precautionary measures. He specifically reports that the adulterous wife enjoys excellent health and a robust constitution. She no longer suffers, but only previously suffered, from tuberculosis. *This* infection is explicitly and completely cured, or "healed up," and continues to play a certain role only and exclusively as a "memory." And it is entirely certain that this memory operates purely as an extortionate means to a psychological end. Tuberculosis serves only as a tactic in the war of the sexes, even if he acknowledges ironically that she resorts to it "only in case of need." But this also means *nota bene* that the disease can no longer be employed as a motivation or justification for the infidelity of this further and particularly notorious adulteress.

It is through this comparison with and these differences from *I'm Not Stiller* that *Gantenbein* marks the end of a process during which tuberculosis, as a disease and a cause of death, gradually removed itself from the inventory of collective fears – a process which is mirrored precisely in Frisch's three most famous novels. In *I'm Not Stiller*, tuberculosis appears within the narrated time proper, and comparatively close to the plot's centre of gravity, at first harmlessly, but then seriously enough to more or less determine the novel's unhappy ending. Then in *Homo faber* tuberculosis is still characterised as a serious and fatal disease, but this characterisation belongs in the deepest prehistory of the narrated time, and on the very periphery of the narrative. In *Gantenbein*, finally, tuberculosis plays next to no role at all: it is simply an illness which can be and has been cured completely, and which is not even simulated with any conviction, but which at most might manifest itself fleetingly in the narrated present as a casual reminder of a past which has been left behind entirely, and a reminder *that* the past has been left behind entirely.

Of course, the gradual disappearance of tuberculosis – and with it of the great 'plagues' – from Frisch's repertoire of motifs did not mean the disappearance of death, nor even of illness, as literary themes in his novels. In exactly the same proportion as consumption declined in the novels, an entirely new type of illness flourished. This overtook tuberculosis, which had dropped to second place, in the Swiss (Eidgenössisches Statistisches Amt 1947, 124; Stiner 1934, 114) and then the German (Hunziker 1933, 7) mortality statistics in the second half of the 1920s – that is, no more than a year or two after Walter Faber's very first sexual experience, after the act of adultery by a consumptive woman which has the earliest narrative date in Frisch's œuvre.

Faber's *Report* is of course characterised quite literally in terms of that 'new' illness – an illness which was not mentioned in *I'm Not Stiller* at all. But on the other hand, that illness was probably part and parcel of an experimental arrangement made in the next novel, *Gantenbein* (Frisch 1967, 132–147). *Homo faber*, however, is consistently, among other things, the *Report* of a cancer patient and the notes about a cancer case.

In Frisch's novels, cancer no longer attacks 'only' female characters or the 'female' side of the body. On the contrary, it always occurs in men. Initially, in *Jürg Reinhart* (1934) and its sequel, *J'adore ce qui me brûle oder Die Schwierigen*, (1943), cancer is confined to *secondary* male characters, and through them held at a distance in both time and space, relegated to the prehistory of the plots, and moreover banished abroad, to Greece, Germany or Austria (Frisch 1986, 1: 338, 363, 429). But then, in *Homo faber*, it strikes no lesser characters than the protagonist and his "role model," his university teacher and prospective *Doktorvater*, who remained an "example" [Vorbild] (Frisch 1986, 4: 103) throughout the protagonist's life and indeed until his death which distinguishes this professor from his predecessor, the high-school "professor" who was supplanted by his pupil in the bed of the tubercular nymphomaniac.

The stomach cancer to which Faber succumbs only two-and-a-half years after Julika Stiller succumbs to her tuberculosis of the lungs thus influences the plot of the *Report* as definitively, or almost as definitively, as Julika's tuberculosis influences the ending of *I'm Not Stiller.* In other words, Frisch's novels do not only testify to the way that the old fears of infection were gradually overcome during the author's lifetime. More importantly, the novels could provide an answer to the question of what replaced those fears and of what filled the vacuum which was left behind by those fears, or perhaps more accurately which was not left behind.

References

Blair, Rhonda L. "Homo Faber, Homo Ludens, and the Demeter-Kore Motif." *Germanic Review* 56.4 (1981): 140–150.

Brandt, Allan M. "Sexually Transmitted Diseases." *Companion Encyclopedia of the History of Medicine.* Eds. William F. Bynum and Roy Porter. Vol. 1. London, New York, NY: Routledge, 1993. 562–584.

Bundesamt für Statistik. "Sterbefälle und Sterbeziffern wichtiger Todesursachen, Männer." *Statistisches Jahrbuch der Schweiz 2010.* Zurich: Neue Zürcher Zeitung, 2010. 331.

Condrau, Flurin. "Lungenheilstätten im internationalen Vergleich. Zur Sozialgeschichte der Tuberkulose im 19. und frühen 20. Jahrhundert." *Historia Hospitalium. Zeitschrift der deutschen Gesellschaft für Krankenhausgeschichte* 19 (1993–1994): 220–234.

Condrau, Flurin. "Patienten von Lungenheilanstalten 1890–1930: Deutschland und England im Vergleich." *Krankenhaus-Report 19. Jahrhundert. Krankenhausträger, Krankenhausfinanzierung, Krankenhauspatienten.* Eds Alfons Labisch and Reinhard Spree. Frankfurt a. M., New York: Campus, 2001. 427–448.

Douglas, Mary. *Purity and Danger: An analysis of concepts of pollution and taboo.* New York, NY: Praeger, 1966.

Eidgenössisches Statistisches Amt. "Statistik der Sterbefälle in der Schweiz nach Todesursachen seit 1902." *Statistisches Jahrbuch der Schweiz 1946.* Basel: Birkhäuser, 1947. 123–127.

Eidgenössisches Statistisches Amt. "Statistik der Sterbefälle in der Schweiz nach Todesursachen seit 1901." *Statistisches Jahrbuch der Schweiz 1956.* Basel: Birkhäuser, 1957. 108–113.

Frisch, Max. *A Wilderness of Mirrors.* Trans. Michael Bullock. London: Methuen, 1967.

Frisch, Max. *Gesammelte Werke in zeitlicher Folge.* Ed. Hans Mayer. 7 vols. Frankfurt a. M.: Suhrkamp, 1986.

Frisch, Max. *Homo Faber: A Report.* Trans. Michael Bullock. San Diego, New York, and London: Harcourt Brace, 1994a.

Frisch, Max. *I'm Not Stiller.* Trans. Michael Bullock. San Diego, New York, London: Harcourt Brace, 1994b.

Frisch, Max. "The Writer and His Partners / The Function of Literature in Society." *Schwarzes Quadrat. Zwei Poetikvorlesungen.* Ed. Daniel de Vin. Frankfurt a. M.: Suhrkamp, 2008. 47–76.

Gilman, Sander L. *Franz Kafka, the Jewish Patient.* New York, NY, London: Routledge, 1995.

Hieronimus, Marc. *Krankheit und Tod 1918. Zum Umgang mit der Spanischen Grippe in Frankreich, England und dem Deutschen Reich.* Berlin: Lit, 2006.
Hunziker, H[ans]. "Wissen, Glaube und Aberglaube in der Krebsfrage." *Bulletin der Schweizerischen Vereinigung für Krebsbekämpfung* 1.1 (1933): 5–24.
Jessen, F[riedrich]. *Lungenschwindsucht und Nervensystem.* Jena: Gustav Fischer, 1905.
Kinsey, Alfred C., Wardell B. Pomeroy, Clyde E. Martin, and Paul H. Gebhard. *Sexual Behavior in the Human Female.* Philadelphia, London: Saunders, 1953.
Latimer, Dan. "Erotic Susceptibility and Tuberculosis: Literary Images of a Pathology." *Modern Language Notes* 105.5 (1999): 1016–1031.
Mann, Jonathan M. "AIDS – A Global Perspective: The World Health Organization's Global Strategy for the Prevention and Control of AIDS." *The Western Journal of Medicine* 147.6 (1987): 732–734.
Mann, Thomas. "Tristan." *Stories of Three Decades.* Trans. H[elen] T[racy] Lowe-Porter. New York, NY: Knopf, 1936. 133–166.
Mann, Thomas. *Gesammelte Werke.* 13 vols. 2nd ed. Frankfurt a. M.: Fischer, 1974.
Mann, Thomas. "Tristan." *Death in Venice and Other Stories.* Trans. David Luke. Toronto, New York: Bantam, 1988. 93–132.
Mann, Thomas. "Tristan." *Death in Venice and Other Stories.* Trans. Jefferson S. Chase. New York, NY: Signet Classic, 1999a. 11–54.
Mann, Thomas. "Tristan." *Death in Venice and Other Tales.* Trans. Joachim Neugroschel. New York, NY: Penguin, 1999b. 103–149.
Mann, Thomas. *Große kommentierte Frankfurter Ausgabe. Werke – Briefe – Tagebücher.* Eds Heinrich Detering et al. 13 vols. to date. Frankfurt a. M.: Fischer, 2002–.
The Nobel Foundation. *The Nobel Prize in Physiology or Medicine 1945.* http://www.nobelprize.org/nobel_prizes/medicine/laureates/1945/ (9 June 2011).
Porter, Roy. "What is Disease?" *The Cambridge Illustrated History of Medicine.* Ed. Roy Porter. Cambridge, New York, NY, and Melbourne: Cambridge University Press, 1996. 82–117.
Rohner, Melanie. *'Whiteness' und 'non-whiteness' in Max Frisch's "Stiller" und "Homo faber"* [to be published 2014].
Schütt, Julian. *Max Frisch. Biographie eines Aufstiegs. 1911–1954.* Berlin: Suhrkamp, 2011.
Stiner, Otto. "Die Verbreitung des Magenkrebses in der Schweiz in den Jahren 1901–1930." *Bulletin der Schweizerischen Vereinigung für Krebsbekämpfung* 2.1 (1934): 114–130.
Thalmann, Hans. *Die Grippeepidemie 1918/19 in Zürich.* Zurich: Juris, 1968.
Weygandt, W[ilhelm]. "Der Seelenzustand der Tuberkulösen." *Medizinische Klinik* 8.3 (1912): 91–95, 137–140.

Priscilla Wald

Afterword

The prehistory of *Contagionism and Contagious Diseases: Medicine and Literature between 1880 and 1933* is the late nineteenth-century technological revolution that enabled medical researchers for the first time to identify microbes and begin to understand their role in contagion. The identification of disease-causing microbes contributed significantly to a changing world about which the literature of Western Europe tells a compelling story. But the premise of this book is that the idea of contagion marks the intersection between science and culture. Ideas were "contagious" long before the identification of disease-causing microbes (Sperber, 1996), although the transmission of disease had of course long been cause for speculation. The transportation and communication revolutions of the mid-to-late nineteenth century brought the world into closer contact. Bacteriology explained why and how that contact might be dangerous, while widespread aesthetic experimentation attested to the rapid transmission of ideas.

"Men are more definitely and variously aware of each other than ever before," observed Albion Small in the first issue of the *American Journal of Sociology* (1895), of which he was the founding editor. They are also more promiscuously perplexed "by each other's presence," he mused. "Whatever modern" men's theory of the social bond, no men have ever had more conclusive evidence that the bond exists (Small 1895, 2).

With "promiscuous *perplexity*," Small signalled the confusion characteristic of rapid dramatic changes, but he also marked the unprecedented intermingling that came with the urban growth and increased travel of the turn of the twentieth century. This social promiscuity resulted in the new perspectives and shifting attitudes evinced in cultural forms. Disease-causing microbes added a material dimension, providing conclusive physical evidence of the bond, as they demonstrated the often dangerous consequences of contacts of which people were often unaware. The distinctions among the scientific, social, and cultural registers blurred as the idea of contagion circulated conceptually among them.

Contagion articulates a worldview: an ecological understanding of the interconnections of society. With defiance of boundaries as one of its chief attributes, the concept sounds the alarm of promiscuity, as in the warning issued by New York City's Commissioner of Health Cyrus Edson in an 1895 issue of *The North American Review*, just months after the appearance of Small's journal. "We cannot separate the tenement-house district from the portion of the city where the residences of the wealthy stand, and treat this as a separate locality," Edson cautioned. "The disease we find in the tenement-house threatens all alike, for a hundred avenues afford a way by which the contagion may be carried from the tenement to the palace." Tracing "the microbes or their spores" from the ghetto as they effortlessly "pass the heavy curtains on the windows of the mansion to find their prey inside" (Edson 1895, 425), he showed how they challenged the distinctions ostensibly enforced by social spaces.

The social transformations that Small noted were already underway prior to the new theories of contagion, but those theories altered social practices and conventions that, in turn, changed the way people understood their interactions and responsibilities as well as the role of the state. For Edson, "disease binds the human race together as with an unbreakable chain," which "the industrial development of the world has enlarged [...] until now all nations are embraced within its band" (Edson 1895, 423). Individuals and the state alike ignored these bonds at their peril, with the threats of disease and revolution equally lurking outside the mansion. Although no advocate of socialism, Edson recognised contagion as capturing its "germ idea [...], that all members of the body politic are theoretically and should be practically joint partners in one great co-operative state" as well as the "[s]ocialistic side of the microbe [which] is to be found [...] in the fact that we may only fight diseases in a community by meeting it everywhere" (*ibid.*, 425). Disease-causing microbes were more than metaphoric for him; they actually constituted social bonds, as they wound their way through an ever-enlarging map of human byways and increasingly promiscuous spaces.

These observations attest to the conceptual power of contagion. Martina King and Thomas Rütten note the longstanding use of contagion to configure the traffic of germs and ideas, its vagueness, and its uneasy position between the literal and the metaphorical. Its increasing precision in the sciences following the identification of disease-causing microbes led at once to renewed efforts for a more scientific study of society. The connections between social and psychic contagion and physical contagion runs through this volume. Writing in the *American Journal of Sociology* in 1896, Small's former classmate, the sociologist Edward A. Ross, defined social influence as "the contagion of emotions, ambitions, desires" that "results from the contact and intercourse of men as individuals" (Ross 1896, 518). For him and other investigators in this new field, cultural influence worked on the same principle as germs and had to be theorized accordingly. The term conveyed a material change of some kind.

In the same journal nearly two decades later Small's University of Chicago colleague Robert E. Park would formalise the concept in the term "social contagion" (Park 1914–15). Although he could not draw on the technology of the microscope, the field of epidemiology offered Park another technology in the form of maps. If the microscope identified the specific microbe responsible for an outbreak, epidemiological maps chronicled the spaces and routes of contagion. Park drew explicitly on his journalistic experience mapping such outbreaks when he argued that it was possible similarly to map the spread of culture. The distinctive neighborhoods of Chicago – the ethnic enclaves and ghettos – offered him a unique opportunity to document the formation, disintegration, and reformation of groups, and he and his students took Chicago as their principal laboratory in which to map and thereby track the contagion of culture.

For these sociologists, the contagion of culture was the mechanism of assimilation, a topic that was much debated in the U.S. national media and sociological literature during the years covered by this volume. In recent years, Park in particular has been criticized for his advocacy of assimilation, which critics read as an affirmation of the superiority of the dominant culture. He based his theories about assimilation on work in botany and zoology where assimilation represented the last stage in a process in which a plant or animal species "invaded" the terrain of another species, underwent a struggle for resources and survival, and finally either won or lost the battle or – most typically – settled into some kind of new relationship. Park argued that human beings manifested the same pattern, and spoke against the nativism and immigration restrictions for which many of his colleagues, including Ross, advocated in the early decades of the twentieth century. He and his associates recognised the particular challenge posed by the massive influx of immigrants, who dangerously swelled the ranks of the tenements and who typified "the conditions imposed by city life," as Park identified them, "in which individuals and groups of individuals, widely removed in sympathy and understanding, live together under conditions of interdependence, if not of intimacy" and in which "the conditions of social control are greatly altered and the difficulties increased" (Park 1914–15). But they also stressed the ecological benefits – the richness and possibility for productive transformation – that immigrants and strangers generally brought to closed groups. For Park, assimilation was an inevitable process when identifiable groups began to encounter each other in shared spaces. Assimilation was also mutual, although typically the smaller group's metamorphosis was more dramatic than the larger one. These changes revealed the intrinsic communicability of culture, what I have elsewhere called "a communicable Americanism" (Wald 2002, 675).[1]

The idea of communicable culture unifies the essays in this volume. Whether chronicling the changing aesthetic dimensions and metaphoric connotations of

1 I have drawn my discussion of the sociologists and early public health officials from Wald 2008, ch. 3.

contagion (Anz, Briese, Gradmann, King, Rousseau) or exploring its use in literary works (Elsaghe, Käser, Montiel, Rütten, Saul), all of the essays describe a change in the understanding of cultural transmission that can be associated with both microbes and modernism. It is a concept that demonstrates how concepts travel among disciplines, mutually inflecting the ideas that shape lived experience. And it explains what literary and cultural critics have to contribute to the study of contagion in all of its manifestations. The idea of communicable culture – specifically, communicable Americanism – was central to the work of a highly influential figure in the history of American letters, the composition and literary scholar Barrett Wendell, who taught Harvard University's first American literature classes at the turn of the twentieth century. His influence in the fields of American literary study and composition studies in the early twentieth century again attests to the importance of the topic addressed in the essays in *Contagionism and Contagious Diseases*.

Wendell did not share Park's celebration of the melting pot, and contagion for him marked the danger immigrants posed to the cultural as well as physical health of the American body politic. The Harvard literature professor supported immigration restriction wholeheartedly, although his devoted students over the years included such figures as Gertrude Stein, W. E. B. Du Bois, and Horace Kallen, a journalist well known for his coinage of the term "cultural pluralism." In a letter to Kallen, Wendell expressed his concern about the mass immigration in the early decades of the twentieth century. "We are submerged," he wrote, "beneath a conquest so complete that the very name of us means something not ourselves [...] I feel as I should think an Indian might feel, in the face of ourselves that were" (Kallen 1956, 7). There is of course a grisly irony in Wendell's identification with a culture (or rather cultures) that had been destroyed by the very culture that now, in his view, faced destruction in turn, but the analogy expresses a threat that was fairly wide-spread at the turn of the century: at the very moment that America was emerging as a world power, American culture was under sufficient attack to face outright destruction.

Wendell's interest in identifying and promoting the distinctive Americanism he believed to be at risk motivated both his design and teaching of American literature classes. Central to that design was his belief in what he called "literary contagion" (Wendell 1909, 174). While much has been written on the sociological concept of social contagion, "literary contagion" was not a term that caught on, but it was an important concept to this powerful figure. The conceptual shifts studied in this volume find unique expression in that term, and they infuse many of the assumptions that underpin the methods and approaches of language and literary study. We might say that the idea of literary contagion "haunts" the study of language and literature because it is at once formative and largely forgotten.

Like many nativists, Wendell, whose wife worked for the quarantine movement in Boston, turned to microbes to depict the threat faced by American culture in material terms, but, in turn, he fashioned the concept of literary contagion into a methodological paradigm. He believed not only in great literature, but also in the classroom as an important site of socialization. There American values were transmitted and Americans made. The stakes could hardly be higher. "Nationality is generally conceived to be a question of race, of descent, or blood," he wrote in the introduction to his *Literary History of America*, "and yet in human experience there is a circumstance perhaps more potent in binding men together than any physical tie [...] In a strange, subtle way each language grows to associate with itself the ideals and the aspirations and the fate of those peoples with whose life it is inextricably intermingled" (Wendell 1900, 3). And language, of course, was the stuff of literature; great literary works could teach his students how properly to use that language, thereby shaping their character. Learning to express oneself effectively and appropriately was, for Wendell, central to the development of character and, by extension, to the responsibilities of citizenship. Conversely, misuse of that language – as, for example, by immigrants and the lower classes – threatened the very fabric of culture and the social structures that depended on it. Words, he explained in his composition textbook, were tangible and material, but they had no meaning beyond common consent. He deplored the "barbarous use of foreign or of new words" (Wendell 1899, 49) and considered the corruption of language to be a prominent social danger. The Tower of Babel was, to him, a cautionary *social* tale with relevance in his own moment.

At stake for Wendell was nothing less than national unity. Language and the values it embodied were contagious, and literary works were carriers, for good or ill. Culture – Americanism – was communicable through these works, and the educator's job was to ensure that the right kind of culture was communicated. Thus he conveyed his sense of the dangerous power of literature, of cultural transmission and cultural volatility. In a piece entitled "The Study of Expression," for example, he defined "the ideal of expression," which he also labelled "literary contagion," as "a momentary fusion of what the writer means with what the reader thinks and feels" (Wendell 1909, 188). Originally delivered as a commencement address in 1909 at the College of Charleston (in South Carolina), this piece manifested Wendell's conviction that an effective use of rhetoric could literally bind the nation. He has always wished, he says, "to know something of the South – not as a student, or a traveler, but as a human being, mingling for a little while with Southern fellow-countrymen in their habit as they live" (*ibid.*, 137). And he is gratified that "in calling [him] from Harvard College to address men who have loyally pursued their studies in the College of Charleston," they "have done something more than a friendly act from men to man, from colleagues to colleague or from institution to institution;" rather, they "have happily urged that for a little while, at a moment such as often lingers long in the memory of those in whose lives it marks an epoch, Massachusetts should speak to South Carolina, Boston to Charleston" (*ibid.*, 138).

With his reference to their "loyalty," Wendell summoned the sectional conflict that inevitably remained in the historical memories of his listeners, and he implied the lingering of the conflict in attachments to local institutions – their loyalty witnessed by their attending the College of Charleston instead of, say, the northern – read national – institution of Harvard. But if, at this epochal and also lingering moment, Massachusetts speaks to South Carolina, Boston to Charleston, with the efficacy he outlines in the address, then he has presumably complicated that loyalty with an act of literary contagion transmitting his (Boston) thoughts and sensibilities to their (Charleston) minds. "The chief end of life," he notes, as he begins to wrap up, "is to put together and to bind together what without us might stay forever separate" (*ibid.*, 193). Thanking them again for the invitation, he concludes with the Lincolnesque *trust* that they will understand "the friendship now so happily binding together your college and mine, your state and mine, your future and mine, in the happy concord of our common country" (*ibid.*, 194).

American literature as he conceived and taught it was both nationalising and contagious, suffused, that is, with a communicable Americanism that it was his job to elucidate. Wendell was instrumental in institutionalizing the move from philology to literary criticism, and he preceded the New Critics by a generation. He was not, on the surface, so radically different from the gentlemen of letters that Gerald Graff and Michael Warner align as "critics" against the philologist "scholars" (Graff and Warner 1989, 5). But Wendell was also not an easy heir of Longfellow and Lowell, and his work makes apparent his interest in a *scientific* study of literature, distinguishing him from the belletrists and the philological literary historians (the students of influence). His conception of literary works as carriers of culture and his sense of their potential danger were hardly new. But from his understanding of the culture they carried he developed a literary critical methodology that is more influential than is generally recognized. Although overshadowed by subsequent figures, such as Cleanth Brooks, Robert Penn Warren or F. O. Matthiessen, his methods of literary critical inquiry and language study stem from a view of culture – implicit in the concept of contagion – that remains a governing, if unrecognized, trope in language and literary study.

The metaphors of infection that abound in his and his students' work offer culture as a volatile and infectious agent, producing positive as well as negative effects, but always dangerous and always in need of control. Literary contagion was not just superficial, but fundamentally institutional, a force that could not only transform individuals, but could also change and even constitute communities. Literary contagion was, for him, the glue of national culture, and it underscored the need for experts who, through their reading practices and rhetorical strategies, could monitor this spread of culture and turn the literary "carrier" into a bearer of an appropriately communicable Americanism that it was his job to elucidate. Wendell insisted that the great writers invariably gave voice to a national sensibility, writing in such a way as to constitute the thoughts, perceptions, even dreams of their readers. But it was the task of the great teacher to foster this literary contagion – to combat the students' immunity to it. It is not surprising that he offered the nation's earliest American literature classes and that, more than a century later, contemporary investments in curriculum *and* approach remain so strong and are so powerfully contested.

Contagionism and Contagious Diseases: Medicine and Literature between 1880 and 1933 comes out of the idea that contagion was a transformative concept in the modernist moment in ways that literary and other cultural works can elucidate. It shows how the concept – uniquely – offered a way of thinking about the transmission of culture as well as disease. But the timing of this volume is also significant. In the past century, globalization has accelerated the world-shrinking processes in ways that would have stretched the imagination of even the most forward looking among the writers treated in this volume. The 1990s witnessed a veritable obsession with contagion narratives in popular culture and the mainstream media, which is not surprising considering the impact of the HIV/AIDS pandemic on every facet of society worldwide. The pandemic, however, was but one of the events that called attention to a changing world. Global networks – virtual and material – have put humankind in unprecedented contact, with all of the dangers and possibilities that implies. Similarly, as the Arab spring made apparent, the cinders of revolution can spread to a conflagration almost as quickly as a packet of information can traverse the worldwide web. And the counter forces can move at an equal pace. The resurgence of interest in the idea of contagion as evinced in the veritable industry of books, articles, and films on this topic is, therefore, not surprising. Interest in contagion surfaces, as *Contagionism and Contagious Diseases: Medicine and Literature between 1880 and 1933* suggests, when rapid global changes reinvigorate humankind's promiscuous perplexity about itself. It is at such heightened moments that the project of inquiry opens itself for inspection, and it is the claim of this volume that the idea of contagion in all of its manifestations offers particular insight into that process.

References

Basler, Roy P. *The Collected Works of Abraham Lincoln*. 8 vols. New Brunswick, NJ: Rutgers University Press, 1953.
Edson, Cyrus. "The Microbe as Social Leveller." *North American Review* 161.467 (1895): 421–426.
Gelder, Ken, and Sarah Thornton (Eds). *The Subcultures Reader*. London: Routledge, 1997.
Graff, Gerald, and Michael Warner. *The Origins of Literary Study: A Documentary History*. London: Routledge, 1989.
Kallen, Horace. *Cultural Pluralism and The American Idea*. Philadelphia: University of Pennsylvania Press 1956.
Park, Robert E. "The City. Suggestions for the Investigation of Human Behavior in the City Environment." *American Journal of Sociology* 20 (1914–15): 577–612.
Ross, Edward Alsworth. "Social Control." *American Journal of Sociology* 1 (1896): 513–535.
Small, Albion W. "The Era of Sociology." *American Journal of Sociology* 1 (1895): 1–15.
Sperber, Dan. *La contagion des idées. Théorie naturaliste de la culture*. Paris: Jacob, 1996.
Wald, Priscilla E. "Communicable Americanism: Contagion, Geography, Fictions, and the Sociological Legacy of Robert E. Park." *American Literary History* 14 (2002): 653–685.
Wald, Priscilla E. *Contagious: Cultures, Carriers, and the Outbreak Narrative*. Durham, NC: Duke University Press, 2008.
Wendell, Barrett. *English Composition. Eight Lectures Given at the Lowell Institute*. New York, NY: C. Scribner's Sons, 1899.
Wendell, Barrett. *A Literary History of America*. New York, NY: C. Scribner's Sons, 1900.
Wendell, Barrett. "The Study of Expression." *The Mystery of Education and Other Academic Performances*. Ed. Barrett Wendell. New York, NY: C. Scribner's Sons, 1909. 137–193.

Notes on Contributors

Thomas Anz was born in Göttingen in 1948. He studied German Studies, Linguistics and Sociology. PhD 1976, Habilitation 1987 in Munich. 1981–1982 editor of the feature pages of the *Frankfurter Allgemeine Zeitung*; 1982 to 1990 lecturer and Privatdozent in Munich; 1990 to 1998 Professor of Modern German Literature at the University of Bamberg, since 1998 at the University of Marburg. From 2004 to 2007, he was the president of the German Association of Scholars of Germanic Studies (DGV). For a semester in 2009 to 2010, he was a guest professor at the "cluster of excellence 'Languages of Emotion'" at the FU Berlin. His chief scholarly interests are: Literary Modernism, contemporary literature, history of literature, medicine, and psychology since the 18th century, psychological aesthetics, theory of literature, literary criticism. Among his monographs are: *Literatur der Existenz. Literarische Psychopathographie und ihre soziale Bedeutung im Frühexpressionismus* (1977); *Gesund oder krank? Medizin, Moral und Ästhetik in der deutschen Gegenwartsliteratur* (1989); *Franz Kafka* (1989); *Literatur und Lust. Glück und Unglück beim Lesen* (1998); *Literatur des Expressionismus* (2002); *Psychoanalyse in der literarischen Moderne* V.1 (2006); and *Handbuch Literaturwissenschaft*, 3 Vols (2007).

Olaf Briese is Privatdozent (unsalaried Associate Professor) at the Department of Cultural Studies of Berlin's Humboldt University, after having held positions as assistant professor of Religious Studies at the FU Berlin and as visiting full professor at Berlin's FU and Humboldt University. He is the author of a wide range of interdisciplinary books on modern German cultural history, including *Steinzeit. Mauern in Berlin* (2011); the four-volume *Angst in den Zeiten der Cholera* (2003); *Konkurrenzen. Zur philosophischen Kultur in Deutschland 1830–1850* (1998); *Die Macht der Metaphern. Blitz, Erdbeben und Kometen im Gefüge der Aufklärung* (1998); and *Der Anspruch des Subjekts. Zum Unsterblichkeitsdenken im Jungen Deutschland* (1995). He has also edited three collective volumes and published over a hundred essays in academic journals, such as *Zeitschrift für Geschichtswissenschaft, Zeitschrift für Religionswissenschaft, Internationales Archiv für Sozialgeschichte der deutschen Literatur, Zeitschrift für deutsche Philologie, Kant-Studien*, and *Medizin, Gesellschaft und Geschichte.*

Yahya Elsaghe was born in Nuremberg in 1960. Studies in Classics and German philology at the Universities of Zurich, Munich and Freiburg i. Br.; various research and teaching positions at Zurich, UC Berkeley, The University of Queensland and the FU Berlin. In 2000 Junior Professor at the University of Zurich.

Since 2001 professor of Modern German Literature at the University of Berne. He is currently completing a book on Max Frisch: *Max Frisch und das zweite Gebot. Relektüren von "Andorra" und "Homo faber"*. He has published three books on Thomas Mann: *Die imaginäre Nation: Thomas Mann und das "Deutsche"* (2000); *Thomas Mann und die kleinen Unterschiede: Zur erzählerischen Imagination des Anderen* (2004); and *Krankheit und Matriarchat: Thomas Manns "Betrogene" im Kontext* (2010). Further publications include books on Goethe and Hölderlin as well as articles on, among others, Christian Reuter, Eduard Mörike, Theodor Storm, Gottfried Benn, Bertolt Brecht and W. G. Sebald.

Christoph Gradmann is professor in the history of medicine at the University of Oslo in Norway. He has published widely on the history of infectious diseases, medical bacteriology and medical biography, 19th and 20th century. After receiving his doctorate in history at the University of Hannover 1991, he has held positions in Hannover, Heidelberg and Berlin, and has moved to Oslo in 2006. Some recent publications are: "Magic Bullets and Moving Targets: Antibiotic Resistance and Experimental Chemotherapy 1900 – 1940," *Dynamis* 31 (2011): 29 – 45; (Ed. with Jonathan Simon) *Evaluating and Standardizing Therapeutic Agents 1890 – 1950* (2010); "Robert Koch and the Invention of the Carrier State: Tropical Medicine, Veterinary Infections and Epidemiology around 1900," *Studies in History and Philosophy of Biological and Biomedical Sciences* 41 (2010): 232 – 240; *Laboratory Disease: Robert Koch's Medical Bacteriology* (2009); and "Locating Therapeutic Vaccines in 19th Century History," *Science in Context* 21 (2008): 145 – 60.

Rudolf Käser (born 1953) teaches German literature and language at the University of Applied Sciences and Arts Northwestern Switzerland, School for Teacher Education, in Brugg-Windisch. He is also titular professor for modern German literature at the University of Zurich. He is the author of *Arzt, Tod und Text. Grenzen der Medizin im Spiegel deutschsprachiger Literatur* (1998); *Wie und zu welchem Ende werden Epidemien erzählt?* (2004); and *Die Schwierigkeit, ich zu sagen. Rhetorik der Selbstdarstellung in Texten des "Sturm und Drang"* (1987). With Vera Pohland, he edited *Disease and Medicine in Modern German Cultures* (1990), with Beate Schappach *Krank geschrieben. Gesundheit und Krankheit im Diskursfeld von Literatur, Geschlecht und Medizin* (forthcoming, 2013).

Martina King studied Medicine, Modern German Literature and Philosophy in Munich. She is a trained paediatrician and has worked in clinical medicine for 20 years. In 2009, she published her PhD in German studies entitled *Pilger und Prophet. Heilige Autorschaft bei Rainer Maria Rilke*. Since then, she has been teaching in Munich, Göttingen, Durham and, as a lecturer in Medical Humanities, in Glasgow; her main field of research is 'Literature and Medicine,' with a focus on contagionism and the intellectual history of Modernism. Currently, she is writing her Habilitation entitled *Die Ambivalenz des Infektiösen. Mikroben und Mikrobenjäger in der Literatur- und Kulturgeschichte der Moderne 1880–1930* as a DFG-Fellow at the University of Berne.

Luis Montiel is Doctor in Medicine, History of Medicine Professor at the *Universidad Complutense*, Madrid, Spain, and former President of the *Sociedad Española de Historia de la Medicina* [Spanish Society of the History of Medicine]. His main lines of research focus on the philosophic medicine of German Romanticism, the history of Animal Magnetism, the history of psychology, and the interface between medicine and literature. His last publications in these domains are: *El rizoma oculto de la psicología profunda. Gustav Meyrink y Carl Gustav Jung* (2012); (with Elvira Arquiola) *La médecine en révolution. Sciences et philosophie de la nature au tournant du XVIIIe et du XIXe siècle* (2012); (Ed. with Nicole Edelman and Jean-Pierre Peter) *Histoire sommaire de la maladie et du somnambulisme de Lady Lincoln* (2009); *Magnetizadores y sonámbulas en el romanticismo alemán* (2008).

George Rousseau has taught at many universities, including Harvard, UCLA, Aberdeen, and, most recently, Oxford. His books include a trilogy entitled *Pre- and Post-Modern Discourses: medical, scientific, anthropological* (1991); (with Roy Porter) *Gout: The Patrician Malady* (1998); *Framing and Imagining Disease in Cultural History* (2003); *Nervous Acts: Essays on Literature, Culture and Sensibility* (2004); *Marguerite Yourcenar: A Biography* (2004); *Children and Sexuality: The Greeks to the Great War* (2007); *The Notorious Sir John Hill: The Man Destroyed by Ambition in the Era of Celebrity* (2012), and a forthcoming 'nostalgia memoir.' His interest in the discourses of contagion developed within ongoing wonder about the intersections of literature and medicine.

Thomas Rütten is Newcastle Director of the Northern Centre for the History of Medicine, after having held academic posts at Princeton's Institute for Advanced Study, at the universities of Münster and Paris VII, and at the Herzog August Library in Wolfenbüttel. The licenced physician (1986) holds a PhD in Medical History (1991) and a Habilitation in Theory and History of Medicine (1995) from the University of Münster. He has published the monograph *Demokrit – lachender Philosoph und sanguinischer Melancholiker* (1992); the exhibition catalogue *Hippokrates im Gespräch* (1993); and the CD-ROM *Geschichten vom Hippokratischen Eid* (2007). He is the editor of the collective volume *Geschichte der Medizinge-*

schichtsschreibung (2009); co-editor of two more collective volumes; author of numerous articles on ancient and early modern medicine ranging from Hippocrates to Christian Thomasius and Johann Georg Zimmermann. Since 2000, he has published 9 articles on Thomas Mann and Medicine and has unearthed and edited Thomas Mann's letters to Adolf v. Grolmann. He is the sole editor of the book series *Studies in the History of Medical History and Medical Historiography* and co-editor of the the journal *Early Science and Medicine*. In collaboration with Anne Oommen-Halbach, he is currently preparing a richly annotated edition of the correspondence between Karl Sudhoff and Tibor Győry.

Nicholas Saul is Professor of German at the University of Durham, England. He has held Guest Professorships at the University of Cologne and the University of Vermont, and his chief scholarly interests are Romanticism, Realisms, Classical Modernism, Romanies and literary Darwinisms. He has published essays on writers from Wilhelm Bölsche to Wilkie Collins, Frederick the Great of Prussia, Goethe, Wilhelm Raabe, Bram Stoker and Zacharias Werner, also on the problem of suicide, on death and on utopias. Some recent books are *German Philosophy and Literature 1700–1990* (2002); *Gypsies and Orientalism in German Literature and Anthropology of the Long Nineteenth Century* (2007); *The Cambridge Companion to German Romanticism* (2009); (with Simon J. James) *The Evolution of Literature* (2011) and (with Dirk Göttsche) *Realism and Romanticism in German Literature* (2013). He is writing a monograph on German literary Darwinisms 1859–2008 and will be leading a project at the Durham Institute of Advanced Study on *The Emergence of Literature* in 2014–2105.

Priscilla Wald is Professor of English and Women's Studies at Duke University, North Carolina. She is the author of *Constituting Americans: Cultural Anxiety and Narrative Form* (1995) and *Contagious: Cultures, Carriers, and the Outbreak Narrative* (2008). She is currently at work on a book-length project that considers the reconfiguration of the human at the intersection of evolutionary theory, the changing geopolitics, and the emergence of biotechnology in the years following the Second World War.

Index of Names and Works

Bei Fragen zur Produktsicherheit wenden Sie sich bitte an:
If you have any questions regarding product safety,
please contact:

Walter de Gruyter GmbH
Genthiner Straße 13
10785 Berlin
productsafety@degruyterbrill.com